The Rheumatology Handbook

The Rheumatology Handbook

edited by

Margaret Callan

Imperial College, London &
Chelsea and Westminster Hospital, UK

ICP

Imperial College Press

Published by

Imperial College Press
57 Shelton Street
Covent Garden
London WC2H 9HE

Distributed by

World Scientific Publishing Co. Pte. Ltd.
5 Toh Tuck Link, Singapore 596224
USA office: 27 Warren Street, Suite 401-402, Hackensack, NJ 07601
UK office: 57 Shelton Street, Covent Garden, London WC2H 9HE

British Library Cataloguing-in-Publication Data
A catalogue record for this book is available from the British Library.

THE RHEUMATOLOGY HANDBOOK

ISBN-13 978-1-84816-320-1
ISBN-10 1-84816-320-7

Typeset by Stallion Press
Email: enquiries@stallionpress.com

Printed by FuIsland Offset Printing (S) Pte Ltd Singapore

Preface

Rheumatology concerns the management of disorders that affect bones, muscles and connective tissues. It is a rewarding specialty in which intellectual, clinical and practical skills are as important as each other. Rheumatic diseases affect individuals of all ages and are a significant cause of pain and disability in the developed world. Disorders are varied in their presentation and multi-system involvement is common. Disease pathogenesis is diverse and may involve inflammation, autoimmunity, abnormalities within biochemical pathways and degeneration. Progress in molecular and cellular biology has led to increased understanding of disease processes and thereby to development of novel therapies targeting specific molecules. Disease scoring systems facilitate use of both novel and conventional drugs in a more effective, goal-directed manner. These advances have resulted in very significant improvements in expected outcome for patients with many different rheumatic disorders.

This book provides clear and concise explanations of relevant basic science and disease pathogenesis. These are combined with comprehensive descriptions and photographs of clinical presentations and up-to-date information about options available for investigation and treatment. A well-illustrated section on common soft-tissue and joint injections is included. Each chapter has been compiled by a Consultant Rheumatologist with relevant subspecialty interest from a major teaching hospital in the United Kingdom and Ireland. Whilst this is a practical guide to management of patients with common rheumatic disorders, it is also a book that seeks to enhance understanding and minimise list learning; it aims to encourage doctors to think rather than memorise.

The Rheumatology Handbook is appropriate for medical students but is sufficiently detailed to be useful for trainees in general practice or in general internal medicine. It may also be of interest to more senior clinicians wishing to update their knowledge of this rapidly moving specialty.

Margaret Callan

Contents

Contributing Authors

Sonya Abraham, MBBS BSc MRCP PhD FHEA, Kennedy Institute of Rheumatology, Imperial College, London.

Maha Azeez, BSc MB MRCPI, Mater Misericordiae University Hospital, Dublin Academic Medical Centre, Dublin.

Andrew Barr, MBBS BSc MRCP, Charing Cross Hospital, Imperial College Healthcare NHS Trust, London.

Shweta Bhagat, MBBS MD MRCP, Addenbrooke's, Cambridge University Hospitals, Cambridge.

Simon Bowman, PhD FRCP, Selly Oak Hospital, Birmingham.

Alexander Brand, MBBS MRCP, Chelsea and Westminster Hospital, London.

Rachel Byng-Maddick, MBBS MRCP, Whittington Hospital, London.

Margaret Callan, MA BM BCh DPhil FRCP, Chelsea and Westminster Hospital, London and Imperial College, London.

Mary Connolly, BSc PhD, St Vincent's University Hospital, Dublin Academic Medical Centre, Dublin.

Michael Doherty, MA MD FRCP FHEA, School of Clinical Sciences, University of Nottingham.

Suzanne Donnelly, MB MRCPI, Mater Misericordiae University Hospital, Dublin Academic Medical Centre & School of Medicine and Medical Sciences, University College Dublin.

Sally Edmonds, MBBS MD FRCP, Stoke Mandeville Hospital, Aylesbury and Nuffield Orthopaedic Centre, Oxford.

Paul Eggleton, PhD, Institute of Biomedical and Clinical Sciences, Peninsula College of Medicine and Dentistry, University of Exeter.

Amel Ginawi, MBBS MRCP, Addenbrooke's, Cambridge University Hospitals, Cambridge.

Frances Hall, MA FRCP DPhil, Addenbrooke's, Cambridge University Hospitals, Cambridge.

Pille Harrison, MRCP DPhil, Nuffield Department of Orthopaedics, Rheumatology and Musculoskeletal Sciences, University of Oxford.

Jeremiah Healy, MA MB BChir FRCP FRCR FFSEM, Chelsea and Westminster Hospital, London and Imperial College, London.

Alison Jordan, MRCP, Selly Oak Hospital, Birmingham.

Eoin Kavanagh, MB BCh BAO MRCPI MSc FFR RCSI, Dublin Academic Medical Centre & Mater Misericordiae University Hospital, Dublin.

Andrew Keat, MD FRCP, Northwick Park Hospital, London.

Sophia Khan, MRCP MMedEd, Solihull Hospital, Heart of England NHS Foundation Trust, Solihull.

Jason Last, MB AFRCSI FFSEM, School of Medicine and Medical Science, University College, Dublin.

Justin Lee, BSc MBBS MRCS FRCR, Chelsea and Westminster Hospital, London.

Paul MacMullan, BComm BSc (Physio) MRCPI, Mater Misericordiae University Hospital, Dublin Academic Medical Centre, Dublin.

Bina Menon, MBBS, BSc MRCP, Nothwick Park Hospital, London.

Anne Miller, MRCGP DRCOG DPCR, Nuffield Orthopaedic Centre, Oxford.

Emma Moberly, Mansfield College, University of Oxford.

Ellen Moran, PhD, St Vincent's University Hospital, Dublin Academic Medical Centre, Dublin.

Elena Nikiphorou, MBBS, BSc MRCP, Norfolk and Norwich University Hospital, Norwich.

Leena Patel, MBBS BSc MRCP, Chelsea and Westminster Hospital, London.

CYH See, Addenbrooke's, Cambridge University Hospitals, Cambridge.

Maliha Shaikh, MRCP, Cambridge University Hospitals, Cambridge.

Nick Shenker, PhD FRCP, Addenbrooke's, Cambridge University Hospitals, Cambridge.

Peter Taylor, MA PhD FRCP, Kennedy Institute of Rheumatology, Imperial College, London and Charing Cross Hospital, Imperial College Healthcare NHS Trust, London.

Tonia Vincent, MRCP PhD, Kennedy Institute of Rheumatology, Imperial College, London.

Pippa Watson, MA MBBS, Addenbrooke's, Cambridge University Hospitals, Cambridge.

Fiona Watt, MBBS BMedSci PhD MRCP, Kennedy Institute of Rheumatology, Imperial College, London and Charing Cross Hospital, Imperial College Healthcare NHS Trust, London.

Richard Watts, MA DM FRCP, University of East Anglia School of Medicine, Norwich and Ipswich Hospital NHS Trust, Ipswich.

Bryan Whelan, MD MSc MMedSci MRCPI MFSEM, Our Lady's Hospital, Manorhamilton.

Nick Wilkinson, MBChB MRCP MRCPCH DM, Nuffield Orthopaedic Centre, Oxford.

Paul Wordsworth, MA FRCP, Nuffield Department of Orthopaedics, Rheumatology and Musculoskeletal Sciences, University of Oxford.

Chapter 1

Basic Science for Rheumatology

Editor: Suzanne Donnelly

Mary Connolly, Suzanne Donnelly, Paul Eggleton, Eoin Kavanagh, Jason Last, Ellen Moran, Bryan Whelan

1.1. Introduction

Rheumatology is a broad discipline that encompasses the non-surgical management of disorders involving the musculoskeletal system. Chapters in this book are dedicated to the four major classes of rheumatic disease: joint disease, multi-system inflammatory disease, disorders of bone and connective tissue and regional pain syndromes (Table 1.1). Rheumatic conditions relevant to paediatric practice are considered separately. The initial chapters provide an overview of basic science and assessment of patients, further chapters cover injection techniques and drugs commonly used in management and a final chapter provides a collection of illustrative case histories.

Many different pathophysiological processes underpin diseases of the musculoskeletal system. These include degeneration, trauma, abnormalities in biochemical pathways, auto-immunity and inflammation. Genetic polymorphisms contribute to susceptibility to many of the conditions, and environmental influences may be important as disease triggers. Information relating to pathogenesis of the individual rheumatic conditions is given throughout the book. This first chapter provides a brief introduction to anatomy, biochemistry, immunology, molecular biology and genetics as relevant to the study of rheumatic diseases.

1.2. Anatomy of Bones and Joints

The human skeleton is formed by 206 bones that are linked to each other at joints. Collagen is the most abundant protein in the human body and is a major

Table 1.1. Rheumatic disorders in adults.

Joint disease	Multi-system inflammatory disease	Disorders of bone and connective tissue	Regional pain syndromes
Rheumatoid arthritis	Systemic lupus erythematosus	Osteoporosis	Shoulder pain
Spondyloarthritis	Anti-phospholipid syndrome	Osteomalacia	Neck pain
Osteoarthritis	Sjögren's syndrome	Paget's disease	Back pain
Crystal arthritis	Scleroderma	Inherited disorders of bone and connective tissue	Neural entrapment
Septic arthritis	Myositis		Tendon disorders
	Sarcoidosis		Plantar fasciitis
	Takayasu's arteritis		Bursitis
	Giant cell arteritis		Morton's neuroma
	Polymyalgia rheumatica		Ganglions
	Wegener's granulomatosis		Overuse syndromes
	Churg–Strauss syndrome		Fibromyalgia
	Microscopic polyarteritis		
	Henoch–Schönlein purpura		

component of both bones and joints. Within collagen, amino acids form helical sequences of more than 1,000 residues in length, with glycine at every third amino acid in the sequence. Three such helices bind together to form the 300 nm long superhelical form of tropocollagen. Many tropocollagen molecules bind to form 1 um long fibrils which bind together to form 10 um long fibres (Fig. 1.1). These fibres cross-link to provide an insoluble latticework or three-dimensional mesh immersed in a proteoglycan milieu. Type I collagen is most abundant in bone, tendons and ligaments, and type II collagen forms most of the collagen within hyaline cartilage.

1.2.1. *Bones*

Bones consist of a combination of organic matter such as collagen and cellular material, together with inorganic matter including calcium, phosphate and magnesium.

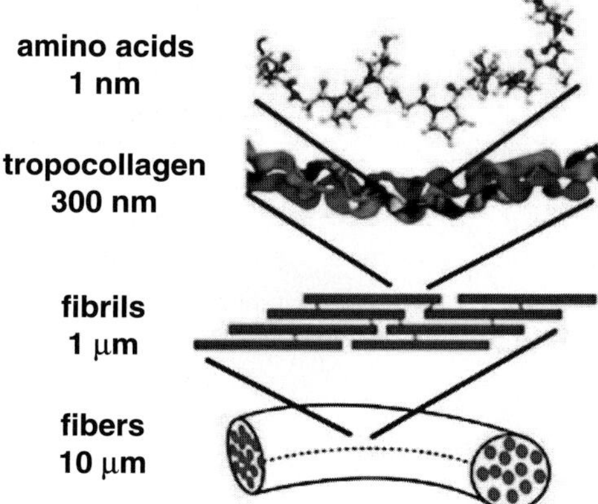

Fig. 1.1. Structure of collagen. Three helical amino acid chains form tropocollagen which binds to form fibrils and fibers of collagen. Reproduced with kind permission Markus J Buehler, Massachussets Institute of Technology. *Proc Natl Acad Sci USA* 2006 **103**: 12285–90. Copyright (2006) National Academy of Sciences USA.

Development of Bones

During embryonic life, clusters of cartilage-forming cells called chondroblasts form cartilaginous templates, each destined to become a bone through the process of endochondral ossification. The ossification sequence is well-characterised and for a typical long bone will involve the formation of a primary ossification centre in the centre or shaft (diaphysis) of the bone and secondary ossification centres within the ends (epiphyses). Cartilage and bone formation remains active around the perimeter of the shafts and in the space between the diaphysis and epiphyses; here the plate of cartilage is called a physis or growth plate.

Microstructure

There are two major cell types within bone. The osteoblasts are derived from osteoprogenitor cells and synthesise the osteoid matrix (predominantly type I collagen) which mineralises to form bone. Osteoblasts mature into osteocytes; these cells are found in lacunae interspersed between layers of osteoid in a pattern referred to as lamellar bone. Osteoclasts are derived from haematopoietic cells. They are found on osteoid surfaces and have a role in bone resorption.

Bone is typically classified into compact or cortical bone and trabecular or cancellous bone. In compact bone, the lamellar bone is found in repeating

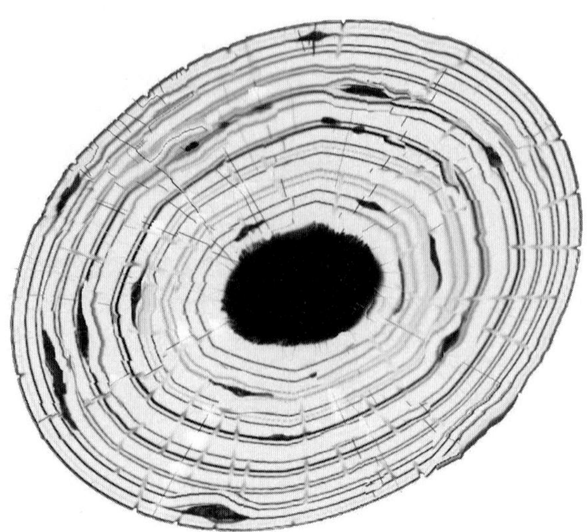

Fig. 1.2. Representation of an osteon or Haversian system. Concentric rings of bone called lamellae surround a central Haversian canal that contains blood vessels. Small channels called canaliculi allow bone cells located in lacunae (the darker spots) to communicate. The bone cells located in the lacunae are called osteocytes. Many Haversian systems will be arranged in parallel to make compact bone.

architectural units known as osteons or Haversian systems. An osteon consists of a neurovascular canal surrounded by concentric cylinders of mineralised osteoid (Fig. 1.2). Each unit may be several millimetres in length and a fraction of a millimetre in diameter. Compact bone is found in the outer layer of all human bones and is therefore often referred to as cortical bone. Although this bone accounts for 85% of the human skeleton, there is a significant proportion of more loosely organised lamellar bone known as trabecular or cancellous bone, found in abundance within ends of long bones and within the bodies of vertebrae.

Surrounding the outside of a bone is a tough membrane known as the periosteum. It comprises an outer fibrous layer and an inner cambium layer; the latter includes osteoblast progenitors which play a role in promoting healing following fracture. The periosteum is rich in vessels and nerves. It is anchored to cortical bone by collagenous Sharpey's fibres and is absent from the articular surfaces of bone.

Macrostructure

Bones are classified according to shape into five groups.

- Long bones, including the humerus and femur, consist of a shaft with two enlarged ends. Smaller bones such as the phalanges also fit this description.
- Short bones include the small bones of the wrist or ankle.
- Flat bones are found in the skull and sternum.
- Irregular bones include most of the facial skeleton and vertebrae.
- Sesamoid bones are the minute bones located within some tendons.

Surface Features of Bones

The outer surfaces of all bones demonstrate morphological features; some of these confer strength and others are the tell-tale signs of tendon or ligament attachment. One expanded end (epiphysis) of a bone is often called the head. The neck (metaphysis) links the head to long rod-like portions of bone termed shafts (diaphyses). Defined raised regions may be tuberosities, trochanters or ridges. The flared end of a long bone is a condyle, and the tip of this is an epicondyle.

Bone Turnover

In order for bone to fulfil its mechanical and biochemical functions, bone turnover must occur in a regulated fashion. Bone responds to areas of weakness or changes in mechanical stress exerted on it by remodelling to maximise the support provided. It also responds to the biochemical stress of hypocalcaemia by mobilising calcium stored in inorganic bone matrix. The normal mechanisms that facilitate these processes involve the bone multi-cellular unit (BMU), which consists of osteoclasts and osteoblasts. Osteoclasts are attracted to sites of bone remodelling and resorb bone; the resorbed surface attracts osteoblasts that lay down new matrix, which is subsequently mineralised. Whether the activity of the BMU results in net bone loss or gain is determined by control of differentiation and activation of the constituent cells and this is heavily dependent on an important signalling pathway known as the Wnt pathway. Wnt proteins are a family of cyteine-rich glycoproteins that are produced ubiquitously in all multicellular organisms and act on the cell through the frizzled receptors, atypical G protein coupled receptors. Wnt signalling leads to osteoblast formation and maturation. In embryonic development the Wnt pathway inhibits osteoclast production, resulting in net bone formation. In later life, the inhibition of osteoclast function is overcome, leading to balanced bone turnover. Dysregulation of this balanced state occurs in conditions such as osteoporosis (OP) and rheumatoid arthritis (RA) where osteoclast activity dominates.

Modulatory effectors of osteoblast function

Osteoblasts have receptors for factors that influence bone remodelling through direct effects on mature cells. The receptors include those for parathyroid hormone (PTH), 1,25-dihydroxyvitamin D, glucocorticoids, sex hormones, growth hormone, thyroid hormone, interleukin (IL)-1, tumour necrosis factor (TNF)-α and prostaglandins. Stimulation or inhibition of any of these factors can lead to a change in the balance between bone formation and bone resorption.

Modulatory effectors of osteoclast function

Osteoblasts, amongst other cells, secrete macrophage-colony stimulating factor (M-CSF) and receptor activator nuclear factor kappa B ligand (RANKL), both of which are required for development of osteoclasts. This cross-talk between osteoblasts and osteoclasts is important for maintaining balanced bone turnover. RANKL binds to the RANK receptor on osteoclasts; this interaction can be inhibited by a soluble protein, namely osteoprotegerin (OPG), which acts as a decoy receptor for RANKL. A monoclonal antibody specific for RANKL, known as denosumab, has been developed for treatment of OP and acts by blocking RANKL-mediated stimulation of osteoclasts.

1.2.2. *Joints*

Classification and Function

The chief purpose of all joints is the union of one element of the human skeleton with another. Bones may be connected to each other with connective tissue or via synovial joints (Table 1.2).

Table 1.2. Types of joints.

Synarthrosis	Diarthrosis
Synostosis, e.g. sutures of skull Synchondrosis, e.g. symphysis pubis or vertebrae	Synovial joint, e.g. hip joint, shoulder joint, knee joints

Where they are connected via connective tissue, little movement is allowed; such joints are called synarthroses. The bones may eventually fuse forming a synostosis, as occurs for the bones of the skull. Alternatively they may remain separated, often by fibrocartilage, as occurs at the symphysis pubis or between vertebral bodies; such joints are termed synchondroses. In contrast, connection via a synovial joint allows greater range of movement and is referred to as a diarthrosis. The following discussion refers to features of synovial joints.

Articular Surfaces

The ends of two adjacent bones taking part in a synovial joint retain a shell of cartilage around those aspects of the epiphyses where apposition occurs. This cartilage is hyaline where the articulating bones are formed through endochondral ossification. There are some bones that take part in synovial joints that develop through intramembranous ossification. In these cases, including the temporomandibular joints and the sternoclavicular joints, the articular cartilage is fibrous.

Cartilage

Like bone, cartilage is a form of connective tissue, with sparsely dispersed cells known as chondrocytes bound in lacunae within an extracellular matrix of collagen and ground substance (Fig. 1.3). Articular hyaline cartilage in histological

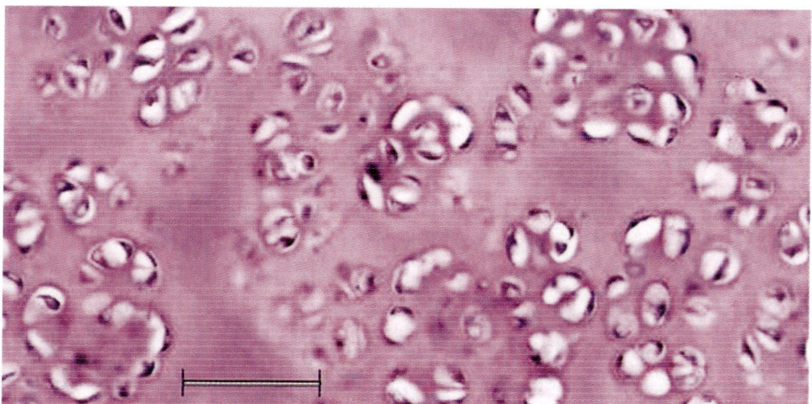

Fig. 1.3. Light micrograph of articular hyaline cartilage. Chondrocytes are seen within an extracellular matrix of type II collagen and ground substance.

section is tightly linked to the underlying bony end plate; it contains no blood vessels and it has no perichondrium. Instead, the outermost layer of the articular cartilage consists of cell-free type II collagen, followed by a layer of flattened inactive chondrocytes. The chondrocytes appear more rounded and become progressively more organised in the deeper layers.

Cartilage thinning occurs with ageing and is also a feature of osteoarthritis; in the latter, collagen degradation leads to development of fissures that can extend down to bone and to breaking away of loose fragments of cartilage. The synovial fluid comes into contact with bone and damages it resulting in formation of the characteristic subchondral cysts. The lack of blood supply and inability of chondrocytes to easily migrate contribute to the failure of cartilage to repair well if damaged. Chondrocytes tend to proliferate at the joint margins, forming chondrophytes, which ossify to become osteophytes, a further feature of osteoarthritis.

Fibrous Capsule

The fibrous capsule of a synovial joint is a sleeve of collagenous fibres that completely envelopes the articulation. The capsule often originates from the surface of the bone that is closest to the edge of the articular cartilage, has fibrous thickenings to support it, and is lined by synovial membrane. The capsule is pierced by nerves and blood vessels. It varies in size, laxity and strength to provide a balance between stability and mobility for each joint and is variably supported by accessory ligaments and tendons.

Capsules may tear on trauma, resulting in pain and joint instability. 'Capsulitis' describes inflammation and stiffness of a joint capsule that results in pain and restricted movement; adhesive capsulitis at the glenohumeral joint is a well-recognised cause of shoulder pain.

Synovial Membrane

The synovial membrane lines the surfaces found within the capsule, except the articular surfaces. It is highly vascular, with capillaries responsible for the plasma dialysate portion of normal synovial fluid and the intra-articular haemorrhage associated with joint injury. The membrane consists of an outer layer of loose stroma containing blood vessels and lymphatics, and an inner layer (adjacent to the joint cavity, often referred to as the lining) that contains two types of synoviocytes; macrophage-like synoviocytes specialised for phagocytosis and fibroblast-like synoviocytes responsible for secreting hyaluronic acid, a major component of synovial fluid. Both types of synoviocytes are also capable of expressing cytokines and degradative enzymes. The synovium is flat in some parts of the joint, and folded in others. The folds are often referred to as villi and appear more frequently in the presence of joint inflammation.

In inflammatory arthritis leukocytes migrate from the blood vessels into the synovial lining and engage in a process of reciprocal activation involving the indigenous cell populations. The inflammatory mediators and enzymes released during these cellular interactions result in synovial inflammation (synovitis) and can also lead to irreversible damage to cartilage and bone.

Synovial Fluid

Synovial fluid is a straw-coloured or colourless viscous fluid. It is found within synovium-lined joint capsules, around tendons in their sheaths and inside bursae. It consists of capillary transudate and the specialised secretions of lining cells including hyaluronic acid. It also contains white cells, although the number of white cells in a normal joint aspirate would be less than 200/ml. Increased volume and cellularity of synovial fluid are features of inflammatory arthritis. Organisms may be seen or cultured from synovial fluid aspirated from patients with septic arthritis.

Ligaments

Ligaments join bone to bone and, like tendons, consist mostly of collagen type I fibres in parallel array, with small amounts of elastin, all within a proteoglycan milieu. They may be categorised as follows:

- Extra-capsular ligaments: Extra-capsular ligaments are associated with synovial joints but lie outside the capsule. The majority of ligaments fall into this category. The medial and lateral collateral ligaments at the knee joint and calcaneofibular (lateral) ligament of the ankle are good examples (Fig. 1.4).
- Intra-capsular ligaments: These occur within the fibrous articular capsule but outside the synovial cavity. The cruciate ligaments within the knee joint are good examples as they are excluded from the synovial space by a fold of synovial membrane.
- Intra-articular ligaments: One example of an intra-articular ligament is found at the costovertebral joints of rib pairs two to nine. Here, a ligament extends from the line between the two articular facets of the head of the rib to the intervertebral disc, dividing a single joint space into two separate synovial cavities.

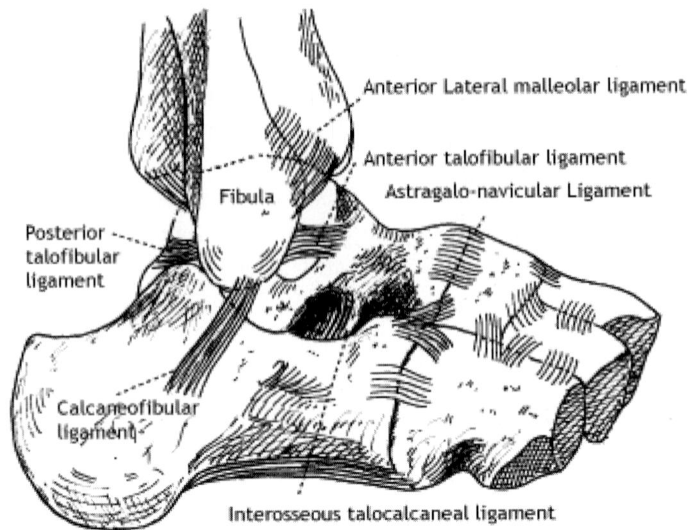

Fig. 1.4. Lateral view of the ankle. Multiple ligaments provide additional stability for tibiotalar, subtalar and midfoot joints. Ankle inversion injuries commonly involve the anterior talofibular and calcaneofibular ligaments. Reproduced with kind permission from Department of Anatomy, University College Dublin.

Ligament strains or tears are common injuries following trauma, resulting in acute pain and sometimes in longer-term instability at the joint; the calcaneofibular ligament of the ankle is vulnerable in ankle inversion injuries and the collateral and cruciate ligaments of the knee are often damaged in sporting injuries. Wrist ligament injuries are also common.

Intra-Articular Structures

Some articular surfaces have a morphology that is modified by the presence of intra-articular fibrocartilage, often in the form of menisci or discs. Here, the fibrocartilage is anchored at its perimeter to the approximated fibrous capsule and, occasionally, to more defined ligaments. A complete disc can help to create two joints in parallel or series within a single capsule. An incomplete disc is called a meniscus. The menisci of the knee, for example, are thought to help create a greater concavity on the tibial plateaus for the femoral condyles, therefore distributing the weight of the body over a wider surface area and also increasing the stability of the knee (Fig. 1.5). Meniscal tears may be a feature of ageing or may be due to trauma and can result not only in pain

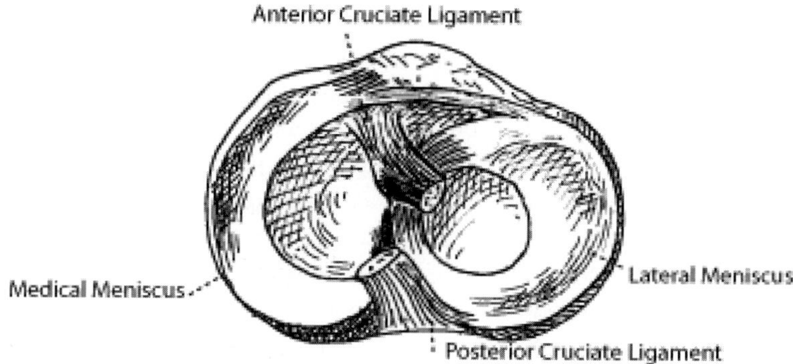

Fig. 1.5. Cross sectional view of a knee joint. The anterior and posterior cruciate ligaments provide additional anterior–posterior stability. The menisci are incomplete discs of fibrocartilage that help to distribute load evenly. Reproduced with kind permission from Department of Anatomy, University College Dublin.

and inflammation but in 'locking' or inability to completely straighten the knee joint.

A further important fibrocartilaginous intra-articular structure is a labrum. Found classically in association with the hip joint and the glenohumeral joint, it is adherent to the perimeter of the acetabulum and glenoid fossa, and helps to deepen the concavity for the head of femur and head of humerus respectively. Again, labral tears may be degenerate or traumatic in origin.

Movement at Synovial Joints

The range of movement permitted at individual joints will be determined by the shape of the articular surfaces and by the restricting influence of stabilising structures including capsules, ligaments and muscles.

- Hinge joint: The shapes of the articular surfaces involved allow movement in only one plane. An example is the interphalangeal joints. Typically ligaments will be found lateral to the axis of movement and are called collateral ligaments.
- Pivot joint: Where a bony process articulates with a ring-like socket, and only rotation is permitted, the joint is said to be a pivot joint. The odontoid process of the axis has a pivot relationship with the atlas. In this case, the ring of tissue into which the odontoid process inserts consists of a transverse ligament posteriorly and the anterior arch of the atlas anteriorly. The movement achieved is rotation of the atlas on the axis.

- Condyloid joint: The term 'condyle' is derived from the Greek word for 'knuckle' and is a rounded bony projection. In a condyloid joint, the rounded bony projection articulates with a concave elliptical surface to allow movement in more than one plane but no axial rotation. The metacarpophalangeal joints are excellent examples, permitting flexion, extension, abduction and adduction and circumduction without axial rotation.
- Saddle joint: In a saddle joint one saddle-shaped surface articulates with a reciprocal saddle-shaped surface. This occurs between the trapezium and first metacarpal, and permits a versatility of movement.
- Ball and socket joint: A distal bone containing a proximal spheroidal head articulates with a proximal bone with a reciprocal concavity. The distal bone is capable of movement in an infinite number of axes. The hip and glenohumeral joints are both examples, but note that the greater the concavity of the socket, the more mobility is limited and stability is enhanced.
- Gliding joint: Apposing surfaces are near planar, and a limited amount of movement occurs in the same plane as the articular surfaces. This form of translational movement occurs at the joints between the articular facets of consecutive vertebrae.

1.3. Biochemistry of Crystal Formation

1.3.1. *Sodium Urate Crystals*

The purine nucleotides guanosine monophosphate (GMP) and adenosine monophosphate (AMP) are both degraded to form xanthine. This is oxidised by oxygen and xanthine oxidase to form uric acid ($C_5H_4N_4O_3$). Unlike some other animals, humans do not possess the uricase enzyme and the uric acid is not further metabolised but is excreted in urine and faeces. Within the kidneys, uric acid is filtered in the glomeruli but may be reabsorbed in exchange for other ions by the ion transporter URAT1. Polymorphisms within the gene encoding URAT1 account for some cases of familial gout. Within the gut, uric acid is converted by bacterial uricases to allantoin.

Uric acid forms a monosodium salt which has a saturation point of 360 umol/l. If sodium urate concentrations rise beyond this point, either as a result of increased production or reduced excretion of uric acid, then crystals may form, particularly in and around joints and this underpins development of gout.

1.3.2. *Calcium Salt Crystals*

Deposition of two types of calcium salt crystals is associated with development of inflammation in and around joints.

Calcium pyrophosphate dihydrate $(Ca_2O_7P_2)\cdot 2H_2O$ crystals form when the ionic product of calcium and pyrophosphate concentrations exceeds saturation. This may occur in conditions with high calcium and/or high pyrophosphate levels such as hyperparathyroidism or hypomagnesaemia. Other conditions such as osteoarthritis affect the balance between local promoters and inhibitors of crystal formation and favour calcium pyrophosphate dihdrate crystal deposition. The crystals tend to deposit within cartilage and account for episodes of acute inflammation known as pseudogout.

Basic calcium phosphate crystals, such as those of calcium hydroxyapatite $Ca_5(PO_4)_3(OH)$, form when the ionic product of calcium and orthophosphate exceeds saturation, as in conditions associated with hypercalcaemia, such as hyperparathyroidism or hypervitaminosis D or when there are local imbalances between promoters and inhibitors of crystal formation as occurs in chronic inflammation or fibrosis. The crystals usually form in tendons or subcutaneous tissue as well as in cartilage and may result in acute episodes of calcific periarthritis.

1.4. Innate and Adaptive Immunity

The immune system has evolved to protect the body from infection. If a pathogen is able to break through constitutive barriers such as mucous, resident commensal bacteria and epithelium then it will likely stimulate an immune response. The innate immune system provides the first line of defence, with subsequent activation of the adaptive immune system. Activation of the immune system, whether appropriately by pathogens or inappropriately by self-antigens may lead to damage to the host and this contributes to pathogenesis of many rheumatic conditions (Table 1.3).

Table 1.3. Leukocytes in innate and adaptive immunity.

Leukocyte	Innate Immunity	Adaptive Immunity
Polymorphonuclear cells	Neutrophils Eosinophils Basophils/mast cells	
Mononuclear cells — lymphocytes	Natural killer cells	T cells B cells
Mononuclear cells — other	Monocytes/macrophages Dendritic cells	

1.4.1. *Cells of the Innate Immune System*

Cells of the innate immune system have evolved such that they can recognise pathogens or pathogen-infected cells in a relatively non-specific manner and respond rapidly to infection.

Neutrophils

Neutrophils are members of the polymorphonuclear (deeply lobed nuclei) family of white cells. They are short-lived cells which migrate rapidly from the blood stream to the site of injury. They express a range of 'pattern recognition receptors' including the Toll-like receptors, which are capable of recognising 'pathogen-associated molecular patterns', such as are present in bacterial sugars, lipopolysaccharides, deoxyribonucleic acid (DNA) or ribonucleic acid (RNA). Neutrophils are phagocytes, capable of ingesting and killing pathogens, and are also able to release enzymes from their granules into the extracellular milieu, facilitating degradation of pathogens and injured tissue. They secrete pro-inflammatory cytokines including TNF-α and IL-1 as well as chemokines that serve to attract other immune cells and angiogenic factors, and thereby play an important early role in orchestrating inflammation.

Recruitment and activation of neutrophils are central to joint inflammation in gout and also occur in other forms of inflammatory arthritis. Systemic activation of neutrophils has been implicated in pathogenesis of Behçet's disease. Anti-neutrophil cytoplasmic antibodies (ANCAs), specific for proteinase 3 or myeloperoxidase, are found in patients with Wegener's granulomatosis, microscopic polyarteritis and Churg–Strauss syndrome. These antibodies are capable of binding to and activating neutrophils which in turn damage vascular endothelium, thereby contributing to the pathogenesis of the vasculitis. Activated neutrophils are also found at the site of damage to blood vessels in patients with some other forms of vasculitis.

Eosinophils

Eosinophils are polymorphonuclear leukocytes found in low numbers in blood and in higher numbers in submucosal tissue. They migrate rapidly to sites of inflammation where they are activated by cytokines. Eosinophils degranulate to release proteins including enzymes and histamine and lipid mediators of inflammation. The latter promote smooth muscle contraction and mucous secretion, thereby contributing to bronchoconstriction. Eosinophils also express cytokines, further promoting the inflammatory response. Major basic protein produced by eosinophils activates basophils and mast cells.

Eosinophils are present in very high numbers in the circulation and in involved tissues in Churg–Strauss syndrome and, to a lesser extent, in other forms of vasculitis.

Basophils and Mast Cells

Basophils are polymorphonuclear cells found in low numbers in blood. Mast cells have similar properties to basophils but are found in tissue. Both types of cell can be stimulated by injury or by cross-linking of their immunoglobulin (Ig) E receptors. They degranulate to release inflammatory mediators including histamine, proteases, prostaglandins and leukotrienes. Whilst mast cells are well-known to have an important role in allergic disease, they may also play a role in recruiting inflammatory cells in conditions such as RA.

Monocytes and Macrophages

Monocytes are members of the mononuclear family of white cells and migrate from the circulation into tissues where they differentiate to form macrophages. Macrophages resident within different tissues may be long-lived and are often referred to by specific names (Table 1.4).

Macrophages express 'pattern recognition receptors' including the Toll-like receptors, mannose receptors and scavenger receptors. They also express Fc receptors and so can bind to and take up antibody-antigen immune complexes.

Table 1.4. Tissue macrophages.

Tissue	Macrophage type
Liver	Kupffer cell
Kidney	Mesangial cell
Bone	Osteoclast
Spleen	Sinusoidal lining cell
Lung	Alveolar macrophage
Neural tissue	Microglia
Connective tissue	Histiocyte
Skin	Langerhans cell

Engagement of macrophage receptors will trigger the cells to ingest and break down pathogens and cellular debris. The macrophages act as antigen-presenting cells; they present fragments of pathogen on cell surface human leukocyte antigen (HLA) molecules. These HLA-peptide complexes may then be recognised by antigen receptors on T cells leading to T cell activation. Activated macrophages can express a range of soluble proteins including the cytokines IL-1, IL-6, IL-10, IL-12, IL-18, TNF-α and type I interferons (IFN). Many of these serve to activate other immune cells, thereby amplifying the immune response. Other cytokines expressed by macrophages include transforming growth factor-beta (TGF-β) and IL-10, which have immunoregulatory roles and can negatively regulate or suppress the immune response.

Cytokine expression by cells of the monocyte/macrophage lineage helps to maintain inflammation in some rheumatic conditions; in RA expression of TNF-α by macrophage-like synoviocytes within joints is pivotal to ongoing joint inflammation, and expression of IL-1 and IL-6 are also very important.

Natural Killer Cells

Natural killer (NK) cells are lymphocytes with cytotoxic and cytokine expressing capacity. They are able to destroy some malignant and virally infected host cells and also enhance the long-term adaptive immune response to pathogens. NK cells express receptors that recognise self-HLA molecules; engagement of the receptors transduces an inhibitory signal that prevents NK cell activation. Infected or malignant cells may downregulate expression of self-HLA molecules; NK cells are then activated rather than inhibited and can kill the abnormal cell and secrete cytokines to help amplify the immune response. A subset of NK cells with enhanced capacity to secrete pro-inflammatory cytokines is highly enriched within joints of patients with inflammatory arthritis although their role in promoting inflammation at this site is not yet clear.

Dendritic Cells

Like macrophages, dendritic cells express 'pathogen recognition receptors' and Fc receptors and so are capable of recognising a wide variety of pathogens. Following activation the dendritic cells ingest the pathogen and process it into peptides. The cells mature and migrate to lymphoid tissue where they can present the peptides on their surface HLA molecules to receptors on T cells. Dendritic cells thereby play a critical role in priming the adaptive immune system.

1.4.2. *Soluble Factors in Innate Immunity*

Complement Proteins

Complement proteins (C1–9) are an important component of the innate immune system. They are produced by the liver and circulate in an inactive form. When triggered they are capable of enzymatically activating other complement proteins in a biological cascade. The complement pathway can be triggered in three ways (Fig. 1.6).

- The classical complement pathway is triggered by immune complexes binding to C1 complement with subsequent activation of C4, C2 and then C3 complement.
- The mannose-binding lectin (MBL) pathway is triggered by direct binding of MBL and other collectins or ficolins to microbial cell surface carbohydrates, leading to activation of C4, C2 and then C3 complement.
- The alternative pathway is triggered more directly by binding of C3b to bacterial wall components and involves factors B, I and P.

Cleavage of C3 via any of the three mechanisms results in activation of C5–C9 complement in the final common pathway resulting in the generation of

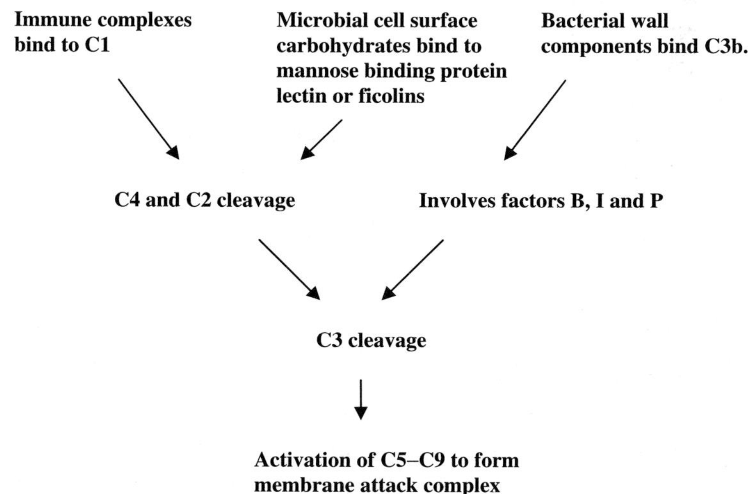

Fig. 1.6. Activation of the complement pathway by three different mechanisms leads to formation of the membrane attack complex.

the membrane attack complex. This complex is capable of generating 'holes' in membranes, leading to cell death. Cleaved complement proteins also serve to attract other cells, thereby amplifying the inflammatory response. They are capable of 'opsonising' pathogens and immune complexes allowing more effective clearance of microorganisms.

The complement cascade plays an important role in systemic lupus erythematosus (SLE). Where patients have the full set of complement proteins, the immune complexes that occur in SLE will trigger the complement pathway leading to inflammation and also to consumption of complement proteins. Levels of C4 and sometimes C3 are therefore usually low in patients with active SLE and may also be low in other conditions associated with circulating immune complexes. However, deficiencies of the early components of the classical complement pathway, particularly C1q deficiency, predispose to development of SLE. This can be explained to some extent by recent evidence indicating that the C1q is important for the recognition and removal of potentially antigenic apoptotic debris from the blood circulation. Failure to clear this debris may be associated with increased risk of developing an immune response to its nuclear components. Patients with deficiencies in other early components of complement C1r, C1s, C2 and C4 are also predisposed to develop SLE, again suggesting an important role for the early part of the classical complement system in preventing autoimmune disease.

Acute Phase Proteins

These are primitive proteins which have been conserved throughout evolution and form part of the innate immune system. Several of the major acute phase proteins found in blood are composed of subunits that form pentagonal structures and are generally referred to as pentraxins. These include C-reactive protein (CRP), serum amyloid P (SAP) and pentraxin 3 (PTX3). The rapid production of CRP and SAP by hepatocytes in the liver in response to inflammation is regulated by pro-inflammatory cytokines (IL-1, IL-6, TNF-α, IFN-γ). In contrast, PTX3 is synthesised in tissue-specific macrophages and dendritic cells and regulated by IL-10. Pentraxins play a role in the activation of complement and in opsonisation.

Measurement of CRP reflects activity in a number of immune-mediated diseases including RA. In contrast, it usually remains low during flares of SLE. Measurement of PTX3 may also provide information about the inflammatory response but is not generally used in clinical practice.

1.4.3. *Cells of the Adaptive Immune System*

Adaptive immunity describes the response of T and B lymphocytes to antigens. There are important differences between the innate and adaptive immune systems.

- Receptor diversity: Antigen receptors on B- and T-cells are created by rearrangement of many different variable, diversity and joining genes, with nucleotides deleted and added at the junctions in a semi-random manner. It has been estimated that this process of gene rearrangement allows for creation of around 10^{11} different receptors. These receptors recognise peptide fragments presented at the cell surface by HLA molecules (Fig. 1.7). Whilst each B- or T-cell expresses only one type of the potential of around 10^{11} receptors, overall there is a potential for recognition of very many different antigens, thus allowing the adaptive immune system to mount a response to any pathogen it encounters.
- Clonal expansion: Recognition of appropriate antigen by a B- or T-cell will result in rounds of cell division, creating an expanded clone of cells expressing the relevant receptor.
- Immunological memory: Whilst some cells within the expanded clones of antigen-specific cells die as infection is controlled, others survive to form a

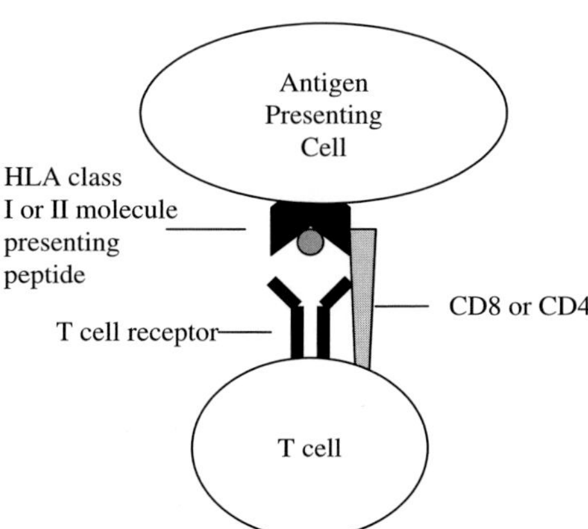

Fig. 1.7. CD4 and CD8 T cells. The T cell receptor engages with an HLA-peptide complex. In the case of CD8 T cells the peptides are usually derived from intracellular proteins and are presented by HLA class I molecules. CD8 interacts with the HLA class I molecule. In the case of CD4 T cells the peptides are generally derived from extracellular proteins and are presented by HLA class II molecules. CD4 interacts with the HLA class II molecule.

pool of 'memory' T cells or B cells or antibody-secreting plasma cells. These cells and antibodies provide enhanced protection against recurrent infection with the same organism.

T Cells

T cells express CD3 on their cell surface and are sub-classified according to their expression of CD4 or CD8. During development they undergo a process of selection in the thymus; positive selection describes the selection of cells with receptors capable of recognising a host HLA molecule loaded with peptides from the thymic environment whilst negative selection describes the deletion of cells with receptors that bind with high affinity to the host HLA-peptide complexes. The threshold for T cell activation is higher in the periphery than the thymus. Therefore, positive selection results in a repertoire of cells capable of mounting an immune response in that host whilst negative selection removes those cells that might be triggered too easily by self and thereby creates a repertoire of cells that is 'tolerant' to self.

Naïve T cells require activation and this has to be tightly controlled in a further effort to avoid auto-immune responses. Consequently, T cells express a number of co-stimulatory molecules which must engage with complementary ligands on antigen-presenting cells before full stimulation occurs. Co-stimulatory molecules found on naïve T cells include CD27, CD28 and CD40L, which bind respectively to CD70, CD80/86 and CD40 on antigen-presenting cells. Prevention of effective T cell co-stimulation has been used as an approach to therapy of immune-mediated disease. Abatacept is a fusion protein of cytotoxic T-lymphocyte antigen 4 (CTLA4) and human IgG; it binds to CD80/86 and thereby inhibits CD80/86 driven co-stimulation of T cells via CD28. It has proven efficacy in treatment of RA.

CD4 T cells

CD4 or 'helper' T cells express antigen receptors that recognise fragments of peptide presented by HLA class II molecules. HLA class II molecules are only expressed on specialised 'antigen-presenting cells' such as dendritic cells and macrophages. These antigen-presenting cells phagocytose pathogens and present peptides derived from these extracellular pathogens on the cell surface, complexed to the HLA class II molecules. Recognition of these HLA-peptide complexes by the CD4 T cells activates them to secrete cytokines. CD4 T cells are sometimes sub-classified according to the range of cytokines they express.

Th1-type CD4 T cells secrete IL-2, IFN-γ and TNF-α, thereby tending to activate macrophages, NK cells and CD8 T cells. Th2-type cells secrete IL-4, IL-5, IL-6, IL-10 and IL-13, tending to suppress macrophage activation and to support the development of the B cell response. Th17-type CD4 T cells are a more recently described subset of CD4 T cells that expresses IL-17. Whilst CD4 T cells are well-recognised for their capacity to express cytokines, a small subset contains cytotoxic granules and is capable of killing target cells.

An emerging concept in T cell biology is that of subset 'plasticity'. CD4 T cells are responsive to a number of programming signals that influence their development into a given subset with capacity to secrete specific cytokines. In some cases a change in the programming signals allows the T cells to revert to another phenotype. Thus a given T cell could play more than one role during the development of an immune response.

CD4 T cells play a central role in protective immunity, being capable of influencing macrophages, CD8 T cells and B cells. They are also often implicated in inflammatory and auto-immune diseases. There are many examples of self-reactive CD4 T cells being found in such diseases; thus CD4 T cells specific for antigens from the thyroid stimulating hormone (TSH) receptor, thyroglobulin and thyroperoxidase have been found in patients with autoimmune thyroid disease, CD4 T cells specific for glutamate decarboxylase 65 (GAD65) have been found in type I diabetes and CD4 T cells specific for collagen and human cartilage glycoprotein 39 (HC gp-39) have been found in patients with RA. However, in many rheumatic diseases it has been difficult to definitively prove that such CD4 T cells play an important role in pathogenesis.

CD8 T cells

CD8 (cytotoxic) T cells express antigen receptors that recognise fragments of peptide presented by HLA class I molecules. HLA class I molecules are expressed on virtually all cell types and are loaded with peptides that derive from intracellular proteins. Thus if cells become infected with an intracellular pathogen such as a virus, fragments of the virus will be presented by the HLA class I molecules on the surface; the HLA-peptide complexes can then be recognised by the antigen receptors on the CD8 T cell. Engagement of these receptors activates the CD8 T cells to kill the target cell and to secrete cytokines. Killing may occur via the release of perforin and granzymes stored in the CD8 T cell granules or via the interaction between Fas ligand (FasL) on the CD8 T cell and Fas (CD95) on the target cell. CD8 T cells are critical for immunity against many intracellular pathogens.

Research into T cell responses in inflammatory and autoimmune disease has generally focused on CD4 T cells. However, CD8 T cells may also be implicated and are present at the site of injury in many autoimmune diseases. CD8 T cells specific for insulin-derived peptides have been found in the pancreas in murine models of diabetes. CD8 T cells specific for peptides from myelin have been found in patients with multiple sclerosis. In both diseases the CD8 T cells could play a role in tissue damage. Furthermore, the capacity of CD8 T cells to kill infected host cells allows intracellular material to become exposed to dendritic cells and other professional antigen-presenting cells, increasing the risk of stimulating a response to autoantigens such as double stranded DNA (dsDNA) or ribonucleoproteins. Consistent with this idea, in animal models of SLE, CD8 T cell deficiency attenuates the development of SLE.

Regulatory T cells

There are several populations of T cells that are capable of regulating the responses of T cells described above. These include a subset of CD4 T cells that expresses CD25 (IL-2 receptor alpha chain) and the transcription factor Foxp3, a subset of IL-10 secreting cells (often referred to as Tr1 cells) and a population of CD8 T cells with regulatory capacity. Regulatory T cells play a role in maintaining unresponsiveness to self-antigens and in suppressing excessive immune responses to foreign antigens that may be damaging to the host.

Abnormalities within regulatory cell populations would be predicted to predispose to development of autoimmune disease and immunopathology. This has been proven by experiments that have depleted regulatory T cell populations in animal models of disease. Abnormalities in frequency and function of regulatory cell populations has been described in a number of diseases in humans including RA, psoriatic arthritis (PsA) and SLE, and manipulation of regulatory cell populations may come to have a place in management of such diseases in the future.

B Cells

B cells are made in the bone marrow and can express surface and secretory Igs. Just as potentially autoreactive T cells are deleted during development in the thymus, B cells that express surface Igs that can bind to self-antigens are deleted during development in the bone marrow. Naïve B cells are exported to the circulation and mature within secondary lymphoid tissue. Engagement of the surface expressed Ig (known as the B cell receptor) with a fragment of extracellular pathogen triggers intake and processing of the receptor/antigen complex; fragments of the antigen are then presented on HLA class II molecules on the B cell surface. Within secondary lymphoid tissue these HLA-peptide complexes may be recognised by CD4 T cells that have been primed by dendritic cells presenting fragments of the same pathogen. The CD4 T cells can then deliver help to the B cells, stimulating them to proliferate and undergo rounds of somatic hypermutation and affinity maturation in which the B cell receptors are further edited and only B cells bearing receptors of optimum affinity survive. At this stage, B cells also undergo 'isotype switching' so that the antibody (a soluble form of the antigen receptor) they secrete changes from the IgM to IgG or another isotype. These B cells differentiate to form 'memory' B cells, capable of responding rapidly to a further infection, or antibody-secreting plasma cells which migrate to reside in the bone marrow.

Secreted antibodies will bind to pathogens and promote their clearance. The B cell response is therefore very important for control of extracellular pathogens.

B cells are thought to play a role in development of several rheumatic diseases; mature B cells interact with other cells of the immune system and may contribute to development of pathology and plasma cells produce antibodies that, in some cases, are specific for self-antigens (see below). Rituximab is a monoclonal antibody specific for CD20, a glycoprotein expressed on the surface of mature B cells but not plasma cells, and is capable of depleting mature B cells. It was developed for treatment of patients with B cell lymphomas but has proven efficacy in management of RA and may also play a role in management of some manifestations of SLE.

1.4.4. *Soluble Mediators of Adaptive Immunity*

Antibodies

Antibodies are secreted by plasma cells and are formed from pairs of Ig heavy and light chains. Two such pairs, forming a Y-like structure, form the basic unit for all antibodies (Fig. 1.8).

There are five different classes or isotypes of antibodies, defined by their heavy chain use as IgM, IgD, IgG, IgA and IgE. Mature circulating B cells express IgM and IgD but following activation by antigen and a germinal centre reaction switch to expressing IgG, IgA or IgE. IgG forms the basis for antibody protection against most pathogens, IgE is secreted in response to helminth infections and in allergy and IgA is found in mucosal tissues. IgG, IgD and IgE exist as monomeric units, IgA exists as a dimer and IgM as a pentamer. There are two different types of light chain: kappa and lambda (Table 1.5).

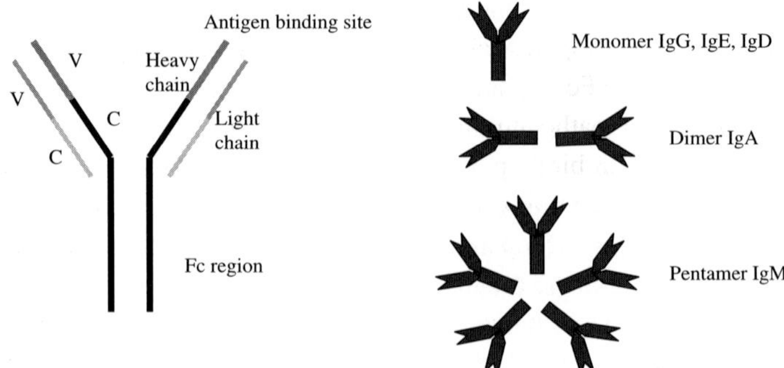

Fig. 1.8. An antibody molecule. An antibody is composed of two heavy and two light chains, each of which have a variable (V) and a constant (C) region. The variable regions of the heavy and light chains contribute to the antigen binding site. The Fc region (stem) is composed of part of the constant region of the heavy chain. IgG, IgE and IgD exist as monomeric structures. IgA is a dimer and IgM is a pentamer.

Table 1.5. The five classes of antibodies.

	Heavy chain	Light chain	Unit	Role of secreted antibody
IgM	M	Kappa or lambda	Pentamer	IgM antibodies secreted early in immune response Complement activation Agglutination of pathogens Neutralisation of toxins
IgD	D	Kappa or lambda	Monomer	Role unclear
IgG	G	Kappa or lambda	Monomer	IgG antibodies secreted in response to most pathogens as response matures Complement activation Agglutination of pathogens Neutralisation of toxins
IgA	A	Kappa or lambda	Dimer	IgA antibodies characteristically found at mucosal surfaces Agglutination of pathogens Neutralisation of toxins
IgE	E	Kappa or lambda	Monomer	IgE antibodies characteristically found in response to helminth infections and in allergy Triggers release of histamine from basophils and mast cells.

The heavy and light chains have a variable region at one end, generated by gene rearrangement forming the Fab or antigen-binding site, and a constant domain at the other, forming the Fc region.

Antibodies bind to pathogens or toxins via their Fab regions and serve to prevent the pathogens from binding to cells and to neutralise toxins. The Fc region of the antibody-antigen complex activates complement via the classical pathway, leading to direct damage to the pathogen, opsonisation (i.e. it facilitates uptake by phagocytic cells) and solubilisation of the immune complex, as well as serving to attract other immune cells. The Fc region of the antibody–antigen complex binds to Fc receptors on macrophages and thereby stimulates these cells to ingest and destroy the pathogen.

Antibodies specific for self-antigens have been found in a wide range of diseases. In organ-specific autoimmune diseases the self-reacting antibodies are directed at tissue-specific antigens and are often clearly important in pathogenesis of disease. Thus antibodies specific for the TSH receptor are capable of activating the receptor and underpin the development of hyperthyroidism in Graves' disease. Antibodies specific for the acetylcholine receptor in myasthenia gravis block signalling via this receptor at the post-synaptic neuromuscular junction, leading to weakness characteristic of the disease. In rheumatic diseases the antibodies are usually directed at more widely expressed nuclear or cytoplasmic antigens rather than organ-specific antigens but may also be important in pathogenesis. Thus in SLE, antibodies specific for dsDNA form complexes with their antigen; these complexes circulate and deposit in blood vessels where they stimulate a local inflammatory response. In other cases antibodies specific for self-antigens are found in patients with rheumatic diseases but may not play a role in causing the pathology; the presence of such antibodies may, however, be useful diagnostically. Thus antibodies specific for topoisomerase (SCL-70) are highly specific for diffuse cutaneous systemic sclerosis but may not cause the clinical manifestations of disease.

1.4.5. *Autoimmunity*

Failure of Tolerance

A range of processes operates to minimise the risk of B- and T-cells reacting to self-antigens. Central tolerance describes the deletion of potentially autoreactive T cells in the thymus and B cells in the bone marrow. Peripheral tolerance describes the mechanisms that exist to prevent autoreactive T and B cells that have escaped central tolerance from reacting with self-antigens in the periphery.

Nevertheless, autoimmunity is a common phenomenon: in SLE alone over 100 different autoantibodies have been described.

Failure of central tolerance

Central tolerance may fail for a number of reasons:

- Self-antigens may be expressed at specific sites so that developing cells within the bone marrow and thymus are not exposed to them.
- Self-antigens may be modified by radiation, drugs, infection or post-translational mechanisms to create novel antigens capable of stimulating immune responses. As an example, exposure of proteins to free radicals which may be generated during inflammation can lead to a number of post-translational modifications including glutathiolation, transglutamination, citrullination and oxidative modification which may enhance the antigenicity of a protein. In RA antibodies specific for citrullinated proteins are characteristic.

Failure of peripheral tolerance

The likelihood of activating T and B cells that have 'escaped' central tolerance and have specificity for self-antigens could be increased by a number of factors:

- T and B cells may be triggered by infectious antigens with similar sequence or structure to a self-antigen (a process termed molecular mimicry). A classical example relates to rheumatic heart disease where group A streptococcus M protein triggers a population of B cells that also recognises cardiac myosin.
- Dietary and environmental factors can contribute to the pathogenesis of autoimmune disease. In the case of coeliac disease, a CD4 T cell response is mounted against gliadin, a component of dietary gluten, a 'foreign' antigen. Gliadin is processed by and so is found in association with the enzyme transglutaminase. The gliadin-specific CD4 T cells can provide help for B cells that recognise the transglutaminase/gliadin complex, resulting in production of antibodies specific for transglutaminase, a self-protein.
- Failure to remove apoptotic debris generated during inflammatory episodes may increase the load of self-antigens, particularly nuclear antigens, thereby increasing the likelihood of generating antibodies directed at nuclear components. The abnormal processing of dying cells, particularly neutrophils,

is believed to play a role in the pathogenesis of SLE, where there is development of anti-nuclear antibodies as well as antibodies specific for a number of proteins (C1q, CRP, SAP) which bind to and recognise apoptotic debris.

- B and T cell reactivity can be modified by a number of cell surface receptors and intracellular proteins. FcγRIIb is known to inhibit B cell activation; in animal models deficiency of this molecule leads to spontaneous lupus-like disease whilst over-expression protects against development of some immune-mediated diseases including collagen-induced arthritis or SLE.
- Inflammation signals danger and effectively decreases the threshold for activation of cells of the adaptive immune system. Whilst this has a beneficial effect in terms of supporting development of responses to foreign antigens, it may also facilitate development of responses to self-antigens. This 'danger model' theory of autoimmunity emphasises the role of environmental factors in triggering autoimmune disease.

Hypersensitivity, Immunopathology and Autoimmunity

Whilst activation of the immune system leads to control of infection it may also result in damage to host tissues. Classically, pathologists have defined four different types of 'hypersensitivity' reactions to describe patterns of damage to host tissue (Table 1.6).

Table 1.6. Gel and Coombs classification of hypersensitivity.

Type	Mechanism	Example with self-antigen	Example with foreign antigen
Type I	Triggering of mast cells by IgE	Eczema	Eczema, asthma, insect bites
Type II	Antibody recognition of surface antigens with activation of complement and cell damage	Goodpasture's disease	Hyperacute rejection of transplant
Type III	Deposition of antibody–antigen complexes in host tissue	Systemic lupus erythematosus	Serum sickness
Type IV	Mediated by T cells and cytokines	Psoriasis	Some forms of contact dermatitis

Immunopathology, defined as damage to the host resulting from the immune response, is a feature of all the reactions listed in Table 1.6. However many of these hypersensitivity reactions are triggered by foreign or by unknown antigens rather than by self-antigens. Autoimmunity, defined as an adaptive (T- or B cell) immune response directed against self, is only a feature of some types of hypersensitivity. In some cases, whilst autoimmunity can be demonstrated, it is not clear that it is leading to immunopathology; i.e. autoantibody-production may be a 'bystander' phenomenon in some diseases. It should be noted that other cell types including B cells (independent of antibody formation) and NK cells may contribute to immunopathology and are not included in the Gel and Coombs classification.

- Type I reactions are usually associated with allergic reactions to environmental antigens although recent work has suggested that IgE may recognise self-antigens in some patients with conditions such as eczema.
- Type II hypersensitivity reactions are usually autoimmune (except where foreign cells have been introduced into the host as in transplantation). As an example, in Goodpasture's disease, antibodies are directed against self-basement membrane resulting in damage to cells within the lungs and kidneys.
- Type III reactions may be autoimmune in origin if the antigen within the antibody–antigen complex originates from self. In SLE complexes of antibodies and dsDNA deposit within the kidney and underpin the development of glomerulonephritis. In contrast, a serum sickness reaction involves complexes of antibodies with foreign antigen (e.g. components of drugs).
- Type IV hypersensitivity reactions are often directed against foreign antigens as in some forms of contact dermatitis in response to nickel. However, it is presumed that diseases such as psoriasis, where there are features of type IV hypersensitivity, are autoimmune although the putative self-antigens involved are not known.

More than one type of hypersensitivity reaction may be a feature of some diseases: in RA, roles for mast cells, B cells and T cells in contributing to immunopathology have all been proposed.

1.5. Inflammation

Inflammation refers to the localised, protective response of tissues to injury. It is classically characterised by the four features of pain (dolor), swelling (tumor), redness (rubor) and heat (calor). Inflammation serves to sequester the injuring agent and the injured tissue and to initiate tissue healing.

Inflammation is a carefully regulated process that is initiated by indigenous cells such as resident macrophages, dendritic cells and mast cells. Release of inflammatory mediators leads to changes in the local vasculature with exudation of plasma and migration of cells from the blood stream. Plasma carries proteins including complement, kinins, Igs and components of the coagulation cascade and fibrinolysis system, and these all contribute to the inflammatory response. Both indigenous and migrated cells can express cytokines, chemokines and enzymes that further promote inflammation. During the acute phase of inflammation granulocytes dominate the cellular infiltrate. This phase may be followed by healing, sometimes with scarring. Collection of cellular debris within a cavity can result in abscess formation. In some situations inflammation does not resolve but progresses to a chronic phase in which macrophages become more prominent. Within a joint, gout exemplifies an acute, and RA a chronic, inflammatory process.

Details of many of the cells involved in inflammation have been given within the section on the immune response. This section focuses on changes within the vasculature, leukocyte migration and some of the cytokines and chemokines that act as biochemical messengers during an inflammatory response, with emphasis on molecules that may be important in pathogenesis or therapeutics of rheumatic diseases.

1.5.1. *Angiogenesis*

Angiogenesis is the formation of new blood vessels from the existing microvascular bed. Angiogenic factors, such as vascular endothelial growth factor (VEGF), platelet derived growth factor (PDGF), fibroblast growth factor (FGF), angiopoeitins 1 and 2, IL-1, TNF-α, IL-8 and TGF-β, activate the normally quiescent endothelial cells which in turn, produce proteolytic enzymes such as matrix metalloproteinases and plasminogen activators. This results in degradation of the basement membrane and the perivascular extracellular matrix. Endothelial cells then proliferate and sprout from the existing blood vessel into the perivascular area towards the angiogenic stimulus. This is followed by capillary lumen formation, deposition of a new basement membrane, proliferation and migration of pericytes and smooth muscle cells. Anastomosis occurs and the blood flow is established. Vascular reorganisation follows whereby redundant vessels regress by apoptosis of endothelial cells.

In diseases such as RA and PsA the neovascularisation brought about by angiogenesis allows delivery of nutrients needed to maintain expanded synovium as well as migration of leukocytes to synovial tissue to promote inflammation. Agents that are antagonists to angiogenic promoters are currently being examined as possible treatments for arthritis. The anti-VEGF neutralising monoclonal antibody bevacizumab, and vatalanib, a small molecule inhibiting the downstream signals mediated by tyrosine kinase on activation of the membrane-bound VEGF receptor have both shown some effect in arthritis as well as cancer.

1.5.2. *Leukocyte Trafficking*

Leukocyte trafficking from the vessels into inflamed tissue such as synovium is a multistep process. The primary step involves weak adhesion or 'rolling' which occurs within 1–2 hours and is mediated by endothelial E- and P-selectins, leukocyte L-selectin and their ligands. Activation of leukocytes occurs, stimulated by the interactions between chemokines and their receptors on leukocytes. This is followed by firm intercellular adhesion, mediated by integrins; intercellular adhesion molecule (ICAM)-1 and vascular cell adhesion molecule (VCAM)-1 expressed on endothelial cells binding to lymphocyte function associated antigen (LFA)-1 and $\alpha4\beta1$ or $\alpha4\beta7$ on leukocytes. Finally, the leukocytes transmigrate through the endothelium.

Agents that inhibit chemokines or adhesion molecules may be therapeutically useful in conditions such as RA; at present small molecule inhibitors of chemokine receptors are under investigation. However, use of efalizumab, an antibody that targets LFA-1, in patients with psoriasis has been suspended because of concerns about development of progressive multifocal leukoencephalopathy due to John Cunningham (JC) virus in some patients. Natalizumab, a monoclonal antibody specific for $\alpha4$ integrin, may be used in management of multiple sclerosis although it is also associated with a risk of reactivation of JC virus.

1.5.3. *Cytokines and Chemokines*

Cytokines

Cytokines are protein messengers with immunomodulatory properties that convey information between cells via specific cell surface molecules. They are small, non-structural proteins with molecular weights ranging from 8 to 50 kDa, capable of mediating a range of effects including regulation of cell differentiation, replication, function, survival and death, tissue repair and fibrosis. In a locally inflamed tissue, cytokine secretion may act locally in an autocrine (acting on the same cell) or paracrine (on surrounding cells) dependent manner. Cytokines are secreted by and influence function of cells of both the innate and adaptive immune systems.

TNF-α

TNF-α is a potent pro-inflammatory cytokine synthesised by a number of different cell types including neutrophils, activated lymphocytes, NK cells, monocytes, macrophages and fibroblasts. TNF-α, in addition to being an autocrine stimulator, is a potent paracrine inducer of other pro-inflammatory cytokines including IL-1, IL-6, IL-8 and GM-CSF. Furthermore, TNF-α is a potent inducer of angiogenesis, stimulates adhesion molecule expression and lymphoid migration into inflamed synovial tissue. The importance of TNF-α in the pathogenesis of RA was confirmed using the collagen-induced arthritis model of RA, where administration of a monoclonal antibody specific for mouse TNF-α following disease onset ameliorated both joint inflammation and damage. Such studies led to the development of TNF-α blocking agents which have proven efficacy in management of RA and are also effective in management of PsA and ankylosing spondylitis (AS).

The IL-1 superfamily

This family consists of 11 structurally related cytokines, of which several members have been implicated in the pathogenesis of RA. IL-1α and IL-1β along with the natural IL-1 receptor antagonist (IL-1ra) are abundantly expressed in the synovial membrane. Numerous cell types including mononuclear phagocytic cells, endothelial cells, keratinocytes, synovial cells and neutrophils produce IL-1 following cytokine stimulation. This results in IL-1 directed regulation of the inflammatory response including the stimulation of further cytokines and chemokines, the up-regulation of adhesion molecules, and the synthesis and secretion of matrix metalloproteinases and growth factors. Targeting IL-1 and components of the IL-1 receptor has proved efficacious in rodent models of arthritis. Therapeutically, a recombinant human IL-1ra, Anakinra, reduces measures of inflammation and bone erosion in RA patients, although it has not compared favourably with the treatment efficacy of TNF-α directed therapies. Both IL-18 and IL-33 are IL-1-like cytokines that have been found within synovium and are thought to promote the inflammatory response in patients with RA. Antagonising these cytokines may prove effective in managing RA in the future.

The IL-6 family

IL-6 is a potent pro-inflammatory cytokine synthesised by T-cells, B-cells and fibroblasts, and is present in synovial tissue of RA patients. It mediates a number of functions and exerts effects on the maturation and activation of B- and T-cells, macrophages, osteoclasts, chondrocytes and endothelial cells. Blocking IL-6 receptor activity has proven to be beneficial in management of inflammatory arthritis. Tocilizumab, a human monoclonal antibody specific for IL-6 receptor, which prevents IL-6 mediated signalling, suppresses disease activity and erosive progression in patients with RA or systemic-onset juvenile idiopathic arthritis. Other members of the IL-6 family that play a role in the pathogenesis of RA such as oncostatin M and leukemia inhibitory factor may also warrant clinical investigation.

The IL-17 family

IL-17A is a member of the IL-17 family of cytokines. This cytokine is secreted by a subset of T cells known as Th17 cells but can also be produced by neutrophils, CD8+ T cells and NK T cells. IL-17 up-regulates production of pro-inflammatory cytokines, chemotactic mediators and cell surface adhesion molecules, and also up-regulates matrix metalloproteinase and RANKL expression resulting in cartilage and bone erosion. Levels of IL-17 are relatively high in synovial tissue and fluid from patients with RA, and levels of IL-17 mRNA predict progression of joint damage in patients with RA. IL-17 inhibition has been shown to be effective in reducing inflammation and joint damage in animal studies of arthritis and may be a future therapeutic option in patients with RA.

Chemokines

Chemotactic cytokines termed ‘chemokines’ are chemo-attractants. They are induced by other pro-inflammatory cytokines, growth factors and inflammatory stimuli and direct the recruitment of leukocytes in inflammation. Chemokines are involved in leukocyte chemotaxis and migration through the endothelial barrier into the inflamed synovium thereby contributing to the pathogenesis of RA. Two chemokines with well-characterised roles in the pathogenesis of inflammatory arthritis are IL-8 and monocyte chemo-attractant protein (MCP)-1.

Pleiotropy and Redundancy

A given cytokine or chemokine may exert multiple effects on different cells, resulting in a variety of biological responses. Such pleiotropy is important when considering immune-mediated diseases; a genetic effect on production of a single cytokine may predispose to several different diseases, depending on other genetic and environmental factors. As an example, a polymorphism within the TNF-α gene promoter, TNF2, has been associated with development of SLE, RA and primary Sjögren's syndrome.

Redundancy refers to the fact that a number of different cytokines can produce similar effects. From an evolutionary point of view this provides a safeguard so that single mutations within a cytokine gene are less likely to result in failure to mount effective protective immune responses.

In the development of anti-cytokine therapy for autoimmune disease these two concepts are important: pleiotropy can influence safety and redundancy can influence efficacy of the therapy. Careful *in vivo* study is required to fully appreciate the clinical effect of antagonising one cytokine at the level of the whole organism.

1.6. Genes and Proteins in Rheumatic Disease

1.6.1. *Deoxyribonucleic Acid and Protein*

DNA

DNA is the hereditary material that is found within the cell nucleus. It includes four different chemical bases known as adenine, guanine, thymine and cytosine, which are each combined with a deoxyribose sugar and a phosphate to form a nucleotide. The bases form pairs, with adenine pairing with thymine, and guanine with cytosine. Strands of these pairs form a ladder-like structure that is twisted to form a double helix. One strand of the DNA is known as the 'coding strand' whilst the other, complementary piece, is known as the 'template strand'. The DNA is tightly wound around proteins known as histones to form a chromosome, with each chromosome containing the equivalent piece of DNA from each parent. A constriction point along the course of a chromosome is known as a centromere. The shorter arm of the chromosome is designated the p arm with the longer arm being the q arm.

Genes, Transcription and Translation

Genes describe sequences of DNA that encode proteins. With the exception of genes within the X and Y chromosomes, each person inherits two copies of every gene; one from each parent. Whilst some genes are identical in virtually everyone, others show variations; the different forms of the genes are then known as alleles. Creation of proteins from genes involves two processes known as transcription and translation.

Transcription describes the process whereby the information encoded within a gene is transferred to messenger ribonucleic acid (mRNA) which then passes out of the nucleus into the cytoplasm. RNA includes the bases adenine, guanine, uracil and cytosine, each with a ribose sugar and a phosphate moiety.

The initial step in transcription involves binding of RNA polymerase to promoter sequences within the template strand of DNA in the presence of certain transcription factors. The DNA sequence is then read by the RNA polymerase which makes a complementary strand of bases using uracil instead of thymine. This complementary strand of RNA will have the same sequence as the coding strand of DNA, apart from the substitution of uracil for thymine. The RNA may be ribosomal RNA, transfer RNA (tRNA), ribozyme (RNA enzymes) or pre-messenger RNA. The latter subsequently undergoes splicing, generally performed by a spliceosome which is made up of small nuclear ribonucleoproteins. Splicing removes the intron sequences leaving the exon sequences to form mature mRNA. This is exported from the nucleus.

Translation is the process whereby the information encoded within mRNA is used to create a chain of amino acids. Sequences of three bases within mRNA are known as codons and code for one of the 20 amino acids that contribute to formation of proteins. Within the cytoplasm the ribosome induces binding of tRNA to complementary codons within the mRNA. Each tRNA carries the relevant amino acid which is then linked to form an amino acid chain that subsequently folds to form a protein (Fig. 1.9). 'Loading' of the tRNAs with their amino acids is catalysed by an enzyme known as aminoacyl-tRNA synthetase.

Coding strand DNA sequence	CTTCACCTACACGCCCTGCAGCCAGAA
Template strand DNA sequence	GAAGTGGATGTGCGGGACGTCGGTCTT
mRNA sequence	CUUCACCUACACGCCCUGCAGCCAGAA
Amino-acid sequence	L H L H A L Q P E

Fig. 1.9. Transcription and translation of part of the T cell receptor V beta 7.1 gene. The template strand DNA sequence is complementary to the coding strand sequence. Transcription generates an mRNA sequence that is complementary to the template strand and hence similar to the coding strand, with the use of uracil rather than thymine. The mRNA is translated within the ribosome to generate a chain of amino acids; CUU, CUA and CUG encode leucine (L), CAC encodes histidine (H), GCC encodes alanine (A), CAG encodes glutamine (Q), CCA encodes proline (P) and GAA encodes glutamate (E).

Many multi-system immune-mediated diseases are characterised by generation of antibodies specific for dsDNA, ribonucleoproteins or enzymes involved in transcription and translation. Thus dsDNA is a common target for antibodies in patients with SLE. Recognition of the centromere is a feature of patients with limited cutaneous systemic sclerosis. RNA polymerase acts as an antigen in diffuse systemic systemic sclerosis and various ribonucleoproteins are recognised in patients with SLE, Sjögren's syndrome, diffuse cutaneous systemic sclerosis and some forms of inflammatory myositis. The aminoacyl-tRNA synthetase enzymes are targets for antibodies for some patients with inflammatory myositis.

1.6.2. *Genetic Disease*

Monogenic and Polygenic Diseases

Genes provide the DNA template for synthesis of proteins and defective genes may result in proteins that function abnormally. Monogenic diseases occur because of the presence of a single defective gene. Disease inheritance is 'dominant' where only one copy of the defective gene is required for disease; for example in the cases of polycystic kidney disease and Huntingdon's chorea. Inheritance is 'recessive' where both copies of the gene need to be defective as is the case for cystic fibrosis or haemochromatosis. In X-linked disorders such as haemophilia A or Duchenne muscular dystrophy the defective gene is on the X chromosome; males only have one X chromosome and so are more likely to be affected in X-linked recessive disorders. In monogenic disorders the single abnormal gene is necessary and sufficient for development of disease. In contrast, polygenic disorders require the presence of multiple different genetic polymorphisms. These are often common variations in DNA sequence, each of which exerts a small effect and would not in itself cause disease. Furthermore, environmental influences may also be important in determining whether an individual with a 'genetic predisposition' develops a particular condition. This type of multi-factorial aetiology underpins many of the immune-mediated rheumatic diseases.

Genetics in Rheumatic Disease

Despite the difficulties involved in studying polygenic diseases some progress has been made in identifying genes that contribute to pathogenesis of rheumatic diseases.

Establishing heritability in polygenic disease

Heritability describes the extent to which the disease phenotype is attributable to genetic variation. Establishing heritability involves determining whether a disease occurs more frequently in families of affected individuals. This is done by comparing the occurrence of disease between monozygotic and dizygotic twins or between different generations of the same family. One study of RA in twins showed, for example, that if one twin had RA then the second twin also had RA in 15.4% of the monozygotic twins and 3.5% of the dizygotic twins. Sharing the same genes therefore increased likelihood of having the condition but was not in itself sufficient for disease development.

Identifying quantitive trait loci

Having established heritability, research is directed at finding the genes that contribute to the disease phenotype. Single nucleotide polymorphisms are common minute variations in DNA sequence that occur with a frequency of approximately one in every 1,000 bases. They can be used as 'markers' to create genetic maps which show the order of genes on a chromosome and the relative distance between the genes. The aim of studies is to find sets of markers that are significantly more likely to occur in individuals with disease than would occur by chance and hence to identify regions of DNA, termed quantitive trait loci, which are associated with the polygenic disease. For any given polygenic disease such quantitive trait loci may be found on several different chromosomes. In studies of OP 20 different loci associated with low bone mineral density have been identified and in AS five loci on different chromosomes have been associated with disease.

Candidate gene analysis

The identified loci usually include many different genes and further candidate gene analysis studies need to be performed to identify the relevant gene. Candidate genes are usually selected for study based on knowledge of their biology. The genes can be amplified in order to look for polymorphisms and further population based studies performed to determine whether an identified genetic polymorphism associates with disease.

Associations between polymorphisms within the HLA-gene complex and disease have been found in many different rheumatic conditions (see below). Associations between genes encoding other molecules important in the immune response and in immune-mediated rheumatic diseases have also been identified.

Specific examples include the IL-23 receptor and aminopeptidase regulator of TNF receptor-1 (TNFR1) shedding (ARTS1) in AS and a lymphocyte-specific tyrosine phosphatase, PTNP22, in RA.

HLA System and Predisposition to Rheumatic Diseases

HLA molecules are encoded by a series of highly polymorphic genes that form part of the major histocompatibility complex (MHC) region on the short arm of chromosome 6. This 3.6 megabase region includes 140 different genes which, apart from coding for cell surface antigen presenting proteins, also code for many other molecules with important immune functions. The area is a source of much of the genetic susceptibility that exists for immune-mediated disease.

The MHC region is itself divided into three distinct regions based on genomic position. The group 1 region encodes all of the HLA-A, -B and -C proteins and the group 2 region encodes the HLA-D proteins. The group 3 region lies between the other two and encodes other, non-HLA, constituents of the immune system such as complement.

The nomenclature of the HLA system is complex and reflects the development of different technologies to determine the different HLA types. The first method to be used was serological and allowed the definition of HLA classes such as HLA B8 or HLA DR4. Cellular typing using human T cells then allowed for distinction between subtypes of these molecules; thus subtypes of DR4 included Dw4 and Dw10. Molecular typing, developed later, led to the ability to determine further subtypes and to clearer notation; thus HLA DRB1*0401 describes a gene in the HLA DRB1 region known as 0401. This is a subtype of serologically defined HLA DR4. In clinical practice HLA typing at the serological level is often quoted; however, not all possible molecularly defined alleles of a serological type may be disease associated (Table 1.7).

The strength of the linkage between HLA subtypes and immune-mediated disease is highly variable but can be very strong. The risk of developing AS is 100-fold greater in those with certain HLA B27 subtypes than those without. A number of different HLA DRB1 alleles have been associated with susceptibility to RA. These share a peptide sequence, known as the 'shared epitope' in positions 67, 70, 71, 72 and 74 of the DRB1 chain, an area that is important in binding to peptide. The HLA association of disease may vary according to the ethnicity of the population studied and sometimes according to the subtype of disease (as in the inflammatory myopathies). Whilst the examples given above are for disease susceptibility, other HLA molecules may be associated with protection against some diseases.

Table 1.7. Examples of serological and molecular HLA types associated with immune-mediated rheumatic diseases.

Disease	Serological type	Molecular type
Rheumatoid arthritis	HLA DR4	DRB1*0401, DRB1*0404, DRB1*0405, DRB1*0408
	HLA DR1	DRB1*0101
	HLA DR10	DRB1*1001
	HLA DR14	DRB1*1401
Ankylosing spondylitis	HLA B27	B*2702, B*2704, B*2705, B*2707
Systemic lupus erythematosus	HLA B8	B*8
	HLA DR2	DRB1*02
	HLA DR3	DRB1*03
Primary Sjögren's syndrome	HLA DR3	DRB1*03

The Role of Abnormal Genes in the Pathogenesis of Disease

The identification of genetic polymorphisms that are associated with polygenic disease is important because it contributes to the understanding of molecular pathways involved in disease pathogenesis and may open up avenues for exploration with respect to therapeutic intervention. This process is not uniformly rewarding. The association between HLA B27 and AS has been known for very many years; as yet there is no clear understanding of how HLA B27 contributes to the development of disease and no new treatments for the disease have resulted from knowledge about the genetic association. Likewise the basis of the association between the HLA DRB1 shared epitope sequence and RA remains ill-understood. In contrast, genetic studies of OP have yielded results that are contributing to drug development. Deletion mutations of the low density lipoprotein receptor-related protein 5 (LRP5) gene were known to be associated with a rare monogenic disorder of bone called osteoporosis pseudoglioma. Variants of LRP5 were then found to be associated with osteoporosis in the general population. LRP5 is a component of the Wnt-signalling pathway and can be inhibited by sclerostin. Agents that block sclerostin, such as monoclonal antibodies, are now in development for management of osteoporosis.

Chapter 2

Clinical Assessment of Patients with Rheumatic Disease

Editor: Margaret Callan

Alexander Brand, Rachel Byng-Maddick, Margaret Callan, Emma Moberly

2.1. Gait, Arms, Legs, Spine Screen

The GALS (Gait, Arms, Legs, Spine) screen has been developed as a means of making a rapid assessment of the musculoskeletal system and can be incorporated into a routine clerking or general assessment of an individual's health. The patient should be asked three questions:

- 'Do you have any pain or stiffness in your muscles, joints or back?'
- 'Can you dress completely without difficulty?'
- 'Can you walk up and down the stairs without difficulty?'

The clinician should then briefly examine the gait (G), arms (A), legs (L) and spine (S) in turn, taking care to look at the appearance (A) of each region and to ensure that the joints move (M) smoothly through their full range. A normal GALS screen may be recorded in the patient's notes as shown in Table 2.1.

Abnormalities within the GALS screen should prompt a more detailed clinical assessment.

Table 2.1. Recording a normal GALS screen.

Pain 0	Gait ✓	Appearance	Movement
Dress ✓	Arms	✓	✓
Stairs ✓	Legs	✓	✓
	Spine	✓	✓

2.2. History

Presenting Complaint

Most patients will present with pain, stiffness and/or localised swelling, some will present with weakness. In all cases ascertain how long symptoms have been present and whether they started gradually or suddenly. Ask whether there was any preceding trauma or illness that might have acted as a precipitant.

Pain is a common symptom of musculoskeletal disease; determine the site of the pain and, if possible, whether it localises to joints or to soft tissues. Information about whether small joints or large joints are involved and whether the pattern of involvement is symmetrical or asymmetrical is crucial for accurate diagnosis.

Ascertain whether the pain is associated with stiffness and whether it is exacerbated or relieved by rest or exercise; symptoms from inflammatory disease such as rheumatoid arthritis (RA) and ankylosing spondylitis (AS) are worse after periods of rest, with stiffness noted particularly first thing in the mornings ('early morning stiffness' or 'gelling') and tend to improve with use of joints. The converse is true for symptoms due to osteoarthritis (OA). Ask whether the patient has noticed any swelling of the joints; this is a more common feature of inflammatory than degenerative disease. Particularly where the complaint relates to the knee joint ask whether the patient has experienced 'locking' of the joint, which would be suggestive of mechanical damage within the joint.

If the pain does not clearly localise to joints, determine whether it localises to muscles, tendons or their entheses (sites of insertion to bone) or to sites of bursae. Ask further about the nature of the pain and whether it is associated with any numbness, tingling or 'pins and needles', suggesting it results from neural compression.

Where weakness is the presenting complaint ask about its distribution to determine whether it is symmetrical or asymmetrical and proximal or distal. Weakness due to an inflammatory myositis tends to be symmetrical and proximal. A more localised pattern of weakness may be neurological in aetiology or may simply be a consequence of joint pain/pathology (Table 2.2).

Table 2.2. Pain and weakness and their associations with rheumatic disease.

Pain and weakness	Common clinical associations
Joint pain	
Involves small joints	Rheumatoid arthritis, psoriatic arthritis, nodal osteoarthritis, connective tissue disease
Involves large joints	Osteoarthritis, spondyloarthritis
Symmetrical	Rheumatoid arthritis
Asymmetrical	Osteoarthritis, spondyloarthritis
Associated stiffness	Any form of inflammatory arthritis
Associated swelling	Any form of inflammatory arthritis
Mechanical features	Injury or osteoarthritis
Soft tissue pain	
Involves muscles	Injury, inflammatory myositis, polymyalgia rheumatica, fibromyalgia
Involves entheses	Spondyloarthritis or overuse syndromes
Involves bursae	Bursitis
Associated paraesthesia	Nerve compression
Weakness	
Proximal symmetrical	Inflammatory myositis, polymyalgia rheumatica
Distal or asymmetrical	Neurological aetiology, secondary to local joint or muscle pathology

It is important to enquire about associated constitutional symptoms such as malaise, fevers and weight loss; these are common features of inflammatory disease but patients may not consider them relevant or volunteer this information when seeing a rheumatologist. Where multisystem disease is suspected then patients should also be asked direct questions about possible manifestations of connective tissue diseases and vasculitis such as the presence of a rash, oral ulceration, Raynaud's phenomenon, hair fall, swelling of glands and chest pain (Table 2.3).

Past Medical History

Individuals with one autoimmune disease are at risk of developing other autoimmune diseases, likely because of common genetic risk factors. It is therefore important to enquire about a history of conditions such as diabetes or hypothyroidism. A prior diagnosis of psoriasis or inflammatory bowel disease is particularly important as these conditions are themselves associated with development of

Table 2.3. Constitutional and organ-specific symptoms and their association with disease.

Constitutional and organ-specific symptoms	Common clinical associations
Constitutional symptoms	
Fevers Sweats Malaise Weight loss	Constitutional symptoms may be associated with any inflammatory condition including rheumatoid arthritis, connective tissue diseases or vasculitis. The differential diagnosis will usually include infection and malignancy, particularly lymphoma.
Organ specific symptoms	
Photosensitive rash	Systemic lupus erythematosus
Other rashes or skin changes	Psoriasis, dermatomyositis, systemic sclerosis
Raynaud's phenomenon	Systemic lupus erythematosus, systemic sclerosis, inflammatory myositis with overlap features
Dry, gritty eyes	Keratoconjunctivitis in Sjögren's syndrome or rheumatoid arthritis
Red, painful eyes	Iritis in spondyloarthritis, keratitis, scleritis or episcleritis in rheumatoid arthritis
Oral ulcers	Systemic lupus erythematosus, Behçet's disease
Dry mouth	Sjögren's syndrome
Hair fall	Systemic lupus erythematosus
Lymph gland swelling	Systemic lupus erythematosus, Sjögren's syndrome, vasculitis
Pleuritic chest pain	Systemic lupus erythematosus
Breathlessness	Systemic lupus erythematosus, systemic sclerosis, vasculitis
Difficulty swallowing	Systemic sclerosis
Headaches	Giant cell arteritis
Visual disturbance	Giant cell arteritis

arthritis. Likewise a history of viral infections that may be associated with arthritis, such as hepatitis B virus (HBV) or hepatitis C (HCV) virus or human immunodeficiency virus (HIV), should be sought.

Family History

The importance of genetic risk factors is highlighted by the fact that rheumatic diseases cluster in families. It is particularly important to enquire about diagnoses of RA, OA, psoriasis or psoriatic arthritis (PsA), AS, gout and osteoporosis (OP) in family members.

Social History

The smoking and alcohol history should be documented. Tobacco use increases the risk of developing erosive RA and OP. It also increases the risk of cardiovascular disease, already high in patients with chronic inflammatory conditions such as systemic lupus erythematosus (SLE) or RA. A high level of alcohol consumption is a risk factor for OP and may pose problems with respect to prescription of potentially hepatotoxic drugs such as methotrexate for inflammatory arthritis. The patient's occupation may be relevant both in terms of aetiology and because the development of a rheumatic condition impairs ability to work in some capacities. A sexual history should be sought particularly for individuals presenting with a possible reactive arthritis and a travel history may be important in cases of infection-associated arthritis such as Lyme disease (Table 2.4).

Drug History

Drug use can be associated with a wide range of musculoskeletal conditions (Table 2.5). Corticosteroids and other immunosuppressive agents predispose to septic arthritis. Both thiazide and loop diuretics as well as low (but not high) dose aspirin predispose to gout. Patients using warfarin are at increased risk of haemarthrosis. Statins may induce a severe myositis and a number of other drugs including ciclosporin, anastrazole and some anti-retrovirals are associated with development of arthralgias and myalgias. Drug-induced lupus is rare but important to consider.

Table 2.4. Important elements of the past, family and social history.

Past history	Family history	Social history
Autoimmune disease (diabetes, hypothyroidism)	Rheumatoid arthritis	Smoking
	Osteoarthritis	Alcohol
Psoriasis	Psoriasis	Occupation
Inflammatory bowel disease	Ankylosing spondylitis	Sexual history
Chronic viral infection (Hepatitis B, C or human immunodeficiency virus)	Gout	Travel history
	Osteoporosis	

Table 2.5. Common associations between drugs and rheumatic disease.

Drug	Rheumatic disease
Immunosuppressive agents including corticosteroids	Septic arthritis
Diuretics, low dose aspirin	Gout
Warfarin	Haemarthrosis
Statins	Myositis
Ciclosporin, anastrazole, anti-retrovirals	Arthralgias, myalgias
Procainamide, minocycline, hydralazine, chlorpromazine, diltiazem, isoniazid, quinidine and anti-tumour necrosis factor agents	Drug-induced systemic lupus erythematosus

2.3. Examination

The extent of examination undertaken will depend on the history obtained. Many joints are superficial structures and abnormalities are immediately visible, allowing for easy diagnosis. The scheme given below focuses on each region in turn and provides a table listing common rheumatic conditions that affect the given region. A logical approach to examination of each region involves a 'look, feel, move' scheme.

2.3.1. *The Hand and Wrist*

Pathology

A wide range of pathologies can present with symptoms affecting the hands and wrists (Table 2.6).

Compression of the median, ulnar or radial nerve may present with hand pain, loss of sensation or loss of function (Fig. 2.1a and Table 2.7).

Hand and wrist pain may also occur due to more proximal compression of nerves caused by spinal cord lesions, cervical nerve root entrapment, thoracic outlet syndrome or brachial plexopathy.

Examination

General examination traditionally starts with hands and useful clinical signs may be elicited even without localising symptoms. Always examine both hands together for comparison.

Table 2.6. Rheumatic conditions that commonly affect the hands and wrists.

Condition	Characteristics
Osteoarthritis	Commonly affects CMC, PIP and DIP joints in people > 40 yrs. Pain relieved by rest, worse after use or movement or late in day.
Rheumatoid arthritis	Commonly affects wrists, MCP and PIP joints. Pain and stiffness after rest improving with movement. Joint swelling. Reduced movement.
Psoriatic arthritis	Commonly affects PIP and DIP joints. Pain and stiffness after rest improving with movement. Joint swelling. Dactylitis.
Trigger finger	Thickening of flexor tendon sheaths compromises gliding of flexor tendons causing the digit to 'catch' or even lock in flexion.
Ganglion	Cysts arising from joint capsule or tendon sheath. Non tender. Frequently arise from dorsal aspect of wrist joint or DIP joint (mucous cyst).
Dupuytren's contracture	Thickening of the palmar fascia causing painless fixed finger flexion.
Raynaud's phenomenon	Triphasic colour change (blue, white then red) in cold temperatures. May develop digital ulcers or gangrene.
Gouty tophi	Irregular, white, chalky deposits around joints or in soft tissue.
Reflex sympathetic dystrophy	Widespread swelling and sweating over dorsum of the hand associated with poorly localised burning pain.
De Quervain's tenosynovitis	Radial wrist pain, often with swelling along course of affected tendons.
Previous trauma	Ligamentous injury, chronic carpal instability or avascular necrosis.

CMC carpometacarpal, DIP distal interphalangeal, MCP metacarpophalangeal, PIP proximal interphalangeal.

Look

Abnormalities affecting the joints are often obvious with clear swelling or deformity. The distribution of abnormalities and the type of deformities that have developed provide very important clues to diagnosis; there are often clear differences between the two common diagnoses of RA and OA (Table 2.8).

The skin is informative in individuals with connective tissue disease. It may show signs of distal cyanosis or erythema, both of which can be associated with Raynaud's phenomenon. Ulceration or pulp infarcts may occur as a more severe

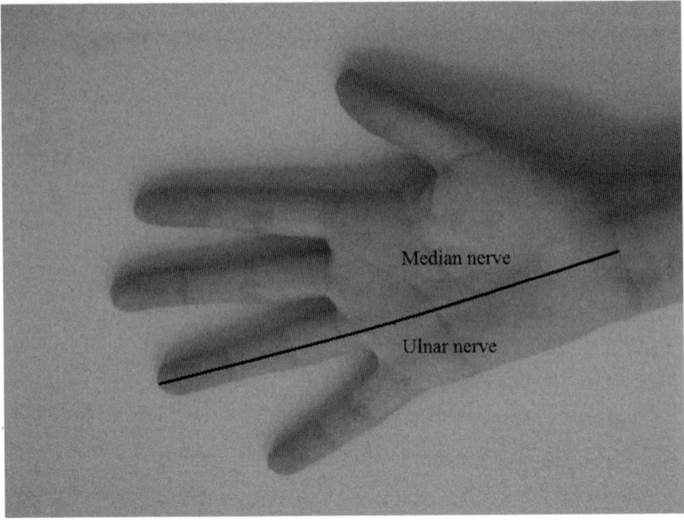

Fig. 2.1a. On the palmar aspect of the hand the median nerve provides sensory innervation to the thumb, index, middle and radial part of the ring finger and the ulnar nerve supplies the ulnar part of the ring finger and the little finger.

Table 2.7. Common features of nerve compression or damage.

Nerve	Sensory symptoms	Motor symptoms
Median nerve usually compressed within the carpal tunnel.	Pain and paraesthesia over thumb, index, middle and radial aspect of the ring finger.	Weakness of thumb flexion and opposition.
Ulnar nerve usually compressed at the elbow or within Guyon's canal at the wrist.	Paraesthesia over little finger and ulnar aspect of ring finger.	Weakness of intrinsic muscles of the hands with weak index and little finger abduction. 'Clawing' of hand (unable to extend little or ring fingers). Weakness of wrist flexion if compression at elbow.
Radial nerve	Minimal sensory loss on dorsum of hand.	Weakness of wrist dorsiflexion (wrist drop).

Table 2.8. Inspection of hands and wrists in rheumatoid arthritis and osteoarthritis.

Rheumatoid arthritis	Osteoarthritis
Multiple joints involved Commonly affects wrists, MCP and PIP joints Always spares DIP joints Ulnar deviation at MCP joints Z-shaped thumb Swan-neck deformity Boutonnière's deformity Dorsal subluxation of distal ulna (piano key sign) Rheumatoid nodules	Any number of joints involved Squaring of thumb reflecting 1st CMC disease Bouchard's nodes (bony swelling dorsal aspect PIP joints) Heberden's nodes (bony swelling dorsal aspect DIP joints)

CMC carpometacarpal, DIP distal interphalangeal, MCP metacarpophalangeal, PIP proximal interphalangeal.

manifestation of poor peripheral perfusion. The presence of roughening and fissuring of the skin, particularly of the palmar aspect of the hands is referred to as 'mechanics hands' and is associated with some forms of inflammatory myositis. Elevated violaceous papules termed 'Gottron's papules' may be found over the dorsal aspects of the metacarpophalangeal (MCP), proximal interphalangeal (PIP) and distal interphalangeal (DIP) joints in patients with dermatomyositis. Calcinosis describes presence of white calcium deposits occurring subcutaneously, often within the fingers, and is a sign of systemic sclerosis (SSc). Tight thickened skin around the fingers referred to as sclerodactyly and telangectasia are also features of this disease. The presence of dilated capillary loops within the nail bed is associated with SSc and dermatomyositis. Nailfold infarcts and splinter haemorrhages suggest a small vessel vasculitis as may occur in patients with SLE. Onycholysis and pitting of the nails both occur in psoriasis. Muscle wasting may be due to neurological or muscular pathology; the distribution of involvement should help determine the cause.

Feel

Feel each joint gently to determine whether it is warm and/or tender; both suggest an inflammatory aetiology. Active synovitis often feels 'boggy'. Squeezing across the MCP joints provides a further crude assessment of synovitis; pain is a positive finding. The fingers may be cool in individuals with significant Raynaud's phenomenon.

Move

A general assessment of MCP and interphalangeal (IP) joint movements can be made by asking the patient to fully extend the fingers and then to make a fist. They should be able to bury their fingernails in the palm of their hand. The range of wrist movements can be evaluated by asking the patient to make a prayer and then an inverse prayer sign. A brief assessment of functional capacity involves assessing the patient's grip and pinch (thumb and forefinger) strength. Passive stretching of an affected tendon usually produces pain in tenosynovitis.

Further examination

It may be relevant to assess motor and sensory function of radial, median and ulnar nerves, and to check that the radial and ulnar pulses are present.

Special tests

Tinel's test for median nerve compression within the carpal tunnel

Tapping over the carpal tunnel may elicit tingling in the distribution of the median nerve in patients with carpal tunnel syndrome (Fig. 2.1b).

Phalen's test for median nerve compression within the carpal tunnel

The patient's wrist should be held in full flexion for at least one minute to provoke tingling or numbness (Fig. 2.1c). The 'reverse Phalen's test' is a further provocation test that involves the patient holding their fingers and wrists in full extension (in the prayer position) for at least two minutes.

Froment's sign for ulnar nerve compression or damage

A piece of paper is grasped between adducted thumb and index finger or palm of hand and then gently pulled away. If an ulnar nerve lesion is present the patient will not be able to maintain hold of the paper and will compensate by flexing the terminal phalanx of the thumb (Fig. 2.2).

Finkelstein's test for De Quervain's tenosynovitis

Flex thumb across palm and wrap the fingers around the thumb. Passively deviate the wrist in an ulnar direction, thereby extending the thumb extensor pollicis brevis and abductor pollicis longus tendons (Fig. 2.3). Patients with De Quervain's tenosynovitis will experience pain.

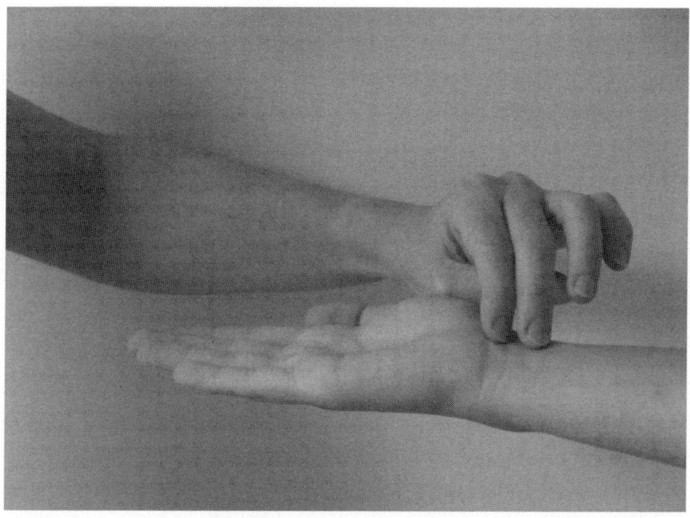

Fig. 2.1b. Tinel's test for carpal tunnel syndrome involves tapping over the median nerve as it passes through the tunnel and is positive if it elicits tingling in the hand/fingers.

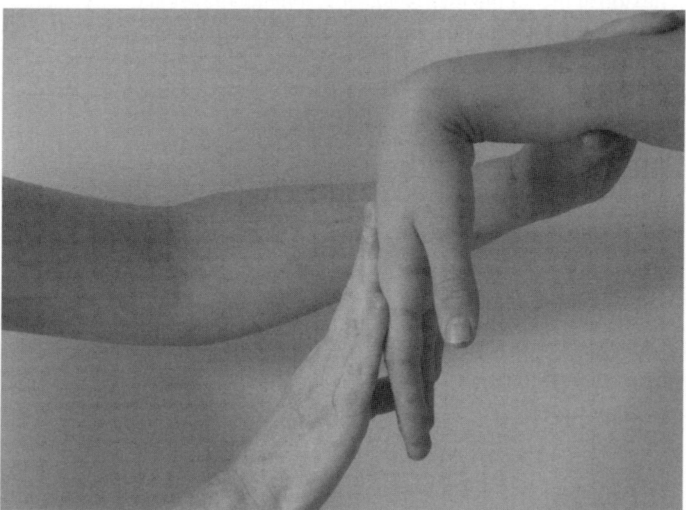

Fig. 2.1c. Phalen's test for carpal tunnel syndrome involves holding the wrist in full flexion for at least a minute to provoke numbness or tingling.

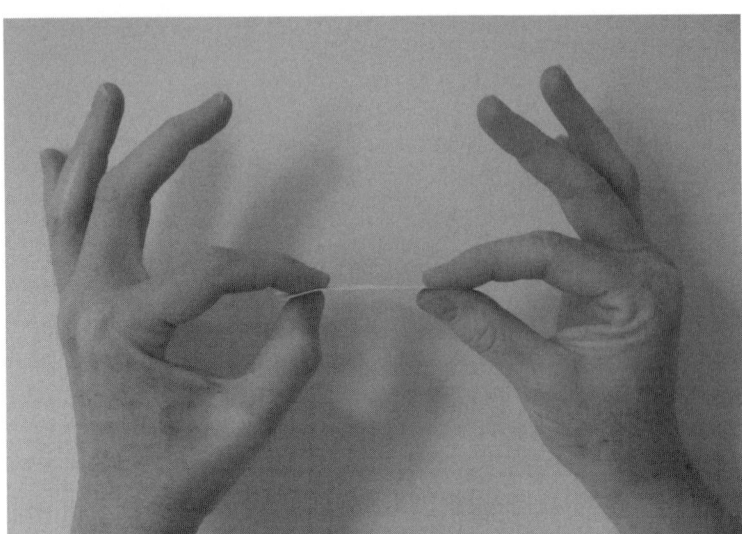

Fig. 2.2. Froment's sign for ulnar nerve compression or damage. A strip of paper is grasped between adducted thumb and palm of hand or index finger. Pulling the paper away will induce flexion at the thumb interphalangeal joint as shown in the left hand above. This is because the long flexor of the thumb substitutes for the thumb adductor.

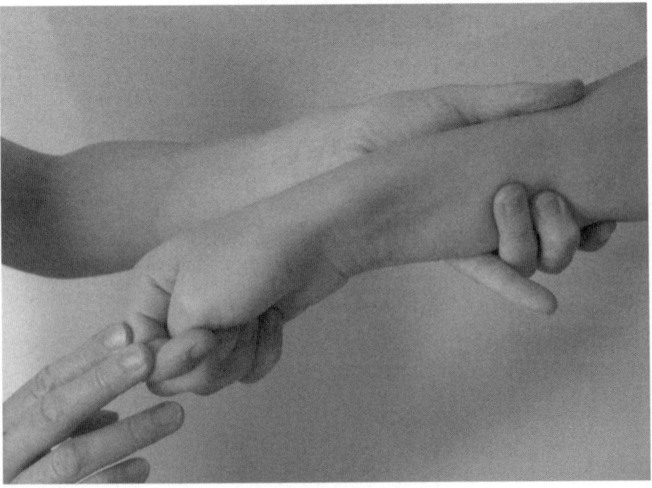

Fig. 2.3. Finkelstein's test for De Quervain's tenosynovitis. The patient's fingers are wrapped around the flexed thumb. The examiner then deviates the wrist in an ulnar direction in order to extend the thumb extensor pollicis brevis and abductor pollicis longus tendons.

2.3.2. *The Elbow*

Pathology

Pathology at the elbow may involve the joint itself, the olecranon bursa or the tendon insertions (entheses) (Table 2.9). Entrapment of the ulnar nerve within the olecranon groove or cubital tunnel may cause elbow and forearm pain but often presents with paraesthesia affecting the little and ring finger and is considered above. Laxity of ligaments, as found in the hypermobility syndromes, may affect the elbow and be associated with joint pain.

Examination

Look

Note the position in which the patient holds the elbow at rest. A joint effusion will feel more comfortable with the elbow in flexion. Conversely, a large olecranon bursa will feel tense in this position and more comfortable with the elbow in extension. Erythema may suggest infection or gout, either within the bursa or

Table 2.9. Rheumatic conditions that commonly affect the elbow region.

Condition	Characteristics
Osteoarthritis	Pain. Worse after movement or at end of day. Reduced movement, commonly with fixed flexion deformity.
Rheumatoid arthritis	Pain and stiffness after rest improving with movement. Joint swelling. Reduced movement, commonly with fixed flexion deformity.
Psoriatic arthritis	Pain and stiffness after rest improving with movement. Joint swelling. Reduced movement, commonly with fixed flexion deformity. May be associated with tendinopathy.
Olecranon bursitis	Swelling over olecranon. Painful and tender if due to infection or gout.
Lateral elbow tendinopathy (tennis elbow)	Pain radiating from lateral elbow to forearm and dorsal wrist/hand. Tender over origin of wrist common extensor muscles on lateral epicondyle.
Medial elbow tendinopathy (golfer's elbow)	Pain radiating from medial elbow to forearm and palmar aspect of wrist/hand. Tender over origin of wrist common flexor muscles on medial epicondyle.
Ulnar nerve entrapment	Pain radiating from medial elbow to ulnar part of hand associated with paraesthesia of little and ring finger.

joint. Traumatic skin lesions that might provide portals of entry for organisms should be noted. The presence of rheumatoid nodules, psoriatic plaques and gouty tophi provide important clues about the underlying diagnosis.

Feel

Palpate the joint and olecranon bursa for warmth and swelling. Gently press on the medial and lateral epicondyles to elicit tenderness suggestive of tendinopathy at muscle origins.

Move

Determine the range of flexion (normally 135°) and extension (normally 0° although women are often able to hyperextend beyond this) and assess the capacity to pronate and supinate (normally 180° range).

Further examination

If no cause for symptoms is identified at the elbow, examine the neck, shoulder and wrist as pain is often referred along the arm. Perform a full neurovascular examination of the forearm and hand.

Special tests

Resisted wrist extension for tennis elbow

The patient should make a fist and extend the wrist against resistance, with the elbow flexed to 90°. Pain at the lateral epicondyle, the site of the common extensor origin, suggests a diagnosis of lateral elbow tendinopathy (tennis elbow).

Resisted wrist flexion for golfer's elbow

The patient should make a fist and flex the wrist against resistance with the elbow flexed to 90° Pain at the medial epicondyle, the site of the common flexor origin, suggests a diagnosis of medial elbow tendinopathy (golfer's elbow).

Tinel's test for ulnar nerve compression at the elbow

Tapping over the ulnar nerve as it runs through the olecranon groove or cubital tunnel may elicit tingling in the distribution of the ulnar nerve in patients with ulnar nerve compression at the elbow.

2.3.3. *The Shoulder*

Pathology

The majority of individuals who present with shoulder or upper arm symptoms have abnormalities within the rotator cuff musculature (tendinopathy or tears) and/or subacromial bursa (bursitis) (Table 2.10). Impingement describes 'rubbing' of the humeral head on the under-surface of the acromion when the arm is raised; this usually occurs if the rotator cuff is damaged or a bony spur has developed on the acromion. Some patients have a capsulitis and a minority have a true arthritis involving the glenohumeral joint. Anterior shoulder pain may be due to OA of the acromioclavicular joint.

Pain felt in the shoulder region can be referred from the cervical spine, exiting cervical nerve roots or brachial plexus. Apical lung or subdiaphragmatic pathology may also present as shoulder pain. Pain from ischaemic heart disease may radiate to the shoulder and arm, particularly on the left. Bony pain at the shoulder may be a presenting feature of leukaemia or lymphoma. Bilateral shoulder pain and stiffness is an important feature of polymyalgia rheumatica.

Examination

Look

View the anterior, lateral and posterior aspects of the shoulder joints, comparing the two sides. Appearances, including the angulation of the scapula should be

Table 2.10. Rheumatic conditions that commonly affect the shoulder region.

Condition	Characteristics
Rotator cuff tendinopathy, impingement, subacromial bursitis	Pain on shoulder movement. Often felt within the upper arm.
Rotator cuff tears	Pain on shoulder movement. Inability to hold arm in abducted position. Commonly affects swimmers and throwers as well as the elderly
Adhesive capsulitis	Movement restricted in all directions.
Glenohumeral arthritis (osteoarthritis, rheumatoid arthritis, crystal arthritis)	Pain, particularly on external rotation.
Acromioclavicular osteoarthritis	Pain over acromioclavicular joint, exacerbated by compression of joint

Table 2.11. Examination of the shoulder.

Condition	Assessed movement	Specific test
Supraspinatus tendinopathy or tear	Shoulder abduction	Empty can test, Drop arm test
Infraspinatus, teres minor tendinopathy or tear	Shoulder external rotation	
Subscapularis tendinopathy or tear	Shoulder internal rotation	
Subacromial bursitis	All movements	
Glenohumeral arthritis	All movements	
Impingement	All movements	Neer's test, Hawkin's test

symmetrical. A joint effusion will manifest as a smooth swelling around the shoulder. Note any muscle wasting.

Feel

Palpate the acromioclavicular and glenohumeral joint margins for tenderness. Exert some pressure laterally between the acromium and humeral head to detect tenderness associated with a subacromial bursitis.

Move

Test active movement first and, if this is impaired, check passive movement. Where a patient has a tendinopathy or muscle tear then active movement will cause more discomfort than passive movement and the muscle or tendon involved can often be deduced from the examination. The supraspinatus acts as a shoulder abductor whilst infraspinatus and teres minor serve to externally rotate, and subscapularis to internally rotate, the shoulder joint. In cases of arthritis, bursitis or capsulitis both active and passive movements, usually in several planes, will be painful and limited (Table 2.11).

Forward flexion is tested by asking the patient to slowly raise their arms in front of them with their elbows straight. Abduction is tested similarly but with arms raised to the side. It is important to examine the full range of abduction; patients with a rotator cuff tendinopathy frequently experience discomfort during an 'arc' of movement with improvement on full abduction. In contrast, patients with arthritis, capsulitis or pain referred from cervical nerve roots experience increasing pain with full abduction. External rotation is crudely assessed by asking the patient to touch the base of their neck posteriorly with their fingertips and to reach down to the upper thoracic spine; internal rotation is assessed by asking the patient to touch their lumbar spine and move their hand up to the mid-thoracic spine. More formal tests of external and internal rotation are usually undertaken with the arm abducted to 90° and elbow flexed to 90° with the palm facing down. Patients should then be able to rotate the forearm upwards (external rotation) or downwards (internal rotation). Shoulder adduction at 90° of flexion, i.e. taking the arm anteriorly across the front of the chest, will cause pain if there is acromioclavicular joint pathology.

Further examination

The cervical spine should be assessed and a neurovascular examination of the upper limbs undertaken.

Special tests

There are a range of provocation tests that may help further in defining the site of pathology.

Speed's test for bicipital tendonitis

The forearm is supinated with the elbow extended and the arm raised in a forward direction to 60°. Further shoulder flexion is resisted by the examiner.

Neer's test for subacromial impingement

The forearm is pronated with the elbow extended and the arm raised in a forward direction with the scapula held stable by pushing downwards on the shoulder.

Pain at 45° of flexion indicates severe impingement with pain at >90° indicating less severe impingement.

Hawkin's test for subacromial impingement

The arm is raised to 90° in a forward direction and the elbow flexed to 90°. The forearm is then rotated in a downward direction to forcibly internally rotate the shoulder joint (Fig. 2.4).

Empty can test for supraspinatus tendinopathy

The arm is abducted with 30° forward flexion and thumbs pointing downwards. The patient is asked to raise the arm against resistance (Fig. 2.5).

Drop arm test for supraspinatus tear

The patient's arm is fully abducted passively and he/she is then asked to actively adduct; the patient will be unable to control the adduction when the arm reaches the 90° position and it will drop.

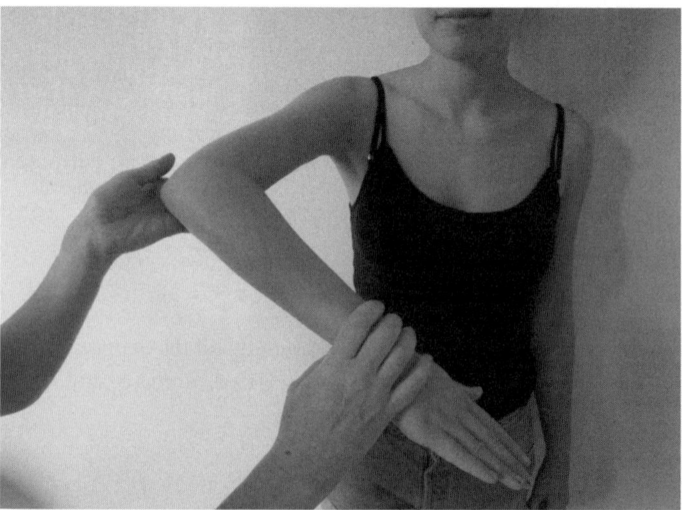

Fig. 2.4. Hawkin's test for subacromial impingement. The arm is raised in a forward direction with the elbow flexed to 90°. The forearm is rotated in a downwards direction to internally rotate at the shoulder joint.

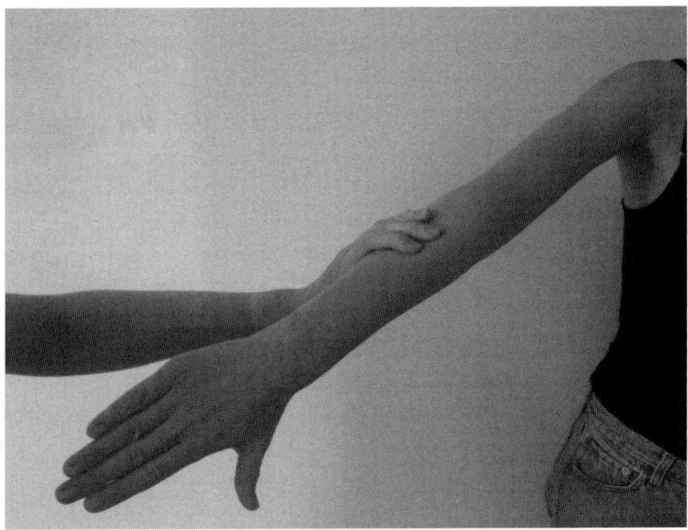

Fig. 2.5. Empty can test for supraspinatus tendinopathy. The arm is abducted with 30° forward flexion and the thumb points downwards. The patient is then asked to further raise their arm against resistance.

2.3.4. *The Hip*

Pathology

The hip joint itself is commonly affected by OA with the characteristic feature of pain that is exacerbated by weight bearing. Of the inflammatory forms of arthritis the spondyloarthritides most typically affect the hip. Bony pathology around the hip may be due to avascular necrosis, occult fractures or malignancy, and presents with mechanical-type pain that is worse on weight bearing. The trochanteric bursa is a common site for bursitis; tendinosis at the site of insertions of the gluteal musculature in this region presents with similar features. Tendinosis at or near the site of the origin of the hip adductors on the pubic rami often follows a sporting injury and is referred to as 'groin strain'.

Pain felt in the hip region may be due to neural compression. Pressure on the lateral cutaneous nerve of the thigh may cause pain and numbness affecting the lateral thigh; this is a purely sensory nerve so there are no associated motor features. Compression of the lumbar nerve roots often results in pain that radiates to the hip region and down the leg; there may be associated motor or sensory features (Table 2.12).

Table 2.12. Rheumatic conditions that commonly affect the hip region.

Condition	Characteristics
Osteoarthritis	Most common pathology >40 years. Pain worse after exercise. Severe disease causes pain at night or constant pain.
Rheumatoid arthritis or spondyloarthritis	Pain worse in early morning and after periods of rest. May progress to secondary degenerative arthritis giving similar symptoms to primary osteoarthritis.
Avascular necrosis	Pain worse on weight bearing. Risk factors include prior trauma, corticosteroid use, high alcohol intake and sickle cell disease.
Occult fracture or malignancy	Pain is exacerbated by weight-bearing or movement.
Trochanteric bursitis or gluteal tendinopathy	Lateral thigh pain often radiating to buttock and lateral aspect of knee with localised tenderness over greater trochanter.
Adductor tendinopathy	Pain in the medial groin, exacerbated by standing or walking on the affected leg. Often follows a sports injury.
Meralgia paraesthetica	Lateral thigh pain with associated paraesthesia or hyperaesthesia. Common in overweight women.
Lumbar radiculopathy	Sharp, shooting pain radiating down leg.

Examination

Look

The hip joint is deep and abnormalities may not be obvious on simple inspection. Attention should, however, be paid to the resting position of the hip joints. Individuals with OA may develop a mild fixed flexion deformity and a consequent exaggerated lumbar lordosis. Patients with synovitis or an effusion will often hold the affected hip in a mild degree of flexion, external rotation and abduction, most easily noted with the patient lying supine. Watching the patient's gait can be informative; an antalgic gait is an important sign of lower limb pathology, a Trendelenburg gait usually suggests weakness of the hip abductor muscles.

Feel

The hip joint itself is best palpated anteriorly, with the patient lying supine, pressing lateral to the femoral pulsation and inferior to the inguinal ligament. This may provoke discomfort in patients with OA or inflammatory arthritis. It is important to palpate over and posteriosuperior to the greater trochanter to elicit tenderness suggestive of trochanteric bursitis or gluteal tendinopathy. Tenderness over the pubic rami may be consistent with adductor tendinopathy following sporting injury or with a fragility fracture in a more elderly or osteoporotic individual.

Move

The majority of the examination takes place with the patient lying supine. The hip should be flexed by bringing the bent knee towards the chest. Internal and external rotation should be tested with the knee bent to 90° and moved medially and laterally respectively. Abduction and adduction are tested with the knee extended by moving the leg laterally and crossing it over the other leg respectively. Extension is less commonly assessed; the patient needs to lie prone and the straight leg is lifted up.

Restriction of internal rotation can be an early sign of OA. More globally restricted movements occur in more severe OA or in inflammatory arthritis.

Further examination

Examination of the back and a neurological examination of the lower limbs may be required if pain referred from the lumbar spine is suspected. Assessment of sensation over the lateral thigh should be undertaken if a diagnosis of meralgia paraesthetica is suspected.

Special Tests

Trendelenburg's test

Ask the patient to stand first on one leg and then on the other and observe the pelvic tilt on the non-weight bearing side. If the hip abductors are weak then the pelvis will drop towards the side of the weak musculature.

Thomas' test for fixed flexion deformity at the hip

With the patient lying supine, place a fist under the lumbar spine and maximally flex the unaffected hip, straightening the lumbar spine, thus squashing the examining hand. If there is a fixed deformity, the opposite leg will rise off the table revealing the amount of flexion present.

2.3.5. *The Knee*

Pathology

A very wide range of pathologies present with pain in the knee region (Table 2.13). It is important to distinguish between intra-articular pathology and pathology affecting soft tissues surrounding the joint. In the former case assess whether the clinical picture is primarily inflammatory or degenerative in nature or due to specific internal derangement, the latter usually being due to trauma.

Pain referred from L5 root and sacro-iliac joint lesions refer down to the popliteal fossa. Pain referred from the hip joint may also be felt in the knee. Both osteosarcoma and Ewing's sarcoma are rare tumours but may occur in bones close to the knee joint and can present as knee pain.

Examination

Look

Observe the patient in a standing position, looking for varus deformity (bow-legged) or valgus deformity (knock-kneed). With the patient supine look at the peripatella dimples, particularly medially; these obliterate with a small increase in synovial fluid. Measure the thigh circumference to document muscle wasting.

Feel

Feel lightly around the joint line for warmth, swelling or tenderness. Initially focus on the knee joint itself; perform a sweep test and attempt to ballot the patella to detect excess synovial fluid (see special tests below). Feel in the popliteal fossa for a Baker's cyst. With the knee flexed palpate the joint lines medially and laterally; localised tenderness can be associated with meniscal injury or OA. Then consider the structures outside the knee joint. Palpate along the course of the medial and lateral collateral ligaments. Feel for enlarged or tender pre-patella, infra-patella and anserine bursa; the latter is located medially over the superior part of the tibia. Palpate over the lateral femoral condyle to detect tenderness suggestive of an ilio-tibial band syndrome.

Move

Ascertain whether the patient is able to fully extend the knee joint and estimate the degree of maximum flexion. It is often informative to palpate over the patella

Table 2.13. Rheumatic conditions that commonly affect the knee region.

Condition	Characteristics
Osteoarthritis	Commonly initially affects medial joint. Pain worse on weight bearing.
Patello-femoral osteoarthritis	Osteoarthritis that affects patello-femoral joint. Pain worse on repeated knee flexion, particularly on weight bearing.
Chondromalacia patellae	Anterior type knee pain, often out of proportion to radiographic changes, due to abnormalities of patella articular surfaces.
Inflammatory arthritis	Rheumatoid arthritis and spondyloarthritis (including psoriatic arthritis) both commonly affect the knee. May be associated with effusions.
Baker's cyst	Cyst within the popliteal fossa that communicates with the knee joint. May rupture into posterior calf muscles resulting in a hot, red, swollen calf.
Septic arthritis	The knee is the most common site for septic arthritis. Systemic features including pyrexia may be present.
Haemarthrosis	Bleeding into the knee joint. Sudden onset of pain and swelling. Associated with injuries such as intra-articular fractures and cruciate ligament tears.
Meniscal tear	Occurs with twisting injuries and often co-exists with osteoarthritis. May cause loss of smooth joint motion or locking.
Cruciate ligament tear	Usually associated with relatively high trauma injury. Effusion may be present. Decreased anterior–posterior stability of knee.
Collateral ligament tear	Associated with valgus/varus injuries. Often involves ligament insertions.
Bursitis	Inflammation of the pre-patella bursa (housemaid's knee), infra-patella bursa (clergyman's knee) or anserine bursa.
Ilio-tibial band syndrome	Aching pain over lateral femoral condyle due to irritation of the ilio-tibial band at this site. Occurs in runners and cyclists.
Osgood–Schlatter's disease	Pain over site of insertion of the patella tendon to the tibial tubercle. Usually occurs in young men and women.
Patella tendinopathy	Pain and tenderness over patella tendon, usually close to insertion to inferior pole of the patella. Known as jumper's knee.

for crepitus when testing the range of movement. Quadriceps strength is assessed by asking the patient to extend the knee against resistance.

Further examination

Examination of the back and a neurological examination of the lower limbs may be required if pain referred from the lumbar spine is suspected. Remember that pain due to hip pathology may be referred to the knee; always examine the ipsilateral hip joint.

Special tests

Sweep test to detect knee effusion

The patient lies supine with the knee extended. Sweep your hand in a vertical direction along the medial peripatella dimple to displace fluid. Then sweep your hand along the lateral peripatella dimple and observe the medial peripatella dimple; the action will displace synovial fluid medially so that a bulge becomes visible on the medial side if an effusion is present.

Ballotment to detect knee effusion

The patient lies supine with the knee extended. 'Milk' any fluid that may be present in the suprapatella pouch into the main knee joint with your left hand and any fluid in the peripatella dimples with your right hand. Then tap firmly on the patella to assess whether it 'ballots' or 'bounces'. This test will be positive if more than approximately 15 mls intra-articular fluid is present and is less sensitive than the sweep test.

Testing integrity of collateral ligaments

The knee should be placed in 20° flexion. Hold distal thigh with one hand to stabilise the leg. Hold calf muscle with other hand. Attempt to adduct the knee to test the lateral collateral ligament and to abduct the knee to test the medial collateral ligament. Elasticity and movement are noted. Pain and laxity may be due to a complete tear or bad sprain or severe articular cartilage damage.

Anterior draw test for integrity of anterior cruciate ligament

Flex knee to 90° and sit on foot to stabilise lower leg. Grasp proximal tibia firmly with both hands and pull forwards. Laxity of greater than 1 cm, pain or abnormal movement suggests a ligamentous tear.

Lachman's test for integrity of anterior cruciate ligament

This test is usually performed in the context of an acute knee injury or where an effusion is present. The knee is flexed to 20°. Hold femur with one hand, applying pressure downwards to stabilise the thigh. Draw the proximal tibia forwards with the other hand and feel for laxity or abnormal movement.

Posterior draw test for integrity of posterior cruciate ligament

This test is performed in the same way as the anterior draw test but the tibia is pushed backwards rather than forwards.

McMurray's manoeuvre to detect meniscal tear

This involves trapping the meniscus between the femur and the tibia. To test the medial meniscus, place fingers of one hand over the medial joint margin and hold the heel with the other hand. Fully flex the knee and apply a varus stress as you extend the knee. A palpable click or popping, sometimes with pain, suggests a meniscal tear. The lateral meniscus may be tested conversely by palpating over the lateral joint margin, fully flexing the knee and applying a valgus stress as the knee is extended.

2.3.6. *The Ankle and Foot*

Pathology

Arthritis, both degenerative and inflammatory, may involve the hindfoot, midfoot, forefoot and toe joints. Pathology involving soft tissues, particularly tendons, ligaments and the intermetatarsal bursae, is also common. Compression of the posterior tibial nerve in the tarsal tunnel may present with pain and paraesthesia (Table 2.14).

Common peroneal nerve injury within the lower leg can cause foot drop due to reduced capacity to dorsiflex or evert the foot.

Table 2.14. Rheumatic conditions that commonly affect the ankle and foot region.

Condition	Characteristics
Osteoarthritis	Most commonly involves the 1st MTP joint but also often affects the midfoot and ankle joints. Pain initially worse on weight bearing.
Rheumatoid arthritis	Most commonly involves the MTP joints and may progress to MTP subluxation. Midfoot and ankle joints may also be involved. DIP joints are spared.
Spondyloarthritis	May involve ankle, MTP and IP joints. Dactylitis of toes is a feature.
Gout	Typically affects the 1st MTP joint. Ankle joint also commonly involved.
Anterior tibial tendinopathy	May occur after using fixed boots (eg skiing, ice-skating) or running on hard surfaces. Usually improves with rest.
Posterior tibial tendinopathy	Tendinosis is common in the elderly with development of flattened longitudinal arch and valgus deformity at ankle. Tenosynovitis may occur in association with inflammatory arthritis.
Achilles tendinopathy	Enthesitis at site of Achilles insertion to calcaneum common in spondyloarthritis. Achilles tendinosis is common and associated with overuse particularly in more elderly athletes.
Plantar fasciitis	Enthesitis at insertion of plantar fascia to calcaneum. Pain worse in morning and on weight bearing. May be associated with spondyloarthritis.
Lateral ligament strain	Lateral ankle pain following inversion injury.
Intermetatarsal bursitis	Common cause of forefoot pain, particularly in elderly women with inappropriate footwear. Pain and tenderness between the metatarsal heads.
Morton's neuroma	Painful swelling of an interdigital nerve, usually in the 2nd or 3rd intermetatarsal spaces. Severe pain on weight bearing with localised tenderness.
Tarsal tunnel syndrome	Compression of posterior tibial nerve within the tarsal tunnel on the medial aspect of the ankle joint leading to foot pain and paraesthesia.

IP interphalangeal, MTP metatarsophalangeal.

Examination

Look

It is very important to observe the patient standing as well as sitting on an examination couch with their knees extended. Look for varus/valgus deformity at the ankle, at the shape of the longitudinal arch for pes planus (flat foot) and pes cavus (high-arched foot), for splaying of the forefoot and for obvious swelling of joints or soft tissues. Wasting of calf muscles is better observed with the patient standing on tip-toe.

Feel

Palpate the individual joints, particularly the ankle and forefoot joints, to detect tenderness or swelling suggestive of an arthritic process. Palpate along the course of the tibial, peroneal and Achilles tendons to detect tendon pathology, over the insertions of the medial and lateral ankle ligaments to detect ligamentous strain, over the intermetatarsal spaces to detect bursitis or a Morton's neuroma, and at the site of insertion of the plantar fascia to the calcaneum to detect plantar fasciitis. If you suspect a metatarsal fracture, palpate along the individual bones to find the site of maximum tenderness.

Move

Assess the range of plantarflexion and dorsiflexion at the ankle and the capacity to invert and evert the foot. The individual midfoot joints each only allow a small amount of movement but together should allow for some rotation. Check that the metatarsophalangeal and interphalangeal joints remain mobile with capacity to flex and extend.

Further examination

A neurological examination of the lower limbs should be performed if neural compression of nerve roots within the spine, common peroneal nerve within the lower leg or posterior tibial nerve within the tarsal tunnel is suspected. Examine the vascular supply to the foot by palpating for the posterior tibial and dorsalis pedis pulses.

2.3.7. *The Neck*

Pathology

Most patients who present with neck pain have degenerative changes within the cervical spine that may involve the discs (dehydration and prolapse) and facet joints (arthritis). These changes are also common in asymptomatic individuals. They may result in stenosis of the spinal canal with consequent myelopathy or in stenosis of the exit foramina with consequent compression of cervical nerve roots. Myofascial pain describes a non-specific syndrome characterised by presence of trigger points and taut bands; these often occur around the neck and upper back. Individuals who experience an abrupt flexion/extension injury, usually in a road traffic accident, may develop a 'whiplash syndrome' with severe pain and stiffness of the neck. It is important to remember that patients with RA may have inflammatory disease of the upper cervical spine with damage to the transverse ligament of the atlas and consequent atlantoaxial instability. Both diffuse idiopathic skeletal hyperostosis (DISH) and severe AS may involve the cervical spine leading to very restricted movement. Torticollis describes abnormal posturing of the neck secondary to severe muscle spasm that may occur as a result of trauma or in response to some drugs (Table 2.15).

Rarely spinal or vertebral malignancies may present with pain. Discitis is unusual within the cervical spine but should be considered if systemic signs of infection are present.

Table 2.15. Rheumatic conditions that commonly affect the neck.

Condition	Characteristics
Cervical spondylosis	Degenerative disease of the cervical spine involving discs and facet joints.
Cervical disc prolapse	May occur as part of degenerative disease or as an isolated phenomenon, particularly after trauma.
Myofascial pain	Tender trigger points and bands, often involving neck and upper back musculature.
Whiplash syndrome	Painful spasm of neck muscles with reduced movement after flexion/extension injury.
Rheumatoid arthritis	Pannus affecting upper cervical spine associated with damage to transverse ligament and consequent atlantoaxial subluxation.
DISH	Florid osteophytes leading to spinal fusion.
Spondyloarthritis	In severe cases cervical spine may be involved with stiffness and restricted movements.
Torticollis	Painful spasm of neck musculature leading to abnormal posturing of neck.

DISH diffuse idiopathic skeletal hyperostosis.

Examination

Look

Note the resting posture of the head/neck and look for the visible muscle spasm that is present in patients with torticollis.

Feel

Palpate along the spinal processes for tenderness and then over the paraspinal and upper trapezius for the presence of trigger points and spasm.

Move

Examine movements of the neck in three planes; forward flexion and extension, rotation and lateral flexion. Abnormalities of rotation are common where pathology involves the upper cervical spine whilst impairment of lateral flexion is more suggestive of lower cervical spine disease.

Further examination

It is essential to perform a neurological examination. Knowledge of myotomes and dermatomes will allow conclusions to be drawn about the level of the pathology within the cervical spine (Table 2.16). The C4 root carries sensory innervations from the shoulder and upper arm, C5 from the lateral upper arm, C6 from the radial aspect of the forearm and hand, C7 from the central forearm and middle finger and C8 from the ulnar part of the hand and forearm. The principal spinal nerve root(s) involved in the biceps reflex are C5 and C6, in the brachioradialis (supinator) reflex is C6 and the triceps reflex are C7 and C8.

Table 2.16. Myotomes of the upper limb.

Action	Principal nerve roots supplying muscles
Shoulder abduction	C4, C5, C6
Elbow flexion	C5, C6
Elbow extension	C7, C8
Wrist flexion	C6, C7, C8
Wrist extension	C7, C8
Finger spreading	T1

If there is concern about the possibility of cervical cord compression then a fuller neurological assessment should take place, including examination of the lower limbs looking for evidence of upper motor neurone signs including hyperreflexia and an extensor plantar response.

2.3.8. *The Thoracic and Lumbar Spine*

Pathology

Most individuals with back pain do not have serious pathology. However, important causes of back pain include the spondyloarthritides, infection, malignancy and vertebral fractures (Table 2.17).

Complications of spinal disease include stenosis of the spinal canal, compression of the spinal cord, cauda equina or individual nerve roots (Table 2.18).

Examination

Look

Examine the patient standing; observe for deformities of the spine including scoliosis (lateral curvature), kyphosis (forward curvature) or abnormalities of the

Table 2.17. Rheumatic conditions that commonly affect the thoracic and lumbar spine.

Condition	Characteristics
Spondylosis	Degenerative disease of the spine involving discs and facet joints.
Disc prolapse	May occur as part of degenerative disease or as an isolated phenomenon, particularly after trauma.
DISH	Florid osteophytes leading to spinal fusion.
Spondyloarthritis (sacroiliitis and spondylitis)	Low back pain and stiffness is characteristic of sacroiliitis. May progress to involve spine.
Discitis or osteomyelitis	Localised pain and tenderness, usually with systemic features of fever and malaise.
Malignancy	Localised pain and tenderness, sometimes with systemic features of anorexia, weight loss and malaise.
Vertebral compression	Localised pain and tenderness. Often due to osteoporosis but may also be secondary to underlying infection or malignancy.

DISH diffuse idiopathic skeletal hyperostosis.

Table 2.18. Neurological complications of spinal disease.

Condition	Characteristics
Spinal stenosis	Back pain and leg pain when walking, relieved by rest (neurogenic claudication).
Cord compression	Variable neurology including upper motor neurone signs in lower limbs and numbness with sensory level.
Nerve root compression	Many different manifestations. Radiating sharp or burning pain. Numbness or weakness corresponding to relevant dermatome and myotome.
Cauda equina syndrome	Weakness of legs, loss of bladder/bowel control, perineal numbness (sometimes termed 'saddle anaesthesia').

usual lumbar lordosis (backward curvature). Look at the skin for scars indicative of previous surgery or trauma.

Feel

The vertebral column should be palpated for tenderness both centrally over the vertebral bodies and the intervertebral discs and slightly more laterally over the facet joints. The sacroiliac joints should also be palpated for tenderness.

Move

The ability of the patient to rotate the thoracic spine should be determined by asking them to 'twist' to the side with their pelvis facing forward. Their capacity to flex the lumbar spine should be assessed by asking them to bend forward and touch their toes. This may be measured more formally using a modified Schober's test as described below. Capacity to laterally flex the spine should also be assessed; a patient should be able move their hand at least 10 cms down the lateral aspect of their legs.

Further examination

If there is suspected leg weakness, paraesthesia or sphincter disturbance a neurological examination of the lower limbs should be carried out. Knowledge of the lower limb myotomes and dermatomes will help to localise the pathology within the spine (Table 2.19). Dermatomes are arranged in approximately diagonal strips, descending lateral to medial. It is helpful to remember that **L3** descends to the **knee** and **L4** to the **floor**. Sensory innervation to the medial aspect of the foot

Table 2.19. Myotomes of the lower limb.

Action	Principal nerve roots supplying muscles
Hip flexion	L2, L3
Hip extension	L4, L5
Knee flexion	L5, S1
Knee extension	L3, L4
Ankle dorsiflexion	L4, L5
Ankle plantarflexion	S1, S2
Great toe dorsiflexion	L5
Great toe plantarflexion	S1

is carried via the L5 root and to the lateral aspect via the S1 root. The knee reflex is mediated by the L3 and L4 nerve roots with the ankle jerk reflex being mediated predominantly by S1 nerve roots.

If there are systemic features look for possible malignancy or sites of infection; remember to examine the breasts in women and prostate in men and to feel for lymphadenopathy.

Palpate the distal pulses (dorsalis pedis and posterior tibial) to rule out significant peripheral vascular disease.

Special tests

Modified Schober's test to assess lumbar flexion

Feel the midpoint of posterior superior iliac spines with patient standing. Mark 10 cm above and 5 cm below. Ask the patient to lean forward to touch toes and re-measure the space between these two points. The distance should lengthen by >5 cm.

Straight leg raise to assess impingement of lower lumbar/sacral nerve roots

With the patient supine passively extend each leg in turn with the knee extended and the ankle dorsiflexed. Pain in the back, buttock or leg on elevation <60° represents a positive result. However, note that pain in the posterior thigh generally reflects tight hamstring musculature rather than neural impingement.

Femoral stretch test to assess impingement of upper lumbar nerve roots

With the patient lying prone flex the knee and gently extend the hip. Back pain suggests compression of nerve roots contributing to the femoral nerve.

2.3.9. *Gait*

There are four phases within a normal gait, with arms moving smoothly with the opposite leg. The heel strikes the ground with the hip flexed and the knee extended and this is followed by the loading/stance phase when the foot pronates. Toe-off occurs with the heel rising and the hip extended, leading to the swing phase when the knee is flexed and the ankle dorsiflexed. If the gait is entirely normal, significant lumbar spine or lower limb pathology is unlikely. Common and easily recognised abnormalities of gait together with their causes are shown in Table 2.20.

2.3.10. *Extra-Articular Features of Rheumatic Disease*

It is important to look for extra-articular features of disease as well as for abnormalities within the musculoskeletal system itself. All types of inflammatory disease may lead to fevers and weight loss. The cutaneous lesions of psoriasis are often obvious over the extensor aspects of elbows and knees but may be more difficult to find around the hairline and at the navel. A facial rash, oral ulceration, lymphadenopathy and signs of serositis are common features

Table 2.20. Abnormalities of gait.

Type	Cause	Gait
Antalgic	Pain in one limb.	Weight-bears for a shorter time on the affected side. Asymmetrical arm swing.
Trendelenburg	Weak abductor, gluteus maximus and minimus muscles or hip joint disease.	Pelvis tilts down to opposite side, the trunk tries to stabilise by swinging over to weakened side.
Stomping	Sensory peripheral neuropathy.	Foot is 'slammed' to the ground due to lack of sensory feedback.
Myopathic (waddling)	Proximal myopathy.	Weakness of proximal muscles results in circumduction rather than usual flexion movement at hip.
High stepping (foot drop)	Common peroneal nerve injury.	Inability to dorsiflex foot requires the knee to be lifted higher before foot is placed on the ground.

of SLE. Tightening of the skin, telangiectasia and calcinosis are signs of SSc, and signs within the respiratory system reflecting interstitial lung disease or within the cardiovascular system reflecting pulmonary hypertension may be present. Keratoconjunctivitis sicca and dryness of the mouth with poor dentition are features of Sjögren's syndrome. Uveitis is associated with the spondyloarthritides and keratitis, scleritis and episcleritis may be features of RA (Table 2.21).

2.3.11. *Miscellaneous Specific Examinations*

Schirmer's Test

Schirmer's test is used to evaluate tear secretion and contributes to diagnosis in Sjögren's syndrome. The tip of a 30 mm strip of filter paper is folded back,

Table 2.21. Extra-articular features of rheumatic disease.

System	Features
General	Well or unwell
	Pyrexia,
	Cachexia
	Lymphadenopathy
Skin	Malar rash of systemic lupus erythematosus
	Psoriasis
	Telangiectasia
	Sclerodermatous changes
	Calcinosis
	Cutaneous vasculitis
Mouth	Dryness
	Poor dentition
	Ulceration
	High arched palate
Eyes	Keratoconjunctivitis sicca
	Conjunctivitis
	Uveitis
	Keratitis
	Scleritis or episcleritis
Heart and Lung	Serositis (pleural or pericardial)
	Pulmonary fibrosis
	Pulmonary hypertension

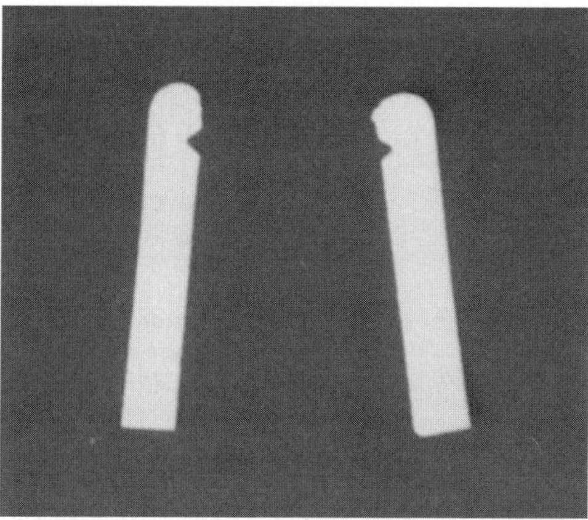

Fig. 2.6a. Schirmer's test for dry eyes. Two small strips of filter paper are used to perform this test.

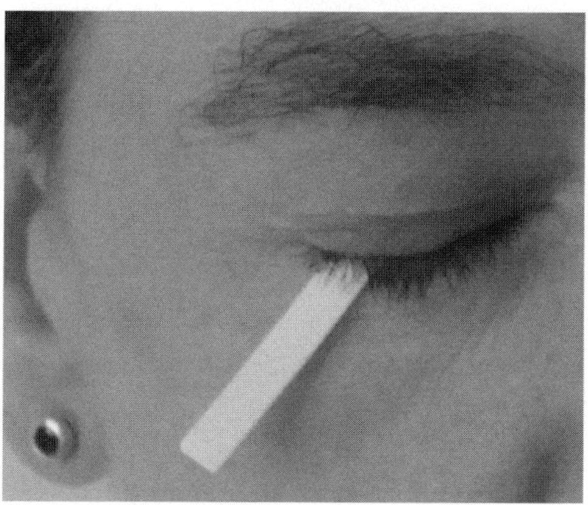

Fig. 2.6b. Schirmer's test for dry eyes. Each strip is inserted inside the lower eyelid and left for 5 mins. The patient will be more comfortable if the eye is closed during this time. The level of wetness along the filter paper is then measured and should be >10 mm.

inserted to inside of lower eyelid and left for 5 mins (Figs. 2.6a and 2.6.b). The level of wetness is then measured and is normally at least 10 mm.

Beighton Score for Hypermobility

This involves testing movement at four pairs of joints and the spine to give a score out of 9. A value of 4 or greater is considered significant (Table 2.22).

Trigger Points for Fibromyalgia

Palpate over 18 (nine symmetrical pairs of) trigger points, applying a force of approximately 4 kg (Fig. 2.7). Tenderness over at least 11 of these sites may signify fibromyalgia.

Table 2.22. Beighton score for hypermobility.

Joint	Abnormal Movement
Little finger MCPs	Passive extension beyond 90°
Wrists	Ability to flex/abduct thumb to touch the forearm
Elbows	Passive extension beyond 10°
Knees	Passive extension beyond 10°
Spine	Ability to flex forward with straight knees to place both palms flat on the floor

MCP metacarpophalangeal.

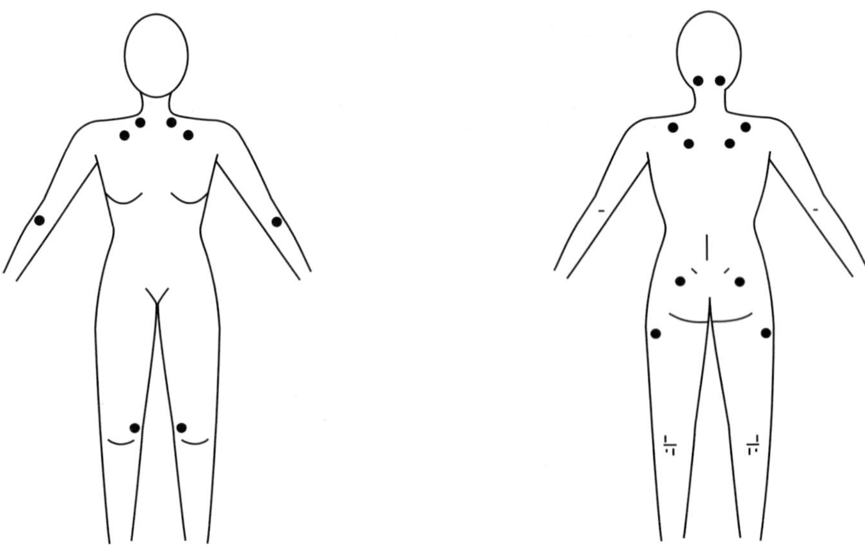

Fig. 2.7. Trigger points in fibromyalgia. Firm pressure should be exerted over each of the 18 trigger points shown above. Induction of pain at a minimum of 11 of these points is part of the diagnostic criteria used for fibromyalgia.

2.4. Investigation of Rheumatic Disease

Throughout the consultation it is important to try and put together the information derived to build a differential so that relevant investigations can be requested and the diagnosis reached as soon as possible. Laboratory tests and imaging studies are frequently helpful in investigation of rheumatic conditions. Neurophysiological tests and histopathological or microbiological studies are also sometimes indicated. Urinalysis to detect protein or microscopic haematuria is a sensitive test for glomerulonephritis and should be performed routinely on patients with SLE or vasculitis.

2.4.1. *Laboratory Tests*

Haematology

Full blood count

A low haemoglobin is a common finding in patients attending rheumatology clinics with the size of the red cells providing clues to the aetiology of the anaemia (Table 2.23).

A leukocytosis, particularly neutrophilia, is a common finding in patients given high doses of corticosteroids. Eosinophilia is characterisitic in Churg–Strauss syndrome and may also be a feature of other forms of vasculitis. Leukopenia may

Table 2.23. Causes of anaemia in patients attending rheumatology clinics.

Type of anaemia	Aetiology	Examples of causes in rheumatic disease
Microcytic	Iron deficiency	Peptic ulceration due to non-steroidal anti-inflammatory agents. Malabsorption as in enteropathic arthritis or underpinning osteoporosis.
Normocytic	Anaemia of chronic disease	Chronic inflammatory diseases such as rheumatoid arthritis or systemic lupus erythematosus
Macrocytic	B_{12} deficiency	Pernicious anaemia
	Folate deficiency	Malabsorption as in enteropathic arthritis or underpinning osteoporosis.
	Drug-induced	Methotrexate Azathioprine Alcohol
Aplastic	Drug-induced	Sulphasalazine Non-steroidal anti-inflammatory drugs

Table 2.24. Abnormalities of white cell and platelet counts.

	White cells	Platelets
High	Corticosteroids (neutrophilia) Churg–Strauss syndrome or vasculitis (eosinophils)	Chronic inflammatory conditions
Low	Systemic lupus erythematosus (lymphopenia, neutropenia) Felty's syndrome (neutropenia) Drug-induced	Anti-phospholipid syndrome Systemic lupus erythematosus Drug-induced

be drug-induced or may be a feature of SLE (lymphopenia or neutropenia) or Felty's syndrome (neutropenia). Thrombocytosis is frequently found in patients with severe inflammatory diseases including RA or vasculitis. A modest thrombocytopenia is often found in patients with an anti-phospholipid syndrome and a more striking thrombocytopenia may be a feature of SLE (Table 2.24).

Erythrocyte sedimentation rate

The erythrocyte sedimentation rate (ESR) quite literally measures the rate at which the red cells sediment (fall in a vertical column) in mm/s. The rate of fall is affected by the presence of fibrinogen (levels of which increase with tissue inflammation) and immunoglobulins (Igs) within the serum. Fibrinogen has a long half-life and so the ESR remains high for some time following resolution of infection or inflammation. A high ESR in the presence of normal biochemical markers of inflammation such as the C-reactive protein (CRP) usually reflects high levels of Igs and should prompt investigation for a connective tissue disease such as SLE or Sjögren's or for myeloma. The normal ESR tends to increase with age so that the upper limit of normal can be calculated approximately as the patient's age divided by 2, with the addition of 5 for a woman.

Clotting profile and the lupus anticoagulant test

A prolonged activated partial thromboplastin time (APTT) or dilute Russel's viper venom time (DRVVT) can be a feature of the anti-phospholipid syndrome. The prolonged clotting time cannot be corrected by addition of normal plasma (to provide clotting factors) but can be corrected by addition of excess phospholipid (to saturate the anti-phospholipid antibodies). Provided no clotting factor inhibitors are present this signifies the presence of a 'lupus anti-coagulant'. The test results cannot be interpreted properly when the patient is taking warfarin.

Biochemistry

Renal and liver function

Baseline studies are often required prior to introduction of potentially toxic drugs. Impaired renal function may be a feature of connective tissue diseases or vasculitis, impaired liver function is more often drug induced.

Bone biochemistry

Vitamin D deficiency is very common and if severe or prolonged will stimulate parathyroid hormone (PTH) secretion in order to maintain serum calcium in the normal range. Correction of the vitamin D deficiency is usually followed by a fall in the PTH to the normal range. Occasionally PTH secretion becomes autonomous resulting in tertiary hyperparathyroidism; the biochemical picture in these patients resembles that found in patients with primary hyperparathyroidism (Table 2.25).

Acute phase reactants

The CRP, serum amyloid A, fibrinogen, ferritin, haptoglobins and alpha 1 antitrypsin all act as acute phase proteins with levels being elevated by inflammation, infection, trauma, infarction and some malignancies. In contrast, albumin and transferrin levels fall in these conditions. The CRP is most commonly measured and used to assess inflammation in rheumatic conditions.

Table 2.25. Vitamin D deficiency and hyperparathyroidism.

Condition	Vitamin D	PTH	Calcium	Alkaline phosphatase
Primary hyperparathyroidism	Normal	High	High	Normal/High
Mild/moderate vitamin D deficiency	Low	Normal	Normal	Normal
Severe/prolonged vitamin D deficiency with secondary hyperparathyroidism	Low	High	Normal	Normal/High
Tertiary hyperparathyroidism (following correction of vitamin D deficiency)	Normal	High	High	Normal/High

It has a short half-life and so can be used to monitor changes in inflammation over time. Unlike the ESR it often remains normal in SLE. Both the ESR and CRP remain normal in OA.

Miscellaneous biochemistry

The serum urate (uric acid) is usually raised in patients who suffer from gout although it may be normal during an acute attack of gout as the acute phase response leads to increased renal excretion of uric acid. The creatine kinase (CK) is raised in patients with myositis and the serum angiotensin converting enzyme (ACE) may be raised in sarcoidosis. The lactate dehydrogenase (LDH) can be elevated in patients with lymphoma, which is often an important differential diagnosis in individuals with constitutional symptoms and multisystem disease.

Immunology

Immunoglobulins and cryoglobulins

A polyclonal increase in serum Ig is seen in many systemic inflammatory conditions and is particularly common in SLE and Sjögren's syndrome. The presence of a monoclonal band of Ig (paraprotein) suggests the expansion of a clone of plasma cells and is found in myeloma or monoclonal gammopathies of unknown significance (MGUS).

Cryoglobulins are monoclonal or polyclonal Igs that precipitate in temperatures $<4°C$ and re-dissolve when warmed. Precipitation causes complement activation and inflammation resulting in vasculitis.

Antibodies associated with rheumatoid arthritis

Rheumatoid factor (RF) describes Ig directed against the Fc portion of autologous IgG. Most assays detect IgM RF although individuals may also have IgG or IgA RFs. The presence of RF has moderate sensitivity and specificity for RA. However, it is important to remember that around 30% of patients with RA may be RF-ve (seronegative) and, conversely, that the presence of RF may be an incidental finding in healthy individuals, particularly in elderly women. RF may also be found in the connective tissue diseases, with high titres being a feature in some patients with Sjögren's syndrome. It can be present, usually transiently, during certain bacterial and viral infections.

Anti-cyclic citrullinated peptide (anti-CCP) antibodies have similar sensitivity but greater specificity for diagnosis of RA compared with RF and are associated with aggressive, erosive disease.

Antibodies associated with connective tissue diseases

The anti-nuclear antibody (ANA) describes reactivity of serum with cells that were originally derived from a human laryngeal carcinoma and are known as Hep-2 cells. Classically the test has been done to detect antibodies that stain the nucleus of the Hep-2 cells and hence the term anti-nuclear antibodies. However, the test can also detect antibodies that stain antigens within the cytoplasm of the cells. A positive ANA has only moderate specificity for connective tissue disease; it is common for healthy women to have low titres of circulating ANA and transient higher levels may be a feature of infection. It does, however, have a relatively high sensitivity (>90%) for SLE and is also very commonly found in other connective tissue diseases such as Sjögren's syndrome, SSc and inflammatory myositis. In many respects it is a screening test; a positive test in the context of relevant clinical features should act as a prompt to request further tests to define the specificity of the autoantibodies in more detail. The staining pattern of the nuclei or cytoplasm of Hep 2 cells can provide clues as to this specificity and laboratories will usually comment as to whether the staining is homogeneous, speckled, nucleolar, cytoplasmic etc. However, the correlation between staining pattern and antigen reactivity is rather variable. Where the ANA is positive, immunology laboratories will generally routinely go on to test for antibodies specific for double stranded DNA (dsDNA) and for the 'extractable nuclear antigens-4' (ENA-4) which are known as Ro, La, Sm and U1RNP. Ro, La and Sm are ribonucleoproteins and were named using the first two initials of the surnames of the patients in whom they were first found whereas U1RNP stands for U1 ribonucleoprotein. All these antibodies may be associated with a diagnosis of SLE although the dsDNA and anti-Sm antibodies are most specific for this condition. Antibodies specific for Ro and La are associated with Sjögren's syndrome and antibodies specific for U1RNP have been associated with an overlap condition sometimes termed 'mixed connective tissue disease'. If there are clinical features of SSc then the laboratory can test for antibodies specific for SCL70 (topoisomerase 1), RNA polymerases I/III or U3RNP (fibrillarin), which are most closely associated with diffuse cutaneous scleroderma or for the presence of antibodies specific for centromere, which are closely associated with limited cutaneous scleroderma. Where staining of

Hep-2 cells is cytoplasmic rather than nuclear, this may be due to the presence of antibodies specific for t-RNA synthetases (Jo-1, PL7, PL12 and others), found in some patients with inflammatory myositis. Antibodies specific for the nuclear antigens Mi-2 (again named after a patient) or signal recognition particle (SRP) are also found specifically in patients with inflammatory myositis. Some patients have inflammatory myositis with features of other connective tissues diseases, commonly scleroderma, and may have antibodies specific for PM/SCL (PM1), Ku, or U1RNP or U2RNP (Table 2.26).

Antibodies associated with the anti-phospholipid syndrome

Antibodies directed against negatively charged phospholipids (anti-cardiolipin antibodies) may be found in some patients with the anti-phospholipid syndrome. Other patients may have antibodies directed against beta-2 microglobulin 1, which is found in association with negatively charged phospholipids. A third test is the 'lupus anti-coagulant test' (see Haematology section). Individuals with the anti-phospholipid syndrome are rarely positive for all three tests but should be positive for at least one of them. The tests should be performed on two separate occasions at least 12 weeks apart as transient responses can be associated with infection.

Antibodies associated with vasculitis

A subset of the vasculitides is associated with the presence of anti-neutrophil cytoplasmic antibodies (ANCA). These antibodies may stain in a peri-nuclear

Table 2.26. Associations between connective tissue diseases and autoantibodies.

Disease	Associated antibodies
Systemic lupus erythematosus	dsDNA, Ro, La, Sm, U1RNP
Sjögren's syndrome	Ro, La
Scleroderma — diffuse cutaneous	SCL70, RNA Polymerase I/III, U3RNP (fibrillarin),
Scleroderma — limited cutaneous	Centromere,
Inflammatory myositis — specific	t-RNA synthetases (e.g. Jo1, PL7, PL12), Mi-2, SRP
Inflammatory myositis as part of 'overlap' with other connective tissue diseases	Pm/SCL (PM1), Ku, U1RNP, U2RNP

(p-ANCA) or cytoplasmic (c-ANCA) distribution. Their specificity should be confirmed by testing for reactivity to myeloperoxidase for p-ANCAs and proteinase 3 for c-ANCAs. Antibodies specific for myeloperoxidase are commonly found in individuals with microscopic polyarteritis and are also found in some patients with Churg–Strauss syndrome and a minority of patients with Wegener's granulomatosis. Those specific for proteinase 3 are most usually found in patients with Wegener's granulomatosis but may be found in some patients with microscopic polyarteritis. p-ANCAs and c-ANCAs that are not found to have specificity for the myeloperoxidase and proteinase 3 antigens are much less likely to be associated with vasculitis and are a common feature of some infections including HIV (Table 2.27).

Complement

Complement C3 and C4 proteins are 'acute phase proteins' and their synthesis tends to be increased in inflammatory disease. However, C3 and C4 complement will be reduced due to consumption when the complement cascade is activated via the classical pathway, either by infection or by activity of autoimmune diseases such as SLE. The C4 complement usually falls first, with the C3 complement falling in more severe disease.

Functional tests of the complement pathways may be helpful in individuals with possible complement deficiencies. The CH50 measures function of the classical pathway whilst the AP50 evaluates function of the alternative pathway; both require the presence of C3 and components of the final pathway (C5–C9). Considering the CH50 and AP50 together will allow isolation of the part of the complement cascade in which the deficit is present; the laboratory can then test specifically for individual complement components. Deficiencies

Table 2.27. Autoantibodies in vasculitis.

Staining pattern	Specificity	Disease association
p-ANCA	Myeloperoxidase	Microscopic polyarteritis Churg–Strauss syndrome Wegener's granulomatosis*
c-ANCA	Proteinase 3	Wegener's granulomatosis Microscopic polyarteritis*

* Less common association.

of C1 complement components such as C1q as well as C2 and C4 are associated with the development of SLE; in these rare patients C3 and C4 levels will not fall with disease activity as is usual in SLE as patients will not be able to activate the classical complement cascade (Table 2.28).

Human leukocyte antigen molecules

Human leukocyte antigen (HLA) molecules present processed peptides from intracellular and extracellular proteins to T cell receptors. Associations have been noted between the presence of particular HLA alleles and the development and/or severity of some autoimmune diseases. The presence or absence of particular HLA alleles is not diagnostic for and neither can it exclude the possibility of a specific autoimmune disease but it may contribute to the overall assessment of the patient. The spondyloarthritides, in particular AS, are strongly associated with the presence of HLA B27 and it is reasonable to test for the presence of this allele where the diagnosis is being considered. However, it must be noted that approximately 8% of caucasion individuals carry this HLA allele and only a small proportion of them will ever develop spondyloarthritis. RA is associated with certain HLA molecules, particularly HLA DR4 alleles. However, this is rarely tested for and clinicians usually gain better information from testing for antibodies and performing imaging studies.

Table 2.28. Investigation of the complement cascade.

Test	Characteristics
C3 complement	Requires C3 to be present. Increases in some forms of inflammation. Decreases in infection and immune complex mediated auto-immune disease.
C4 complement	Requires C4 to be present. Increases in some forms of inflammation. Decreases in infection and immune complex mediated auto-immune disease.
CH50	Requires C1, C2, C4, C3, C5–C9 to be present and functional.
AP50	Requires B, I, P, C3, C5–C9 to be present and functional.

Microbiology and Virology

Microbiology

Gram staining and culture of synovial fluid are mandatory when a diagnosis of septic arthritis is being considered (see below). Blood cultures should also be taken.

Some bacterial infections, particularly gastrointestinal and sexually acquired infections, may lead to the development of a 'reactive' arthritis which normally involves large joints. Stool cultures are rarely helpful in diagnosis of reactive arthritis following salmonella, shigella or campylobacter infection as the infection has usually cleared prior to the presentation with arthritis. Urethral swabs are required for diagnosis of chlamydia infection. Throat swabs and anti-streptolysin O titre (ASOT) are helpful in diagnosis of post-streptococcal arthritis.

Viral serology

A number of virus infections are associated with inflammatory arthritis. Epstein–Barr virus, mumps, rubella, parvovirus B19, alphavirus, adenovirus, enterovirus and HIV seroconversion may all be characterised by a transient arthritis. HBV and HCV may be associated with a more chronic form of inflammatory arthritis. Serological tests for the presence of these viruses can be helpful if other features of virus infection are present.

Urinalysis

Microscopic haematuria and/or proteinuria can be detected on urine dipstick testing. They can be early indicators of renal disease and will usually pre-date an increase in plasma creatinine or urea. Regular urinalysis is therefore mandatory in patients with diseases such as SLE or the vasculitides that can involve the kidneys. Where dipstick testing suggests haematuria, microscopy should be performed to look for red cells or red cell casts; presence of the latter is highly suggestive of glomerulonephritis. The occurrence of red cells without casts may occur in glomerulonephritis but may also be a feature of bladder disease or urethral trauma. Myoglobulinuria may result in a positive urine dipstick for blood but red cells will not be seen. It is a feature of severe myositis, particularly rhabdomyolysis and may be associated with acute renal failure (Table 2.29).

If dipstick testing suggests proteinuria, then quantification of protein excretion should be undertaken, either from a 24-hour urine collection or by calculating the protein:creatinine ratio from a random urine sample.

Table 2.29. Interpretation of urine dipstick testing for blood.

	Dipstick positive for blood	Red cells on microscopy	Red cell casts on microscopy
Glomerulonephritis	+	+	+/–
Bladder lesion or trauma	+	+	–
Myoglobulinuria	+	–	–

Synovial Fluid and Tissue Analysis

Cells

Neutrophils and lymphocytes are commonly present in synovial fluid where there is an inflammatory aetiology. A very high neutrophil count (>90% leukocytes) is a particular feature of gout or infection. The presence of red cells may reflect trauma such as an intra-articular fracture but may also occur with pigmented villonodular synovitis. Low level trauma during the process of aspiration may also lead to a blood-stained fluid.

Crystals

Crystals should be detected using polarised microscopy. Uric acid crystals are 3–20 μm in length, needle-shaped and negatively birefringent (blue then yellow as red plate compensator is rotated through 90°). Calcium pyrophosphate crystals are rhomboid shaped crystals that are positively birefringent.

Gram staining and culture

Gram staining and culture must be performed if there is concern about possible infection. It may also be appropriate to request specific staining for acid and alcohol fast bacilli (AAFB) and prolonged culture to look for evidence of *Mycobacterium tuberculosis* infection.

Synovial biopsy

A synovial biopsy can be performed during open surgery or via an arthroscopic or percutaneous procedure. It is indicated where there is persistent synovitis without clear evidence for a primary inflammatory arthritis in order to exclude atypical infection or other pathologies such as amyloidosis or pigmented villonodular synovitis.

2.4.2. *Imaging Studies*

Plain Film

Plain films provide two-dimensional images and so must be performed in two planes (e.g. antero-posterior and lateral) to obtain an adequate view of a joint (Fig. 2.8). They are very useful for looking at bone pathology and are sensitive for some soft tissue abnormalities. They do not detect early pathology in patients with arthritis but do detect later changes and can be used to monitor development of erosive disease or other joint damage over time. Different types of arthritis have characteristic features on X-ray imaging (Table 2.30).

Computed Tomography

Computed tomography (CT) uses X-rays to produce a series of cross-sectional images. It differentiates bone, muscle, fluid and fat. It is useful for looking at bone pathology, particularly fractures that may be difficult to see on plain films (Fig. 2.9). It is otherwise rarely used in rheumatic disease as it cannot provide appropriate detail about soft tissue structures.

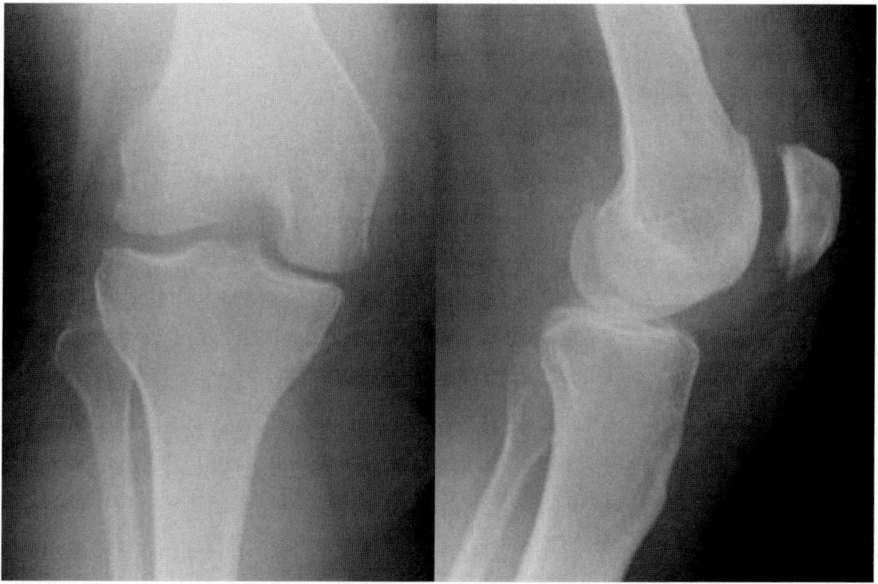

Fig. 2.8. X-rays of a knee joint. Plain films are performed in two planes (anteroposterior and lateral) to obtain an adequate view of the joint.

Table 2.30. Radiographic features of common rheumatic conditions.

Disease	Radiographic features
Rheumatoid arthritis	Joint space narrowing
	Peri-articular osteopaenia
	Peri-articular erosions
	Subluxation
Osteoarthritis	Joint space narrowing
	Peri-articular sclerosis
	Osteophytes
	Bone cysts
Ankylosing spondylitis	
Sacro-iliac joints:	Irregular joint margins
(Sacroiliitis)	Subchondral erosion
	Sclerosis
	Fusion
Spine:	Loss of lumbar lordosis
(Spondylitis)	Squaring of vertebrae
	Romanus lesions (erosion at the corner of vertebral bodies)
	Enthesitis (calcification of tendon/ligament insertion)
	Bamboo spine
Psoriatic arthritis	
Peripheral arthritis:	Peri-articular erosions
	Fluffy periostitis
	Lysis of terminal phalanges
	'Pencil-in-cup' appearance (gross destruction of isolated joint)
Sacro-iliac joints:	Features of sacroiliitis (often asymmetrical)
Spine:	Features of spondylitis (usually mild)
Gout	Large juxta-articular punched-out 'rat-bite' erosions
	Soft tissue shadowing (uric acid deposition)
Paget's disease	Patchy lucency/sclerosis
	Pathological fractures
Osteomyelitis	Patchy osteopaenia
	Loss of bone cortex

Ultrasound

Ultrasound (US) waves reflect at interfaces between different types of tissue and so provide a two-dimensional image of the structures lying below the ultrasound probe (Fig. 2.10). US can prove extremely useful in examining soft tissues, particularly where these are relatively superficial. It is used

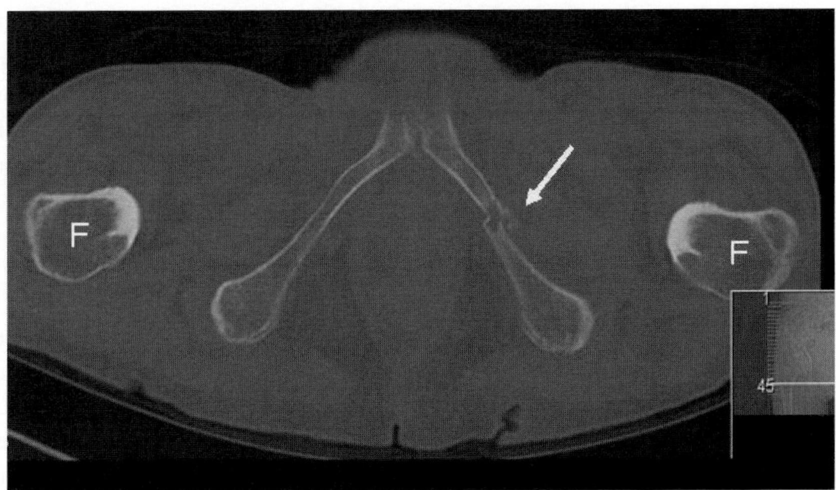

Fig. 2.9. CT scan of pelvis showing a fracture through the left pubic ramus (white arrow). F = cross sections through the proximal femurs.

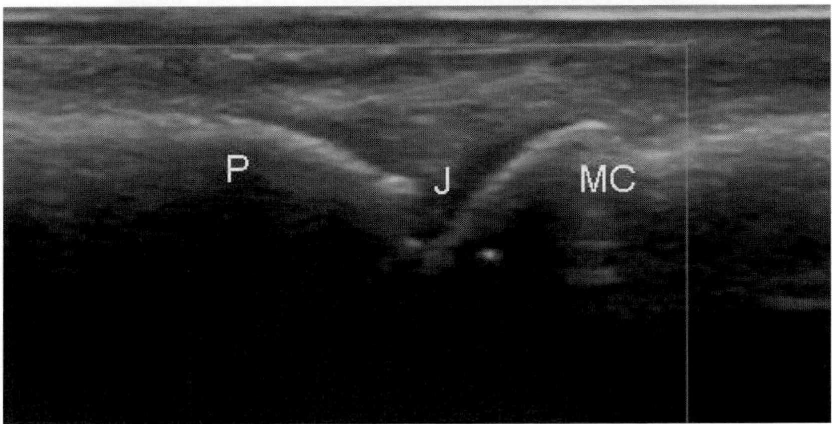

Fig. 2.10. Ultrasound scan of metacarpophalangeal joint. Longitudinal view of dorsal surface. Ultrasound waves are reflected at interfaces between tissues. The surfaces of bone appear dense (white) whilst synovium and synovial fluid are hypodense (dark). MC = metacarpal bone, P = proximal phalanx, J = metacarpophalangeal joint.

increasingly to detect synovitis, effusions or very small erosions within joints, and abnormalities within muscle, ligaments or tendons such as ruptures or tenosynovitis. Use of power doppler allows assessment of blood flow and this further enhances the sensitivity of the technique for detection of early or active synovitis. Imaging with US can facilitate aspiration of or corticosteroid injection into joints.

Magnetic Resonance Imaging

Magnetic resonance imaging (MRI) makes use of a powerful magnetic field to spin hydrogen nuclei (protons); the images obtained reflect the distribution of nuclei in a given tissue and their behaviour in the externally applied magnetic field (Fig. 2.11). Several different sequences may be acquired. T1 weighted images are obtained rapidly and provide good spatial resolution. Fat and haemorrhage or other protein rich fluids are bright but other fluids are dark. In T2 weighted images fluid is bright and because most pathologies involve oedema these images are useful for highlighting pathology. However, the contrast

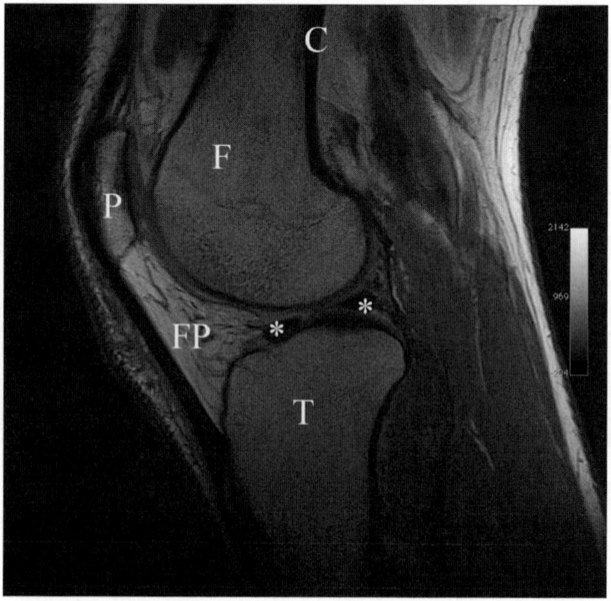

Fig. 2.11. MRI scan of the knee. F = femur, T = tibia, P = patella, C= cortext of bone, FP = fat pad. * show the meniscus.

between fat and fluid may not be very great. Suppression of the signal from fat may be achieved using inversion recovery sequences. MRI provides high resolution pictures of soft tissues. It is helpful in diagnosis of tendon, ligament and cartilage pathology. It is particularly useful for imaging the spine; disc prolapse, cord compression, cauda equina or exiting nerve root compression can all be demonstrated. MRI provides an alternative to US as a means of imaging early arthritis; it is capable of detecting early synovitis and erosive disease and is the modality of choice for detecting early sacroiliitis.

Bone Scintigraphy

Bone scintigraphy is performed using intravenous Technetium-99m labelled substituted diphosphonates. These are taken up by bone, with extent of uptake depending on local blood flow and osteoblastic activity. The sensitivity of the technique for detecting abnormalities within bones and joints is high. It is useful for detection of bony metastases and can demonstrate fractures that may have been missed on plain films. In terms of joint disease the specificity for individual diagnoses is low; most forms of arthritis will result in some increased uptake within affected joints. It can be useful in excluding important joint pathology in patients with widespread arthralgias and no obvious clinical signs but has largely been superseded by other techniques.

Positive Emission Tomography Scanning

Positive emission tomography (PET) scanning uses 18F-Fluorodeoxyglucose (18FDG) to identify cells using an excess of glucose. It is increasingly used, often in conjunction with CT scanning, to image large vessels to help in diagnoses of conditions such as Takayasu's arteritis or giant cell arteritis; increased uptake of 18FDG occurs within vessels affected by active vasculitis.

Dual Energy X-ray Absorptiometry

Dual Energy X-ray Absorptiometry (DEXA) scanning provides an estimate of bone mineral density by assessing the attenuation of the energy of X-ray beams of two different frequencies as they pass through tissues. Results are reported as grams/cm^3 but are also expressed in terms of a T score and a Z score. The T score represents the number of standard deviations of the result from the mean bone density of a healthy population of young women. The WHO have defined a T score of –1 to –2.5 as constituting osteopenia and a

T score of <–2.5 as constituting OP. The Z score considers the result in relationship to individuals of the same age, sex and ethnicity and represents the number of standard deviations from the mean bone density of the relevant population.

2.4.3. *Electrophysiological Tests*

Nerve Conduction Studies

These assess capacity of motor and sensory nerves to conduct action potentials; both the amplitude of the action potentials and the velocity of conduction can be assessed. Abnormalities in the former suggest axonal damage whereas abnormalities in the latter usually reflect damage to the myelin sheath. A focal abnormality of nerve conduction often reflects local nerve compression.

In rheumatology practice nerve conduction studies are very useful for detection of nerve entrapment conditions such as carpal tunnel syndrome. They are also helpful in investigation of vasculitis associated neuropathies such as mononeuritis multiplex.

Electromyogram

An electromyogram (EMG) measures electrical activity in muscles at rest and during contraction. It is particularly useful in evaluation of inflammatory myositis where characteristic findings include increased spontaneous activity with fibrillations, complex repetitive discharges and sharp waves with short duration, low-amplitude polyphasic units occurring on voluntary activation. Such findings are, however, not entirely specific and it may be difficult to differentiate ongoing muscle inflammation due to myositis from steroid induced myopathy. An EMG is also helpful in evaluation of nerve root compression within the spine. Provided the operator has a secure knowledge of muscle innervation it is possible to deduce the level of neural compression from the distribution of muscles involved.

Chapter 3
Arthritis

Editor: Sonya Abraham

Sonya Abraham, Andrew Barr, Michael Doherty, Andrew Keat, Bina Menon, Elena Nikiphorou, Leena Patel, Peter Taylor, Tonia Vincent, Fiona Watt

3.1. Rheumatoid Arthritis

Rheumatoid arthritis (RA) is a systemic condition, best regarded as a syndrome, with its predominant manifestation in peripheral joints. It is the commonest of the inflammatory arthritides with a worldwide prevalence of about 1%, a female preponderance and a peak incidence in the early middle years, although it can present at any stage of life. It is a major cause of disability and unemployment. Although the aetiology remains unknown, there have been considerable advances in understanding of the pathogenesis in the last two decades and these have led to major advances in the pharmacological management of this condition.

Pathogenesis

Cellular pathology

Rheumatoid arthritis is characterised by chronic inflammation of synovial joints that is thought to be a consequence of reciprocal activation between infiltrating leukocytes and cells indigenous to the synovium. Microscopic inspection of RA synovium shows blood derived cells including activated T cells, macrophages and plasma cells as well as proliferation of the synovium.

Prominent vasculature is a feature of RA synovitis; angiogenesis is evident from the earliest stages of disease development and a fine network of vessels is visible over the rheumatoid synovium at arthroscopic inspection. Formation of new blood vessels permits a supply of nutrients and oxygen to the augmented inflammatory cell mass and so contributes to the perpetuation of synovitis.

The synovial tissue becomes markedly hyperplastic and locally invasive at the interface of cartilage and bone with progressive destruction of these tissues in the majority of cases. This invasive tissue is referred to as 'pannus'. The accompanying destruction of bone and cartilage is thought to be mediated by cytokine-induced degradative enzymes, notably the matrix metalloproteinases.

The factors that lead to the development of the observed pathological changes remain poorly understood although evidence suggests that the disease results from a complex interplay between cells of the innate and adaptive immune system and cells normally resident within the synovium (Table 3.1).

Genetic factors

Genetic factors were originally implicated in the aetiopathogenesis of RA following the discovery that, in population studies, there is a small increase in the frequency of RA in first-degree relatives of patients with this disease. In hospital-based population studies of identical twins, concordance rates of disease are around 30%, compared with 5% in non-identical twins. The figures support the

Table 3.1. Importance of cells of the adaptive and innate immune systems in pathogenesis of RA.

Evidence for involvement of T cells	Evidence for involvement of B cells	Evidence for involvement of cells of the innate immune system
Association between RA and HLA DR B1 alleles	Lack of tolerance resulting in production of RF (antibody response to Fc region of IgG)	Presence of activated macrophages within synovium
Association between RA and PTPN22 alleles	Lack of tolerance to citrullinated proteins leading to presence of anti-CCP antibodies	Abundance of cytokines expressed by macrophages within synovial tissue
Presence of activated T cells within synovium	Presence of plasma cells within synovium	Efficacy of drugs aimed at antagonising TNF-α and IL-6 in treatment of RA
Efficacy of abatacept in treatment of RA	Efficacy of rituximab in treatment of RA	

CCP cyclic citrullinated peptide, HLA human leukocyte antigen, PTPN22 protein tyrosine phosphatase non-receptor 22, RA rheumatoid arthritis, RF rheumatoid factor, Ig immunoglobulin, IL interleukin, TNF tumour necrosis factor.

concept of a genetic contribution to disease but argue against the proposition that RA is the result of a dominant single-gene disorder. These and other epidemiological studies have led to the conclusion that RA is a polygenic disease and that non-inherited factors are also of great importance.

Human leukocyte antigen polymorphisms

Genes encoding particular class II human leukocyte antigens (HLA) are among the candidates for involvement in predisposition to RA. This discovery came about with the observation that 60–70% of Caucasian patients with RA are HLA DR4 positive compared with 20–25% of control populations. Furthermore, patients with more severe RA, especially those with extra-articular complications such as vasculitis and Felty's syndrome, are even more likely to be HLA DR4 positive than patients with less severe disease confined to joints. HLA DR1 is a further susceptibility allele. Nucleotide sequencing of HLA DR β1 exons coding amino acid residues 70 to 74 has revealed that HLA DR4 subtypes Dw4, Dw14 and Dw15 share similarities with each other (with a conservative substitution of glutamine with lysine at position 71 in Dw4) and with HLA DRl. This sequence predicts susceptibility to RA and is associated with disease in 83% of Caucasian patients in the United Kingdom (UK). In contrast, negative associations are observed in individuals who are DR4w10, in whom the charged basic amino acids glutamine and arginine in positions 70 and 71 are replaced by the acidic amino acids aspartic and glutamic acid. Molecular modelling studies suggest that amino acid residues 70–74 are located in the α-helix forming the wall of the peptide-binding groove, and thus are likely to be involved in antigen binding. Acidic substitutions could profoundly alter protein structures and thereby alter affinity for peptide antigens. However, molecular mechanisms accounting for HLA associated susceptibility to RA remain to be elucidated. Possibilities include permissive binding of specific peptides such as those on autoantigens or on environmental antigens, initiation of disease by specific binding of superantigens to HLA molecules, or modulation of the T cell repertoire by selection or tolerance. It has also been hypothesised that severity of disease and extra-articular complications are related to HLA DR β1 homozygosity and the density of disease-associated MHC molecules that critically influence the selection of the T cell repertoire and tolerance to antigens.

Protein tyrosine phosphatase non-receptor 22 polymorphisms

A genetic association between RA and an allele of protein tyrosine phosphatase non-receptor 22 (PTPN22) also points to a possible role for T cells in disease pathogenesis. PTPN22 is a lymphocyte specific tyrosine phosphatase that plays a role in suppressing T cell activation. The 1858T allele of the PTPN22 gene has been shown to increase susceptibility to RA and type I diabetes and is also associated with development of other autoimmune conditions.

Autoantibodies

Whilst genetic studies have highlighted a possible role for abnormal T cell responses in RA, serological studies have shown abnormalities of B cell responses. Rheumatoid factor (RF) describes antibodies with specificity for the Fc portion of immunoglobulin (Ig) G that are present in many patients with RA. These are most commonly IgM antibodies although some patients may have IgA or IgG RF, often in addition to the IgM RF. Anti-citrullinated protein antibodies are often found in patients with RA and are directed at citrullinated (deiminated) self proteins. Citrullination (deimination) of proteins occurs at sites of inflammation and involves the loss of an amino group from tyrosine residues. Whilst this process occurs in healthy individuals, the propensity to develop an antibody response to these citrullinated proteins is specifically associated with the development of RA and can predate disease onset by many years.

Cytokines

Cells of the innate immune system, particularly macrophages, as well as the fibroblast-like cells that are normally resident within synovium, play a role in disease development. Cytokines derived from macrophages and fibroblasts are abundant in the rheumatoid synovium. These include interleukin (IL)-1, tumour necrosis factor (TNF)-α, granulocyte macrophage-colony stimulating factor (GM-CSF), IL-6 and numerous chemokines. Many of these factors are important in regulating inflammatory cell migration and activation. There are also a number of cytokines that cause co-stimulation of T cells including IL-7, IL-12, IL-15 and IL-18. However, given the extent of synovial inflammation and lymphocytic infiltration, factors produced by T cells such as interferon (IFN)-γ, IL-2 and IL-4 are surprisingly sparsely expressed, with T helper (Th) 1 cell activity as defined by IFN-γ production showing some predominance over Th2 cell activity. In contrast, IL-17 production by Th17 cells is more prominent.

In support of the concept of cytokine dysequilibrium within the chronic inflammatory state in rheumatoid synovium is the observation that multiple anti-inflammatory mediators are also up-regulated, but at a level insufficient to suppress synovitis. Examples include the abundant expression of IL-10, IL-13

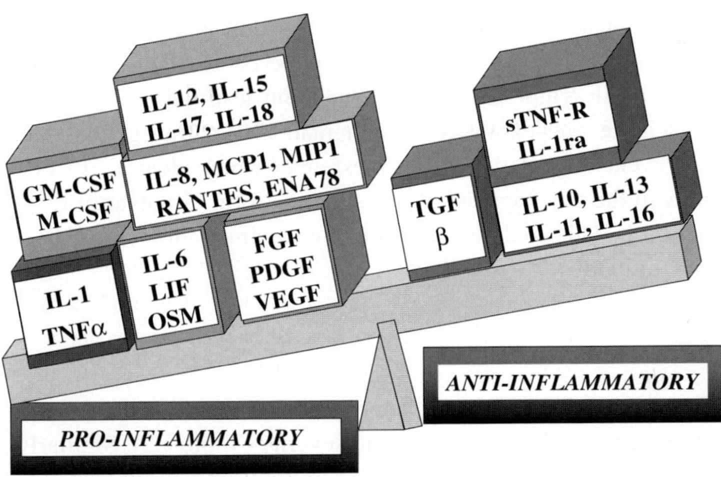

Fig. 3.1. The concept of cytokine dysequilibrium. Many cytokines are detectable in rheumatoid synovial tissues, including some with predominantly anti-inflammatory properties. The net effect is a dominance of pro-inflammatory activity.

and transforming growth factor (TGF)-β both in latent and active form. Naturally occurring cytokine inhibitors, such as IL-1 receptor antagonist (IL-1ra) and soluble TNF receptors, the specific inhibitors of IL-1 and TNF-α respectively, are also up-regulated in the rheumatoid joint (Fig. 3.1).

The extensive range of cytokines that can be detected in RA synovial samples is independent of donor disease duration, severity or even conventional (non-biologic) drug therapy. Pro-inflammatory cytokines continue to be spontaneously produced over several days in dissociated RA synovial membrane cell cultures. This occurs in the absence of extrinsic stimulation, suggesting that the cultures produce one or more soluble factors regulating prolonged cytokine synthesis. Addition of anti-TNF-α antibodies to these cell cultures was observed to strikingly reduce the production of other pro-inflammatory cytokines, including IL-1, GM-CSF, IL-6 and IL-8. In contrast, blockade of IL-1 results in reduced production of IL-6 and IL-8 but not of TNF-α. These observations led to the concept that TNF-α occupies a dominant position at the apex of a pro-inflammatory cytokine network. TNF-α is a pleiotropic cytokine with biological properties that include stimulation of enhanced synovial proliferation and production of prostaglandins and metalloproteinases as well as regulation of other pro-inflammatory cytokines. Its potential as a drug target was demonstrated by a number of independent *in vivo* studies that showed that antibody therapies blocking bioactivity of TNF-α, administered either during the induction phase of murine collagen-induced arthritis or, more importantly, after the onset of disease, were able to ameliorate clinical symptoms and prevent joint destruction. Furthermore, in a murine model, the over-expression of a human TNF-α transgene modified at its 3′ end to prevent degradation of its messenger ribonucleic acid (mRNA) was associated with the development of a destructive form of polyarthritis four to six weeks after birth. This could be prevented by administration of a TNF-α specific monoclonal antibody.

Clinical Features

The clinical presentation of RA is heterogeneous, with a wide spectrum of age of onset, degree of joint involvement and severity (Table 3.2). Similarly, the disease course is variable. The relapsing and remitting nature of RA and the tendency of symptoms to move from one joint area to another, is reflected in the root of the word 'rheumatoid', which is derived from the Greek 'rheum' (ρευμ) meaning 'to flow'.

RA often begins insidiously with joint pain, which may be associated with swelling. Patients frequently report marked stiffness of joints on waking in the morning and also following periods of inactivity. This stiffness often lasts for more than an hour. The joints most commonly involved first are the metacarpophalangeal joints, proximal interphalangeal joints, wrists and metatarsophalangeal joints. There may be only a few joints involved initially with subsequent progression to involvement of multiple joints in a symmetrical distribution over a time period spanning weeks to months. There may be progressive decline in physical

Table 3.2. Spectrum of clinical presentation of RA.

Clinical presentation of RA
Insiduous onset polyarthritis
Acute or subacute polyarthritis leading rapidly to restricted mobility and loss of function
Migratory arthritis that 'flits' from joint to joint and is termed palindromic arthritis
Polymyalgic presentation that is initially indistinguishable from polymyalgia rheumatica
Persistent inflammatory monoarthritis that antedates development of polyarthritis by many years
Diffusely swollen hands and fingers, often with associated carpal tunnel syndrome
Tenosynovitis involving the dorsal extensors of the wrist and the flexors of the fingers in the palm and wrist

function with loss of grip strength and difficulty undertaking simple everyday tasks such as doing up buttons, undoing jar lids or turning on taps. Fatigue and lethargy are common features and there may be an accompanying low-grade fever and weight loss. In most cases, with the passage of time, more joints become involved and the distribution of arthritis becomes permanently established.

In its established phase RA is generally straightforward to recognize and is characterised by a deforming symmetrical polyarthritis of varying extent and severity (Figs. 3.2 and 3.3). The synovitis of joints and tendon sheaths may be associated with articular cartilage loss and erosion of juxta-articular bone. Patients commonly develop swan neck and boutonniere deformities within their fingers, subluxation at the metacarpophalanageal joints with ulnar deviation, collapse of the carpal bones leading to a prominent distal ulnar styloid and fixed flexion deformities of the elbows. They may also develop deformities affecting the feet with subluxation of the metatarsal heads, widening of the forefeet and clawing of the toes as well as a tendency to valgus at the ankles with flattening of the longitudinal arch of the foot. Secondary degenerative changes at the hips and knees are common.

In a proportion of patients, systemic and extra-articular features may be observed during the course of disease (and rarely prior to joint disease). Such features include anaemia, weight loss, vasculitis, serositis, nodules in subcutaneous, pulmonary and scleral tissues, mononeuritis multiplex, and pulmonary interstitial inflammation as well as salivary and lachrymal gland involvement.

In view of the heterogeneous nature of the presentation and course of RA, the American Rheumatism Association developed and revised classification criteria for the diagnosis of RA, based on a hospital population of patients with established active disease. There are seven components to these classification criteria for RA as listed in Table 3.3.

The criteria combine a constellation of clinical, serological and radiological features, and have become widely accepted for epidemiological and clinical studies. By emphasising key features of the syndrome, the criteria help to differentiate RA from other forms of inflammatory arthritis, with a diagnostic sensitivity and specificity of about 90% for established active disease. However, these requirements have a much poorer sensitivity for a diagnosis of RA in the early stages of presentation, where the sensitivity of the classification criteria ranges from 40% to 60%, and the specificity is no better than 80–90%. More recently a new classification system has been proposed by the American College of Rheumatology (ACR) and European League against Rheumatism (EULAR) that takes account of anti-cyclic citrullinated peptide (anti-CCP) and acute phase reactants as well as the pattern and persistence of arthritis and these may prove more useful in the context of early disease (Table 3.4).

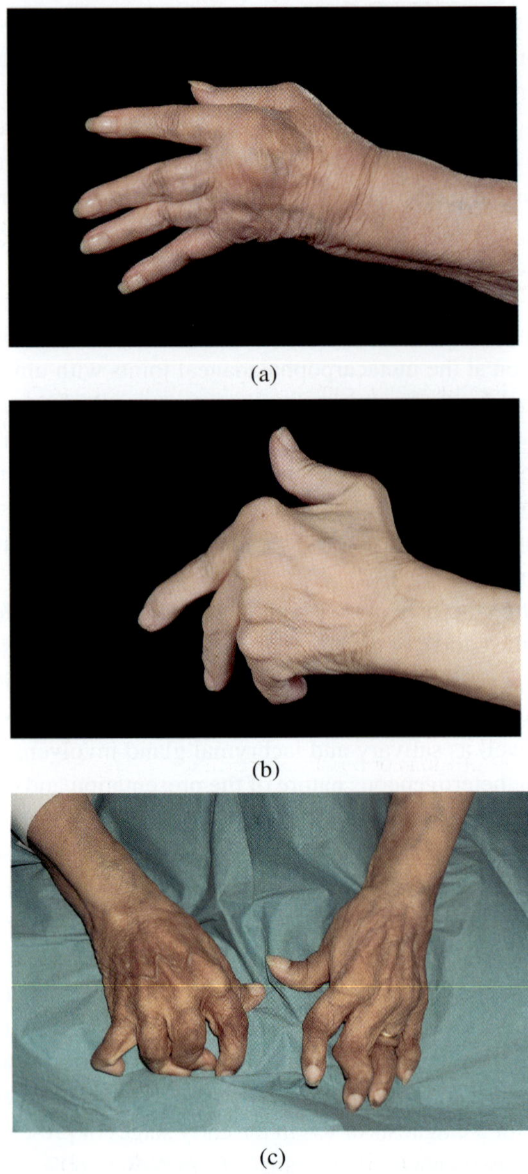

Fig. 3.2. Rheumatoid arthritis. (a) Synovitis of the MCP joints with early swan necking and ulnar deviation. (b) Severe rheumatoid arthritis with Z thumb, swan necking of the index finger and flexion deformities of the 2-5th MCP joints. (c) Advanced rheumatoid arthritis.

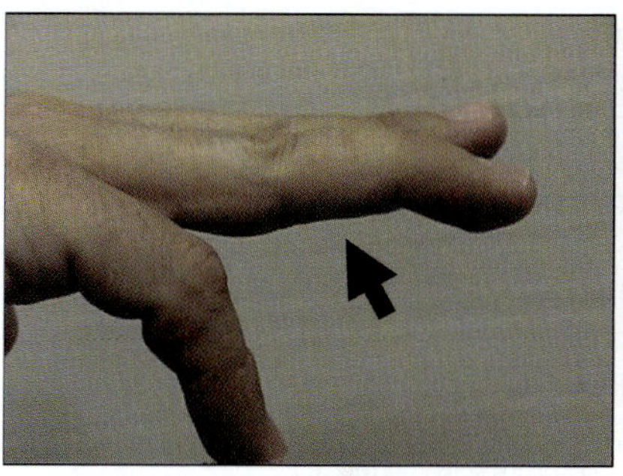

'Swan neck' deformity

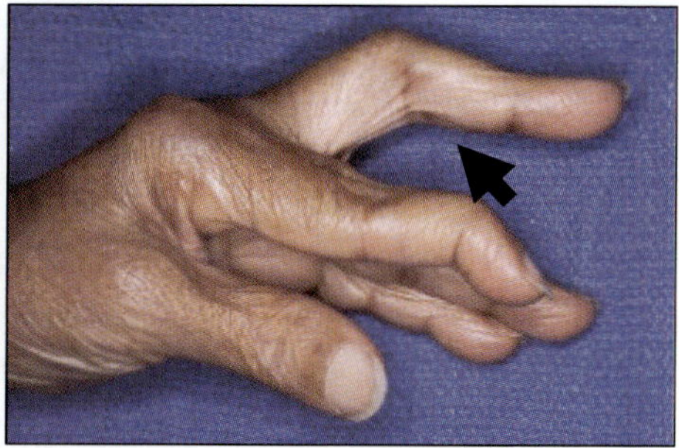

'Boutonniere' deformity

Fig. 3.3. Hand deformities in rheumatoid arthritis. Swan neck deformity describes hyperextension at the PIP joint with flexion at the DIP joint. Boutonniere deformity describes flexion at the PIP joint with hyperextension at the DIP joint.

Table 3.3. American Rheumatism Association 1987 criteria for classification of RA.

Feature	Time Frame
Morning stiffness >1 hour	Present for at least 6 weeks
Swelling of at least 3 joints	Present for at least 6 weeks
Swelling of hand joints	Present for at least 6 weeks
Symmetric joint involvement	Present for at least 6 weeks
Radiographic changes (erosions or bony decalcification)	
Presence of rheumatoid nodules	
Rheumatoid factor in serum	

Rheumatoid arthritis is defined by the presence of four or more criteria.

Investigations

Both laboratory tests and imaging studies play a role in the investigation of patients with RA (Table 3.5).

Laboratory tests

The 1987 classification criteria include only one serological test, namely RF. IgM RF is detectable in the blood in a majority of patients. The prevalence of RF increases with duration of disease: at three months the prevalence is 33%, while at one year it is 75%. Up to 20% of patients remain negative for RF (also known as 'sero-negative RA') throughout the course of disease. Antibodies to CCP have a similar sensitivity to RF but much higher specificity. As in the case of high-titre

Table 3.4. The American College of Rheumatology/European League against Rheumatism 2010 classification criteria for RA.

Feature	Details	Score
A. Joint involvement	1 large* joint	0
	2–10 large joints	1
	1–3 small** joints (+/– large joints)	2
	4–10 small joints (+/– large joints)	3
	> 10 joints (at least 1 small joint)	5
B. Serology	Negative RF and anti-CCP antibodies	0
	Low# positive RF or anti-CCP antibodies	2
	High## positive RF or anti-CCP antibodies	3
C. Acute phase reactants	Normal CRP and ESR	0
	Abnormal CRP or ESR	1
D. Duration of symptoms	< 6 weeks	0
	> 6 weeks	1

Classification criteria are applicable to patients with synovitis in at least one joint without an alternative clear explanation. Joint involvement includes any tender or swollen joint. * Large joints refers to shoulders, elbows, hips, knees and ankles. **Small joints refers to metacarpophoalangeal, proximal interphalangeal, second to fifth metatarsophalangeal, thumb interphalangeal joints and wrists. # Low positive refers to values higher than and up to three times the upper limit of normal. ## High positive refers to values > three times the upper limit of normal.

A score of at least 6/10 is needed for classification of a patient as having definite RA.

CCP cyclic citrullinated peptide, CRP C-reactive protein, ESR erythrocyte sedimentation rate, RF rheumatoid factor.

Table 3.5. Helpful investigations in a patient with rheumatoid arthritis.

Laboratory tests	Imaging
Serological tests for RF, anti-CCP, ANA	X-rays
ESR and CRP	US scan with power Doppler
FBC, C&E, LFT	MRI scan

ANA anti-nuclear antibody, CCP cyclic citrullinated antibody, C&E creatinine and electrolytes, CRP C-reactive protein, ESR erythrocyte sedimentation rate, LFT liver function test, MRI magnetic resonance imaging, RF rheumatoid factor, US ultrasound.

RF, anti-CCP antibodies are associated with persistence and destructiveness of RA. Many patients have anti-nuclear antibodies (ANA), often at relatively low titres. The C-reactive protein (CRP) and erythrocyte sedimentation rate (ESR) provide a measure of disease activity. A full blood count (FBC) may show evidence of anaemia of chronic disease and/or thrombocytosis reflecting the inflammatory state. Assessment of renal function and liver function is important as it may influence choice of treatment.

Imaging

Imaging is of considerable importance in the diagnosis and assessment of RA and is increasingly used to detect soft tissue as well as bony abnormalities. An ultrasound (US) scan can detect synovial thickening and analysis of Doppler signal allows an assessment of blood flow to the synovium as a marker for 'activity' of the synovitis. Magnetic resonance imaging (MRI) also provides detailed information about synovial proliferation. Both US and MRI can detect presence of early erosive damage to the joints. Plain radiography offers only late signs of preceding disease activity and its resulting cartilage and bone destruction (Fig. 3.4). It has a number of limitations including the use of ionising radiation and projectional superimposition that can obscure erosions and mimic cartilage loss as an inevitable consequence of presenting a three-dimensional structure in only two planes. Sequential plain radiographs of hands and feet performed at annual intervals do, however, provide important information about progression of erosive damage over time.

At the present time there is much research interest in standardising newer imaging technologies for the assessment of RA, and in the case of MRI, in determining the pathophysiological correlates of imaging abnormalities. It is very likely that we will see increasing use of these tools in the future in order to better inform management decisions with a view to optimally suppressing synovitis at an early stage and improving treatment outcomes.

Management

A multidisciplinary approach

RA is a chronic disease and the majority of patients will have a long-term relationship with their health care providers. Pharmacological intervention represents only one aspect of the management plan for RA at any given stage of disease, irrespective of its severity. A holistic approach to patient care is dependent on multidisciplinary teamwork and co-ordination of patient care between physicians in primary and secondary care settings and a number of other key health care professionals, including specialist nurses, physiotherapists, occupational therapists, podiatrists, social workers, pharmacists and surgeons. Important aspects of the total

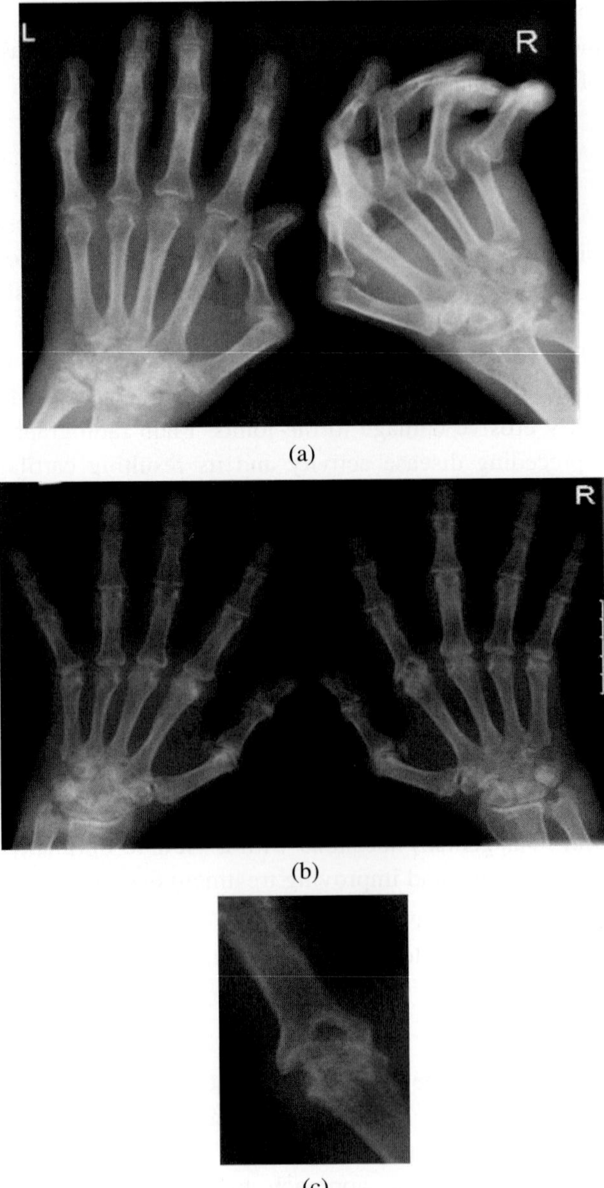

(a)

(b)

(c)

Fig. 3.4. Radiological changes in rheumatoid arthritis. (a) Destructive arthritis at the wrist with erosion of ulnar styloid and partial fusion of carpal bones. Subluxation at the MCP joints on the right with ulnar deviation. (b) Erosive damage at wrists and MCP joints. (c) Enlarged view of erosive disease affecting the right index MCP joint.

management plan include patient education and, where necessary, psychological and employment counselling. The optimum quality of life and functioning can be supported by a realistic evaluation of the most appropriate level of rest and exercise. Appropriate access to splints, aids and adaptations can help preserve function and maintain independence and mobility. Counselling and information about access to social and financial benefits is also of great importance. Appropriate comfortable footwear and proper care of the feet, particularly in those patients with established deformities, can help maintain mobility and comfort. Surgical treatment may also play an essential role in relieving intractable pain and may help restore physical functioning and mobility lost as a result of mechanical damage to joints and associated structures. Surgery may also be invaluable in the treatment of secondary complications of joint disease such as peripheral nerve entrapment at the wrist or elbow and cervical cord compression in relation to instability of the cervical spine.

Pharmacological intervention

Whether the diagnosis is beyond doubt or uncertain, it is very important that such patients are referred to a secondary care specialist at the earliest possible date. In recent years it has become recognised that more favourable clinical outcomes are achieved when synovitis is optimally suppressed early in the course of disease. The approach to treating RA has undergone a major evolutionary change in recent years with a move away from predominantly symptomatic treatment towards much earlier intervention with disease-modifying anti-rheumatic drug (DMARD) therapy and the use of regimes designed to optimally suppress synovitis. Five major classes of drugs are used in the management of RA (Table 3.6).

All patients should be offered simple analgesics and many will also benefit from non-steroidal anti-inflammatory drugs (NSAIDs). Consideration must be given to side-effects of the latter and concomitant prescription of a gastroprotectant may be advisable.

Table 3.6. Classes of drugs used in the management of RA.

Class of drug
Analgesics
Non-steroidal anti-inflammatory drugs
Disease-modifying anti-inflammatory drugs
Corticosteroids
Biologic agents

Disease-modifying anti-rheumatic drugs

Disease-modifying anti-rheumatic drugs form the cornerstone of management of RA and are effective in decreasing synovitis and reducing long-term structural damage to joints. Conventional DMARDs include low dose once weekly methotrexate, sulphasalazine, leflunomide and hydroxychloroquine (Table 3.7).

These drugs act slowly to reduce synovitis and patients should be warned not to expect an effect for two to three months or, in the case of hydroxychloroquine for four to six months. The majority of rheumatologists use methotrexate as a first line agent, often in combination with other DMARD(s). Methotrexate may also be given parenterally (subcutaneously) and is sometimes better tolerated when used in this form. Folic acid is generally given at least once weekly with the aim of reducing some of the side-effects of methotrexate but should not be taken on the same day as methotrexate. Methotrexate is associated with significant risks of toxicity particularly affecting the liver, bone marrow and lungs and requires careful monitoring. The drug is teratogenic and should be stopped three to six months

Table 3.7. Commonly used DMARDs in RA.

DMARD	Dose and route	Important side effects	Monitoring
Methotrexate	10–30 mg weekly po or sc	Hepatic toxicity Bone marrow toxicity Pulmonary toxicity	Blood tests required to assess FBC, renal and liver function
Sulphasalazine	1000–1500 mg bd po	Bone marrow toxicity particularly within first six months of treatment	Blood tests required to assess FBC, renal and liver function
Leflunomide	20 mg od po	Hepatic toxicity Bone marrow toxicity Hypertension	Blood tests required to assess FBC and liver function BP monitoring required
Hydroxychloroquine	200 mg bd po	Retinal toxicity	Monitor visual acuity and refer to ophthalmologist if acuity is impaired or changes

bd twice daily, BP blood pressure, FBC full blood count, po by mouth, sc subcutaneous route.

prior to planned conception. Sulphasalazine or leflunomide may be used as alternatives or in addition to methotrexate. Again, careful monitoring is required because of risks of bone marrow and liver toxicity. A leflunomide washout should be performed using cholestyramine or activated charcoal and a time interval of at least 3 months should be allowed to elapse prior to planned pregnancy. Hydroxychloroquine has more modest clinical efficacy in RA when given as a single agent but is often used in combination with methotrexate.

Corticosteroids

Corticosteroids act rapidly to decrease inflammation and improve symptoms in patients with RA. They play a very important role in early disease where they achieve suppression of synovitis before the slower benefits of DMARDS can be realised. Controversy remains as to the optimum corticosteroid regime in this context and the choice of administration route and dose will depend to some extent on the severity of disease. Corticosteroids may also be used as 'bridging' therapy when DMARD regimes are altered because of inefficacy or toxicity. However, the side effects of this group of drugs argue against prolonged oral use and the aim must be to suppress disease activity in the long term using alternative agents. Corticosteroids may be injected directly into inflamed joints and are of clear benefit when used in this way throughout the course of the disease.

Biologics

'Biologics' is a term used to describe protein-based drugs that have been designed to either inhibit or augment a specific component of the immune system. The major impetus for development of biologic therapies has come from advances in molecular technology that have facilitated identification of cell subsets and cytokines contributing to the inflammatory and destructive components of the disease. At present the drugs target five different pathways involved in pathogenesis of RA (Table 3.8).

- Cytokine modulation

Very considerable progress in understanding the important role of cytokines in the immunopathogenesis of RA has led to two potential approaches to cytokine modulation of rheumatoid synovitis: inhibition of dominant pro-inflammatory cytokines such as TNF-α, IL-1, IL-6 or IL-15, or augmentation of the inadequate anti-inflammatory activity of certain cytokines or naturally occurring cytokine inhibitors as, for example, by administration of soluble TNF receptors or IL-1ra.

Anti-TNF-α therapy, particularly when used in combination with methotrexate, gives rise to substantial improvements in symptoms and signs of disease in

Table 3.8. Biologic agents in RA.

Name	Type of agent	Target	Route
Adalimumab	Monoclonal antibody	TNF-α	sc
Golimumab	Monoclonal antibody	TNF-α	sc
Certolizumab	Monoclonal antibody	TNF-α	sc
Infliximab	Monoclonal antibody	TNF-α	iv
Etanercept	Recombinant protein (TNF receptor p75-Ig)	TNF-α TNF-β	sc
Tocilizumab	Monoclonal antibody	IL-6 receptor	iv
Rituximab	Monoclonal antibody	CD20 on B cells	iv
Abatacept	Recombinant protein (CTLA4-Ig)	CD28 ligands	iv
Anakinra	Recombinant protein (IL-1ra)	IL-1 receptor	sc

CTLA-4 cytotoxic T lymphocyte antigen 4, Ig immunoglobulin, IL interleukin, TNF tumour necrosis factor.

about two-thirds of rheumatoid arthrits patients. Furthermore, this treatment combination protects joints from structural damage in a majority of patients, irrespective of whether a clinical response is achieved or not. Although anti-TNF-α agents are well tolerated and have a good overall safety profile, pitfalls of the use of these drugs apparent with increasing clinical experience include infective complications and, in particular, reactivation of tuberculosis. To date, no statistically significant increase rate of tumour occurrence over that expected has been noted. The overall relative risk of lymphoma is higher than that in the general population but similar to that seen in patients with RA not treated with TNF-α blockade. TNF-α antagonists should be avoided in individuals with moderate or severe heart failure or demyelinating disorders.

Blockade of the biological effect of IL-6 by means of intravenously administered antibodies to the IL-6 receptor (tocilizumab), usually given in addition to background methotrexate therapy, also demonstrates efficacy for reduction in symptoms and signs of RA with acceptable safety.

Clinical trials of IL-1ra show relatively modest anti-inflammatory efficacy but radiographic evidence indicative of retardation of joint damage. Several other pro-inflammatory cytokines represent potential therapeutic targets including IFN-β, IFN-γ, IL-6, IL-15, IL-17 and IL-18 and biological interventions targeting some of these molecules are in clinical trials.

- Targeting T cells

In contrast to the successes of cytokine blockade as a new approach to RA therapy, early randomised, placebo-controlled clinical studies exploring the potential of biological therapies targeting T cells in the treatment of RA have had generally disappointing results. Some anti-T cell agents were non-efficacious whereas other preliminary trials demonstrating some clinical efficacy were terminated due to adverse events, particularly prolonged and profound T cell depletion.

An alternative approach seeks not to deplete or inactivate T cells but to modulate their function in such a way as to reduce their pathogenicity. For example, the co-stimulation blocker abatacept (CTLA4-Ig), which blocks the interaction between CD80 and CD86 on antigen-presenting cells and CD28 on T cells, has efficacy in RA patients with an inadequate response to methotrexate although in general, it takes longer for the maximum benefit to be achieved compared with anti-TNF agents.

- Targeting B cells

The potential of B lymphocyte depletion as an approach to therapy has been confirmed in RA patients seropositive for RF and/or anti-CCP antibodies using the anti-CD20 monoclonal antibody, rituximab. Originally licensed for treatment of B cell lymphomas, this drug effectively depletes B cells but not plasma cells, usually for up to 6–12 months. The loss of B cells is associated with improvement in RA disease activity and patients may be re-treated when the B cell compartment repopulates.

A goal directed approach to management

Several studies have demonstrated that a 'goal directed' approach to management of RA in which physicians regularly perform formal assessments of disease activity and escalate treatment, aiming for remission, significantly improves outcomes for patients. Many rheumatologists use the disease activity score (DAS) 28 score to assess activity in this context. The upper limb joints (excluding distal interphalangeal joints) and knee joints (a total of 28 joints) are assessed for tenderness and swelling and patients are asked for a global assessment of disease activity (GADA) on a visual analogue scale of 0–100 where 0 represents no disease activity. These parameters together with an ESR are entered into a complex formula to provide a score as shown below.

$$\begin{aligned} \text{DAS28} &= 0.56 \times \text{sqrt (tender jt)} + 0.28 \times \text{sqrt (swollen jt)} \\ &\quad + 0.70 \text{ In (ESR)} + 0.014 \text{ GADA} \end{aligned}$$

Computation programmes are readily available on the internet. A DAS28 score of <2.6 represents remission and a score of <3.2 reflects low disease activity. Conversely, scores of >5.1 are consistent with high disease activity and, in the UK, represent the threshold for introduction of biologic agents when conventional DMARDS have failed.

Table 3.9. Minimising the risk of long-term co-morbidity in patients with RA.

Cardiovascular disease	Osteoporosis	Infection
Monitor blood pressure and treat hypertension	Monitor bone density	Vaccination against influenza (annual)
Avoid tobacco use	Avoid tobacco use	Vaccination against pneumococcus
Monitor lipids and treat hyperlipidaemia	Ensure adequate intake of calcium and vitamin D	Educate patients to report relevant symptoms promptly
Encourage regular aerobic exercise	Encourage regular weight bearing exercise	
Avoid obesity	Minimise alcohol use	

Management of co-morbidities of chronic inflammatory disease

An active approach to managing joint synovitis should be matched by an equally active approach to managing the longer-term problems associated with chronic inflammatory disease. Patients are at increased risk of cardiovascular disease, infection and osteoporosis (Table 3.9).

The increased risk of cardiovascular disease is considerable and all patients should be assessed for other cardiovascular risk factors and appropriate measures put in place to minimise these. The heightened risk of developing osteoporosis is related to chronic inflammation, decreased physical activity and use of corticosteroids. Patients should undergo bone density scanning and be advised about lifestyle and offered treatment with a bisphosphonate if appropriate. The infection risk reflects abnormalities in T cell function associated with RA in addition to the effects of the immunosuppressive drugs used in its management. Patients with RA on DMARDs or other immunosuppressive medication should receive vaccinations against influenza and pneumococcus.

3.2. Spondyloarthropathies

The spondyloarthropathy (SpA) family is an interrelated group of disorders that includes ankylosing spondylitis (AS), psoriatic arthritis (PsA), reactive arthritis (ReA) and enteropathic arthritis. In addition, less clearly defined entities fall within the 'family', principally undifferentiated SpA and juvenile idiopathic arthritis (Fig. 3.5).

Spondyloarthropathies are polygenic disorders with a strong association with HLA B27. Approximately 90% of individuals with AS, 70% of enteropathic arthritis patients, 60% of PsA patients with sacroiliitis and 50% of ReA patients possess the HLA B27 gene. The actual mechanism by which HLA B27 promotes

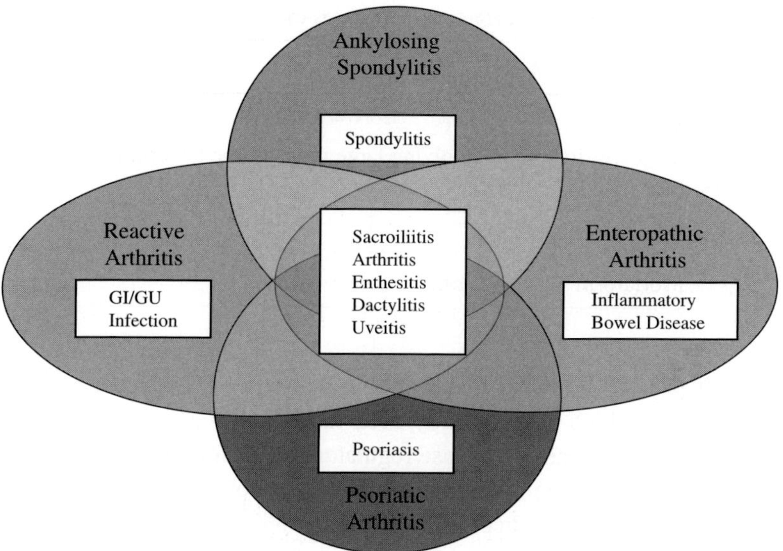

Fig. 3.5. Diagram depicting the overlap between the spondyloarthropathies.

Table 3.10. Possible molecular mechanisms for the association between HLA B27 and spondyloarthropathy.

Putative roles for HLA B27 in predisposition to spondyloarthropathies
Molecular mimicry between a protein from an infective agent and part of the HLA B27 molecule leads to a cross-reactive, tissue damaging immune response.
HLA B27 presents specific bacteria-derived peptide(s) to T lymphocytes, thus inducing a tissue damaging immune response.
HLA B27 facilitates the entry to and/or intracellular persistence of certain bacteria to phagocytic cells. Persistent low grade infection at certain sites promotes local inflammation.
A natural tendency of the HLA B27 molecule to misfold allows it to perform its antigen presentation function abnormally leading to autoimmunity.

HLA human leukocyte antigen.

an inflammatory response is not yet known but several theories have been proposed (Table 3.10). Some evidence for each proposed mechanism exists though their true relevance to disease pathogenesis is unproven.

It is clear that only a small minority (1–2%) of the general population with HLA B27 develop SpA whilst 20% of HLA B27-positive first-degree relatives of

Table 3.11. Characteristic features of spondyloarthritis.

Features of SpAs
Sacroiliitis
Oligoarthritis, often involving large joints of the lower limbs
Enthesitis
Dactylitis
Anterior uveitis
Psoriaform skin changes

people with this condition do so suggesting that other genes must be involved. Two other genes which have recently been identified as associated with AS are ARTS1 (encoding an aminopeptidase regulator of TNFR1 shedding) and IL-23R (encoding IL-23 receptor). Whereas the discovery of the association between HLA B27 and AS has not been informative in terms of disease pathogenesis, these more recently reported associations may be helpful in understanding disease pathogenesis and directing future research into possible therapies.

As well as sharing an association with HLA B27, the SpAs share several clinical features that help to distinguish them from other forms of inflammatory arthritis (Table 3.11).

Sacroiliac joint inflammation and oligoarthritis (inflammation of no more than four joints) are typical. Enthesitis is a hallmark feature; the term describes inflammation at the insertion point of tendons, ligaments and joint capsules into bone. Cellular infiltration by lymphocytes, polymorphonuclear leukocytes and plasma cells occurs at the enthesis, with adjacent bone marrow oedema. This initial phase may be followed by repair with ossification that extends along the tendon, ligament or capsule to form an 'enthesophyte'. Dactylitis is common and refers to the swelling of a whole digit, usually reflecting both synovitis and tenosynovitis. Uveitis may occur, reflecting inflammation of the uveal tract, formed by the iris, ciliary body and choroid. Anterior uveitis (iritis) is most frequent, manifesting as a painful, red eye, sometimes associated with blurring of vision. Prompt treatment is required to reduce risk of permanent visual impairment. Psoriaform skin changes may occur not only in PsA but also in other SpAs, particularly ReA.

AS, ReA and enteropathic arthritis are described in subsequent subsections with PsA being covered in Section 3 of this chapter.

3.2.1. *Ankylosing Spondylitis*

Ankylosing spondylitis affects approximately 0.2% of the Northern European population with a male:female ratio of 3–4:1.

Pathogenesis

The term 'ankylosing spondylitis' is derived from the Greek, *ankylos* meaning 'crooked' and *spondylos* meaning 'vertebra'. In common with other spondyloarthritides the hallmark lesion is enthesitis. Initial lesions usually comprise a combination of enthesitis and synovitis of the sacroiliac joints. Subsequently, the spine may be involved with enthesitis at the discovertebral junction and at the sites of the bony attachment of the longitudinal ligaments. In the early stages erosive changes at the corners of the vertebral bodies can be seen on radiographs and are termed 'Romanus lesions' or referred to as the 'shiny corner sign'. New bone formation at the attachments of the longitudinal ligaments then leads to vertical calcification at the margins of the discs (syndesmophytes) with periosteal new bone formation along the anterior border of the vertebrae leading to an appearance of 'squaring' of the vertebrae. Capsular enthesitis occurs at the facet joints. Synovitis, histologically indistinguishable from that found in RA, may also occur in patients with AS and is characterised by its tendency to involve joints of the lower limb.

TNF-α, a major pro-inflammatory cytokine, has been identified in sacroiliac joint material from patients with AS and is probably present at other sites of inflammation. This cytokine is also present at relatively high levels in the blood of patients. It is capable of promoting inflammation via a number of distinct mechanisms and likely plays a pivotal role in this disease. However, the basis for the anatomical distribution of the inflammatory lesions found in AS remains poorly understood.

Clinical Features

Inflammatory back pain

Symptoms usually begin in early adult life with inflammatory back pain (Table 3.12).

Pain centred on one or both buttocks may radiate to the groin and thigh but not below the knee. Pain is often present at night and the patient tends to wake with spinal aching and stiffness. Pain may be reproduced by direct pressure over the sacrum with the patient lying prone. Symptoms generally, but not always,

Table 3.12. Features of inflammatory back pain.

Features of inflammatory back pain
Improvement with exercise
Pain at night
Insiduous onset
Age at onset <40 years
No improvement with rest

ascend over months or years to involve the thoracic and cervical spine, causing restriction of rotation and flexion. Involvement of the costovertebral joints can lead to restriction of the ribcage and difficulty with breathing. All this must be differentiated from mechanical back pain, which worsens on exercise and improves with rest. Inadequately treated AS results in the loss of lumbar lordosis, exaggeration of thoracic kyphosis and hyperextension of the cervical spine. In severe cases the posture resembles a question mark with thoracolumbar kyphosis and fixed flexion at the hips and knees. Symptoms may range from minimal back stiffness to complete rigidity of the spine (Figs. 3.6 and 3.7). Women are more likely to suffer atypical symptoms, especially isolated sacroiliitis, and less frequently develop spinal fusion.

Peripheral arthritis

Peripheral arthritis occurs in approximately one third of patients with AS and is usually asymmetric and oligoarticular in contrast to the symmetrical polyarthritis

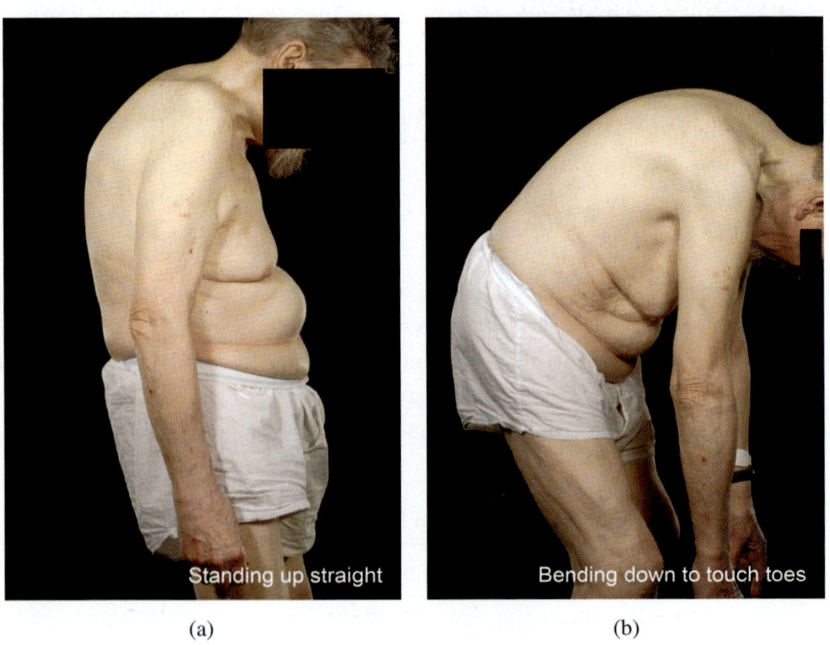

Fig. 3.6. Ankylosing spondylitis. (a) Classical posture of an individual with severe ankylosing spondylitis. (b) Capacity for forward flexion of the spine is limited.

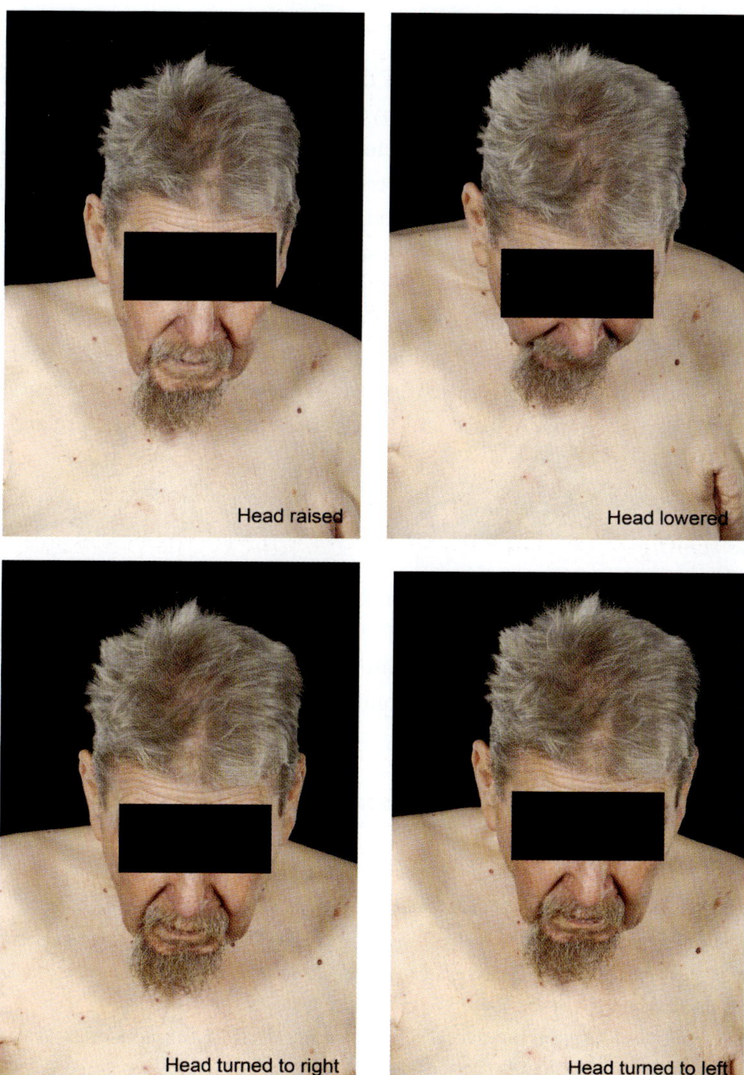

Fig. 3.7. Ankylosing spondylitis. Reduced capacity for neck movements in an individual with ankylosing spondylitis with involvement of the cervical spine.

of RA. Swelling and pain mostly affect the large joints such as the hips and knees but smaller joints, especially within the feet, may be affected. This form of peripheral arthropathy, particularly with knee involvement, may be the presenting complaint.

Extra-articular features

Extra-articular features characteristic of the SpA family are common in AS. The most common of these is anterior uveitis, occurring in 20% of sufferers. Peripheral entheses are typically affected, especially the Achilles tendon and plantar fascia. In the cardiovascular system, aortitis is an infrequent problem but can lead to aortic regurgitation. Cardiac conduction defects may be a feature. More commonly, ongoing inflammation accelerates atheroma formation, the consequence of which is coronary artery disease and hypertension. Chronic inflammation also predisposes to amyloid deposition in the kidneys which can cause renal failure. Rarely, apical pulmonary fibrosis occurs, especially when the rib cage is rigid as a result of costovertebral disease. Osteoporosis occurs in the spine and hips early in the disease and predisposes to vertebral fracture and spinal cord injury.

Disease scoring

Clinical evaluation involves use of a range of standardised composite indices. Chief amongst these are assessment of features of disease activity and function using the Bath Ankylosing Spondylitis Disease Activity Index (BASDAI) (Table 3.13) and Bath Ankylosing Spondylitis Functional Index (BASFI).

Table 3.13. Bath Ankylosing Spondylitis Disease Activity Index.

Patients are asked to rate the following on a visual analogue scale from none to very severe (0–10)
1. How would you describe the overall level of fatigue/tiredness you have experienced? 2. How would you describe the overall level of ankylosing spondylitis neck, back or hip pain you have had? 3. How would you describe the overall level of pain/swelling in joints other than neck, back or hips you have had? 4. How would you describe the overall level of discomfort you have had from areas tender to touch or pressure? 5. How would you describe the overall level of discomfort you have had from the time you wake up? 6. How long does your morning stiffness last from the time you wake up?

The mean of the scores of 5 and 6 is added to the sum of the scores of 1–4 and the total divided by 5 to give the BASDAI with a maximum value of 10. A score of >4 is consistent with significant disease activity.

Table 3.14. The Bath Ankylosing Spondylitis Metrology Index.

	Normal (0)	Moderate (1)	Severe (2)
Cervical rotation (mean of L + R)	>70°	20–70°	<20°
Tragus-to-wall (mean of L + R)	<15 cm	15–30 cm	>30 cm
Lumbar side flexion (mean of L + R)	>10 cm	5–10 cm	<5 cm
Lumbar flexion (modified Schober's test)	>4 cm	2–4 cm	2 cm
Intermalleolar distance	>100 cm	70–100 cm	<70 cm

L left, R right, Scores should be summed to give a composite score with a maximum of value of 10.

Clinical assessment should include posture and hip mobility and measurement of tragus-to-wall distance (spinal flexion deformity), cervical rotation, chest expansion (costovertebral stiffness), lateral spinal flexion, lumbar flexion (Schober's test) and intermalleolar distance (hip restriction). Movements may be expressed in a single composite using the Bath Ankylosing Spondylitis Metrology Index (BASMI) (Table 3.14).

Investigations

Laboratory tests

Blood tests can aid diagnosis but none are conclusive. HLA B27 is present in the majority of AS patients but is also present in approximately 5% of healthy individuals, depending on race. It can be helpful in patients in whom there is a high index of suspicion of AS but where clinical findings are inconclusive. The inflammatory markers CRP and ESR are elevated in some but not all cases. Tests for RF, ANA and anti-CCP antibodies are negative.

Imaging

The key radiographic finding is bilateral sacroiliitis and this forms the cornerstone of the modified New York classification criteria commonly used for diagnosis of AS (Table 3.15).

However, the New York criteria are very insensitive for detection of early disease; it is now recognised that it is only after an average of 6 years of symptomatic sacroiliitis that X-ray changes become detectable (Fig. 3.8). The challenge today is to identify AS before these radiographic changes occur. Increasingly, computed tomography (CT) and MRI are used to image the sacroiliac joints. MRI is now the modality of choice for identifying bone marrow oedema, joint inflammation and

Table 3.15. Modified New York classification of AS.

Classification of AS
Clinical Criteria
1. History of inflammatory back pain for at least 3 months
2. Limitation of lumbar spine movement in both sagittal and frontal planes
3. Reduced chest expansion compared to age-matched peers
Radiographic Criteria
1. Radiographic sacroiliitis (Grade 2 bilaterally or Grade 3 or 4 unilaterally)

At least one clinical criterion must be met together with the radiographic criterion.

cartilage abnormalities before they can be seen on plain films. MRI evidence of sacroiliitis in an individual with back pain contributes to the diagnosis of Axial Spondyloarthritis by the Assessment of Spondyloarthritis International Society (ASAS) criteria. Where disease progresses to involve the spine, squaring of vertebrae and syndesmophytes may be seen on X-ray; changes can be recorded and quantified using the modified Stoke Ankylosing Spondylitis Spinal Score (mSASSS). Late in the course of AS the florid new bone formation in the vertebral column may give rise to the classical appearance of 'bamboo spine'.

Bone density should be measured in all patients since spinal and hip osteoporosis may develop early in the disease.

Management

As with all forms of arthritis, patient education and support are crucial to effective management. All patients should see a physiotherapist for advice on maintaining spinal mobility and some may also benefit from input from an occupational therapist. NSAIDs have been the cornerstone of management for patients with axial disease. Oral prednisolone should be avoided where possible, particularly because of the high risk of osteoporosis in these patients. Intra-articular corticosteroids may, however, be beneficial in management of peripheral arthritis. DMARDS such as sulphasalazine and methotrexate are effective in management of peripheral arthritis but do not have a beneficial effect on axial disease. Anti-TNF-α therapy is highly effective for both axial and peripheral symptom control although its effect on disease progression is unknown. In severe cases referral to orthopaedic surgeons for hip or knee replacement or for spinal osteotomy may be indicated. Bisphosphonates should be used to manage osteoporosis.

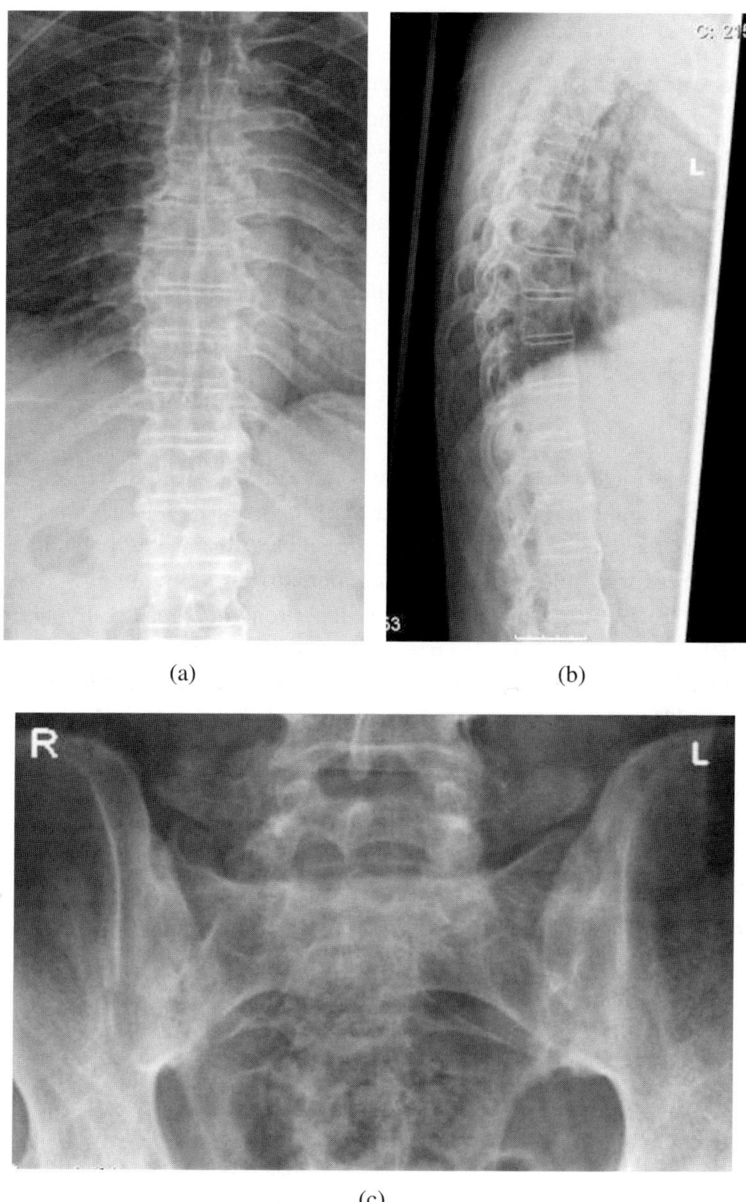

(a) (b)

(c)

Fig. 3.8. Ankylosing spondylitis. (a) and (b) X-ray of thoracic spine showing syndesmophyte formation (c) X-ray of pelvis showing fusion of sacroiliac joints.

3.2.2. *Reactive Arthritis*

Reactive arthritis is an acute SpA associated with an infection elsewhere in the body but without viable organisms being present in the joint(s). Sexually transmitted and gastrointestinal diseases have long been regarded as causal factors and certain respiratory infections may play a similar role. Men and women are equally affected by enteric ReA but males are more commonly affected by the sexually acquired form. The overall prevalence is difficult to determine as mild forms may go undiagnosed. The incidence in Europe is approximately 30 cases in 100,000.

Pathogenesis

A genetic contribution to the pathogenesis is clearly associated with inheritance of HLA B27 in approximately 50% of cases. However, ReA is set apart from the other spondyloarthropathies by the presence of an identifiable preceding infection, the most credible mechanism of pathogenesis involving provocation ('triggering') of ReA by specific bacterial infections in a genetically susceptible individual. The best data are from epidemiological studies in diarrhoeal infections, with arthritis occurring in 1–4% of affected individuals in outbreaks of *Shigella* species, *Campylobacter jejuni*, *Salmonella enteritica* and *Yersinia enterocolitica* infection. Sporadic genital-tract infections with *Chlamydia trachomatis* have also been implicated. Antigens from these micro-organisms have been found in affected synovial tissue but this does not establish causality.

More recently, streptococcal infections have also been implicated as a causal agent in adults. Group A streptococcal infections are well recognised causes of rheumatic fever in children and teenagers but a phenotypically distinct form of arthritis, similar to ReA, has been described, mostly in young adults, after a range of streptococcal infections. Arthritis in these patients does not fulfil the Jones criteria for rheumatic fever and it has been proposed that post-streptococcal ReA is a separate entity.

Clinical Features

Symptoms usually begin with swelling and pain of one or more of the lower limb joints and systemic features of fever, malaise and weight loss may be prominent. A careful history will reveal the antecedent infection. Up to one-third of patients have buttock pain, a sign of sacroiliitis, at presentation. Asymmetrical oligoarthritis involving the knees, ankles, subtalar joints and metatarsophalangeal joints is typical. As with other forms of SpA, dactylitis and tendinopathies are common.

Features of infection including dysuria, urethral or vaginal discharge, diarrhoea or abdominal pain may be present though such clues to underlying infection are sometimes entirely absent. Conjunctivitis or anterior uveitis occurs in up to one-third of patients. Although uveitis is less common it may lead to blindness so that anyone with a painful red eye should immediately seek ophthalmology advice. Cutaneous and mucosal lesions are another hallmark of ReA and range from oral ulcers to keratoderma blenorrhagica, the latter being characterised by hyperkeratotic lesions that typically appear on the palms of the hands and soles of the feet and which are histologically indistinguishable from pustular psoriasis. Circinate balanitis is also a characteristic psoriasiform skin lesion on the glans penis. These lesions may be especially severe in the context of human immunodeficiency virus (HIV) infection. Heel pain due to enthesitis at the Achilles' tendon or plantar fascia attachment may be painful and disabling.

The prognosis is variable; some patients recover after a single episode of arthritis, others develop recurrent episodes and a few develop chronic arthritis. Recurrent or persistent disease is more common following sexually aquired ReA than in enteric ReA. Eye and skin lesions may recur independently of arthritis. HLA B27 is associated with more prolonged episodes of arthritis, extra-articular features, spinal symptoms and a poorer overall prognosis.

Investigation

Diagnosis of ReA is a two-step process: recognition of an SpA, then identification of the likely causal infection. There is no one diagnostic test. An elevated ESR or CRP suggests inflammation. When sexually acquired disease is suspected care should be taken to exclude a wide range of sexually transmitted infections including, where appropriate, HIV infection. There are no specific radiographic findings although unilateral sacroiliitis may be present. Synovial fluid aspiration is important for exclusion of infection or gout.

Management

Where sexually acquired ReA is suspected the patient should be referred to a sexual health service for education, investigation and treatment. Patients with a swollen, painful joint will usually respond well to aspiration of the joint with injection of corticosteroid. NSAIDs will provide symptomatic relief. Where the arthritis persists beyond 3 months then treatment with methotrexate or sulphasalazine should be initiated. Patients should be referred to a physiotherapist for advice and some may also benefit from advice from occupational therapists and an orthotics department.

3.2.3. *Enteropathic Arthritis*

Arthritis associated with inflammatory bowel disease is described as enteropathic when other diagnoses have been excluded. Arthritis is mainly associated with ulcerative colitis and Crohn's disease but may also complicate other bowel disorders, such as coeliac disease or Whipple's disease. Inflammatory bowel disease affects 0.5–1% of the population. Of these, almost one-sixth will develop a SpA.

Pathogenesis

As with other SpAs, genetic and environmental factors are both likely to be involved in the pathogenesis. 70% of affected individuals carry the HLA B27 gene. In addition to the overt inflammatory bowel disease of enteropathic arthritis, a high proportion of patients with other SpAs have subclinical large and/or small bowel disease, suggesting that change in the bowel may be a key feature of SpAs in general. Genetic studies in Icelandic subjects have demonstrated a close link between overt or covert inflammatory bowel disease and AS, emphasising their common genetic background.

Several strands of evidence support, but do not prove, a role for gut microorganisms in the pathogenesis of enteropathic arthritis. In man these include the association of gut infection with ReA and epidemiological evidence of arthritis associated with Whipple's disease and following jejuno-ileal bypass surgery with bacterial overgrowth in blind loops of bowel. In laboratory animals, development of a SpA-like syndrome in HLA B27 positive transgenic rats has been demonstrated with development of arthritis being dependent upon the presence of normal bacterial gut flora. Leukocyte trafficking between the gastrointestinal tract and the joint may be crucial to the link; $CD163^+$ macrophages are seen in the inflammatory lesions of the gut and the synovium in affected individuals and T cells with similar antigen receptor molecules have been found at both sites.

Clinical Features

The patterns of arthritis are similar in both ulcerative colitis and Crohn's disease. Two major types of enteropathic arthritis are recognised. Type 1 involves up to five joints, often knees and ankles, and follows a relapsing/remitting course. Type 2 involves five or more joints, typically with symmetrical small joint involvement. In both types, arthritis and inflammatory bowel disease follow independent courses. In addition, there may be a third subset of patients who develop non-specific arthralgias or a fibromyalgia-like syndrome. Back pain or buttock pain due to sacroiliitis is a frequent presenting symptom. The sacroiliitis of inflammatory bowel disease is usually bilateral and indistinguishable from that in AS. As in other SpAs, enthesitis, dactylitis and anterior uveitis are characteristic. Skin lesions including pyoderma gangrenosum and erythema nodosum may occur in association with inflammatory bowel disease and this is sometimes helpful in pointing to the correct diagnosis. Bowel symptoms usually predate rheumatic features though this is not always so.

Investigation

There is no one diagnostic test for enteropathic SpA. Diagnosis relies upon the recognition of features of a spondyloarthrits and identification of inflammatory bowel disease with exclusion of other forms of arthritis. Blood tests may reflect an inflammatory response. Radiographic changes are similar to those of other SpAs.

Management

Patients will need education about enteropathic arthritis and the management options available to them. Involvement of a multidisciplinary team with input from physiotherapists, occupational therapists and an orthotics department will be required. NSAIDs will provide symptomatic relief although they can provoke flares of bowel symptoms. Intra-articular corticosteroids are helpful in controlling inflammation in individual joints. Oral or parenteral corticosteroids may improve symptoms but must be used with caution because of side-effects. Methotrexate or sulphasalazine are commonly used as DMARDS. Biologic agents have a role and may be indicated for management of the bowel disease itself; in particular infliximab is used for fistulating Crohn's disease. In severe cases referral to orthopaedic surgeons for joint replacement may be required.

3.2.4. *Undifferentiated Spondyloarthropathy*

This term is applied when some of the features of an SpA are present but criteria for any one disease are not fulfilled. Examples include lower limb oligoarthritis or enthesopathy. Many individuals subsequently develop a differentiated form of SpA. Approximately 50% of people with undifferentiated SpA are HLA B27 positive. It is a diagnosis of exclusion and is treated in a similar way to the other SpAs.

3.3. Psoriatic Arthritis

Psoriatic arthritis is a chronic inflammatory joint disease and, as the name implies, has a well-recognised link to psoriasis. Psoriasis affects 1–3% of the population and estimates suggest that approximately 10–20% of these patients will develop arthritis.

In terms of the temporal relationship between skin and joint involvement, approximately two thirds of patients will have skin disease well before the onset of arthritis. In around half of the remaining third the arthritis and skin involvement will first manifest within a year of each other and in the other half the arthritis will precede the skin lesions by more than one year. PsA affects men and women equally, with the usual age of onset being in the second or third decade of life.

Pathogeneis

The aetiopathogenesis of PsA remains to be firmly established although studies have shown that genetic, immunological and environmental factors all play a role in the onset of the disease.

Genetic factors

Approximately 40% of patients with PsA have a family history of psoriasis or PsA in first-degree relatives. Twin studies likewise point to the importance of genetic factors in the aetiology of PsA and population studies show an association between certain HLA genes and disease expression. Whilst HLA B27 is one of these genes, the frequency of HLA B27 in patients with PsA is not as high as it is in AS or ReA. Further genetic links have been identified and these include a genetic locus on chromosome 16q (22-A), class I MHC chain related gene A (MICA), TNF-α and TNF-β polymorphisms on chromosome 6 and loci in the IL family gene cluster on chromosome 2. Many of these genetic links point to aberrant immune responses playing a role in the development of PsA.

Immunological factors

PsA differs from RA in that there is no evidence for development of antibody responses to self-antigens. Despite this difference, studies have shown that the inflammatory response in psoriatic synovial lesions is at times histologically indistinguishable from that seen in RA. An increased level of pro-inflammatory cytokines such as TNF-α and ILs is present in the synovium and synovial fluid in PsA in a pattern similar to that seen in RA. However, CD8 rather than CD4 T cells appear to predominate within the entheses.

Environmental factors

There is interest in the antigens that may be driving abnormal immune responses in patients with PsA and infections have been implicated as possible causative agents for PsA. A study has suggested a link between streptococcal infection and PsA, by demonstrating higher levels of antibody to streptococcal organisms in the sera of patients with PsA. The possible role of bacterial antigens in the pathogenesis of psoriasis and PsA is further supported by the indirect observation of an enhanced humoral and cellular immunity to gram-positive bacteria present in psoriatic plaques. HIV also seems to predispose to psoriasis and PsA. Whether this is due to an altered balance between $CD4^+$ and $CD8^+$ T cells or whether it suggests a viral trigger of PsA remains to be established. More detailed understanding of the immunologic mechanisms that drive the disease will be fundamental for the development of new therapies.

Clinical Features

PsA manifests in a variety of ways and, in common with other SpAs, may involve peripheral joints and/or the axial skeleton with features of synovitis, enthesitis and/or dactylitis (Figs. 3.9–3.11). Five different clinical patterns of joint involvement have been described in the Moll and Wright classification system although it should be noted that patients may show more than one pattern of disease (Table 3.16).

In approximately 50% of patients the disease presents as an asymmetrical oligoarthritis often, but not always, affecting the lower limb. In another 15% of cases the disease begins as an inflammatory polyarthritis which may resemble RA. In 10% of patients swelling at the distal interphalangeal joints of one or both hands occurs. Low back or pelvic pain due to sacroiliitis may be a presenting feature. Subsequently the spine may also become involved although

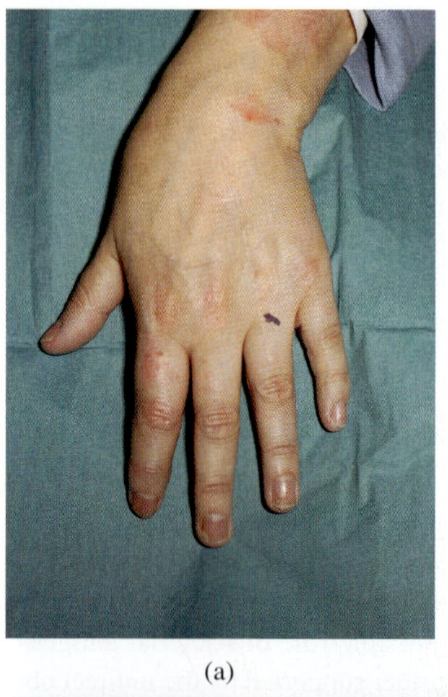

(a)

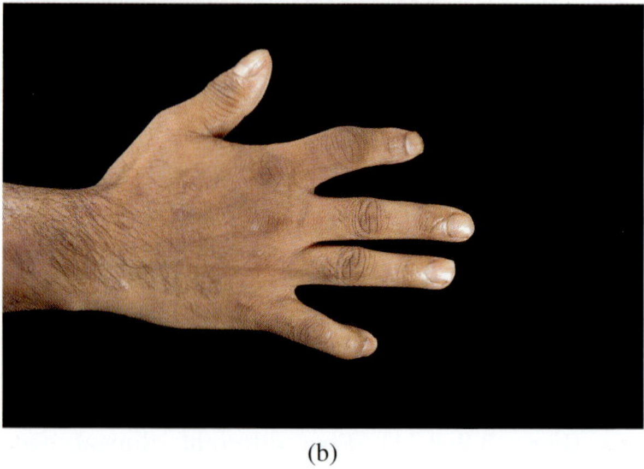

(b)

Fig. 3.9. Psoriatic arthritis affecting the hands. (a) Arthritis of the index PIP joint with nail pitting and cutaneous psoriasis (partially treated). (b) Arthritis of the index PIP joint and little finger DIP joint in an individual with psoriasis.

'psoriatic spondylitis' typically differs from AS by its asymmetric nature and discontinuous involvement of the vertebrae. Arthritis mutilans is the rarest and most destructive form of the disease and may result in telescoping of the digits (Fig. 3.12).

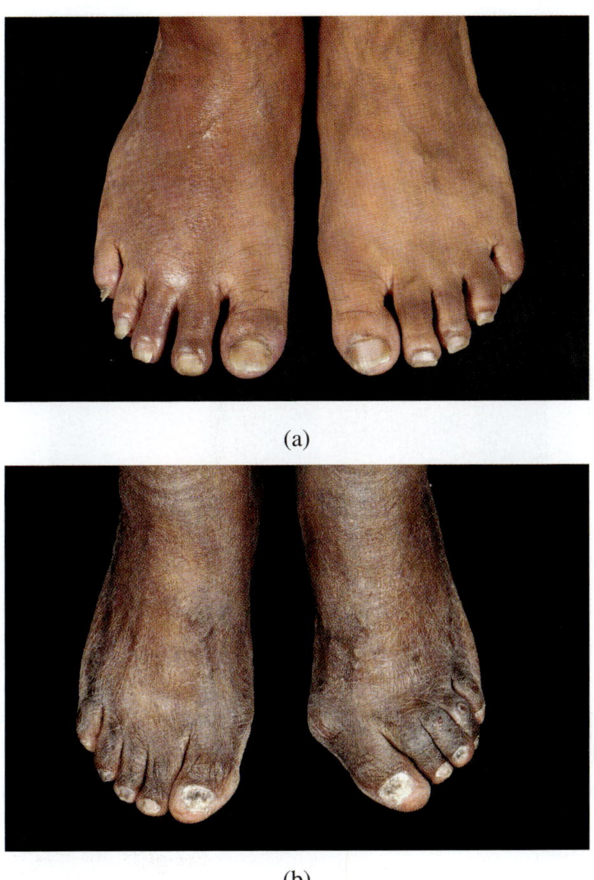

(a)

(b)

Fig. 3.10. Psoriatic arthritis affecting the feet. (a) Dactylitis of the right second and third toes with arthritis affecting other IP joints. (b) Onycholysis of the nails with valgus deformity at the left 1st MTP joint and involvement of the left 2nd to 5th MTP joints associated with clawing of the toes.

The clinical presentation, along with unique radiological features, forms the basis for diagnosing PsA. The Classification of Psoriatic Arthritis (CASPAR) study considered the cases of 588 patients with PsA and 536 patients with other forms of inflammatory arthritis and suggested a set of criteria to help classify a patient as having PsA (Table 3.17).

Finding psoriatic lesions is a key element of the diagnosis. These may be typical scaly hyperkeratotic plaques over the extensor surfaces, scalp, ears, umbilicus or natal cleft, or pustular lesions on the soles of the feet with

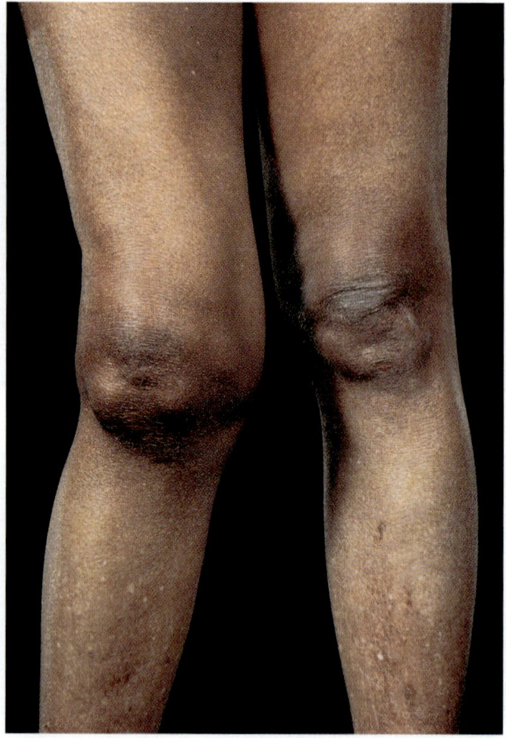

Fig. 3.11. Knee effusion in psoriatic arthritis. Large effusion of the right knee in a patient with psoriatic arthritis and secondary degenerative changes leading to a valgus deformity.

characteristic nail dystrophy. Lesions may not have been recognised by the patient and a rigorous examination may be necessary.

A variety of nail lesions occur in psoriasis and have a strong association with development of arthropathy, particularly that involving the distal interphalangeal joints (Table 3.18 and Figs. 3.9, 3.10 and 3.12).

Even in the absence of cutaneous psoriasis, the presence of typical nail lesions in a patient with distal and asymmetric joint involvement should alert the clinician to the possibility of PsA.

Enthesitis, especially that involving the Achilles tendon, is seen commonly in patients with underlying psoriasis. Enthesitis can also involve the pelvic bones and plantar fascia and may be associated with marked osteitis in the immediately adjacent bone. Tenosynovitis is another feature of PsA and can involve the flexor tendons of the hands or other sites. Tenosynovitis may contribute to the clinical finding of

Table 3.16. Moll and Wright classification system of joint involvement in PsA.

Type	Characteristic features
Asymmetric oligoarthritis	The most common presenting type. No more than four small or large joints affected on either side of the body. Male predominance.
Symmetric polyarthritis	Affects multiple, symmetric pairs of joints, small or large. Similar or at times indistinguishable from RA. Female predominance. More evidence of erosive joint damage in this group.
Distal arthritis	Involvement of the distal interphalangeal joints.
Spondyloarthropathy	Includes sacroiliitis and spondylitis. May be asymmetrical. Stronger link to HLA B27 positivity in bilateral sacroiliitis.
Arthritis mutilans	A destructive and deforming type of PsA. Subluxation of joints and telescoping of digits. Generally long-standing, end stage disease. Female preponderance.

HLA human leukocyte antigen, PsA psoriatic arthritis.

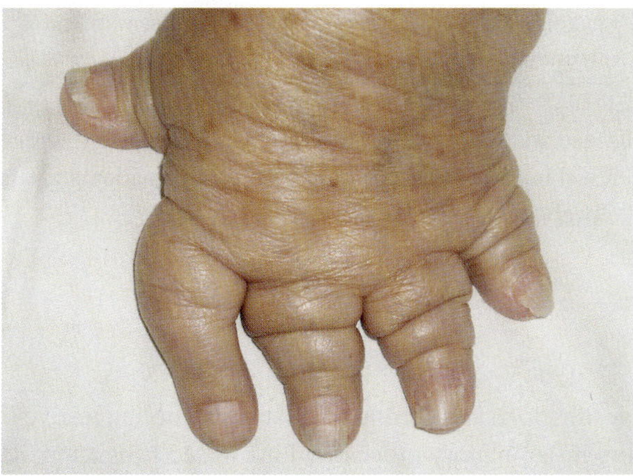

Fig. 3.12. Psoriatic arthritis. Digital shortening (telescopic fingers) due to osteolysis of the phalanges. Note also onycholysis of nails. Image kindly provided by Dr Tom Marshall, Norfolk and Norwich Hospital.

dactylitis, often called 'sausage digit', which is a typical feature of PsA. Ocular inflammation is known to occur in PsA, commonly in the form of anterior uveitis.

The outcome from PsA is very variable but around 20% of patients go on to develop a severely destructive, deforming and disabling form of disease.

Table 3.17. CASPAR criteria for classification of psoriatic arthritis.

Classification criteria for psoriatic arthritis
Musculoskeletal inflammation (inflammatory arthritis, enthesitis or inflammatory back pain) plus three out of the following: 1. Skin psoriasis (current or previous history of psoriasis or a positive family history if the patient is not affected). 2. Nail lesions 3. Dactylitis 4. Negative rheumatoid factor 5. Juxta-articular bone formation on radiography

If current skin psoriasis is present, then only one other feature is required.

Table 3.18. Nail lesions in psoarisis.

Nail plate	Nail bed
Nail pitting	Onycholysis
Nail plate crumbling	Nail bed hyperkeratosis
Leukonychia	Splinter haemorrhages
Lunular red spots	Salmon patches

Polyarticular disease and a high ESR have both been associated with poor prognosis and these features should prompt physicians to ensure patients are treated actively and monitored closely.

Investigations

Laboratory tests

Laboratory investigations are not diagnostic but can be suggestive of the presence of an underlying inflammatory process, with a raised ESR and CRP and a leukocytosis. Anaemia of chronic disease or reflecting gastrointestinal blood loss associated with prolonged use of NSAIDs can also be present. Hyperuricaemia is sometimes evident as a result of high skin cell turnover in association with psoriasis and may result in gouty arthritis.

Imaging

The characteristic radiographic features of PsA include joint space narrowing with development of joint erosions (Fig. 3.13). Bone osteolysis may occur

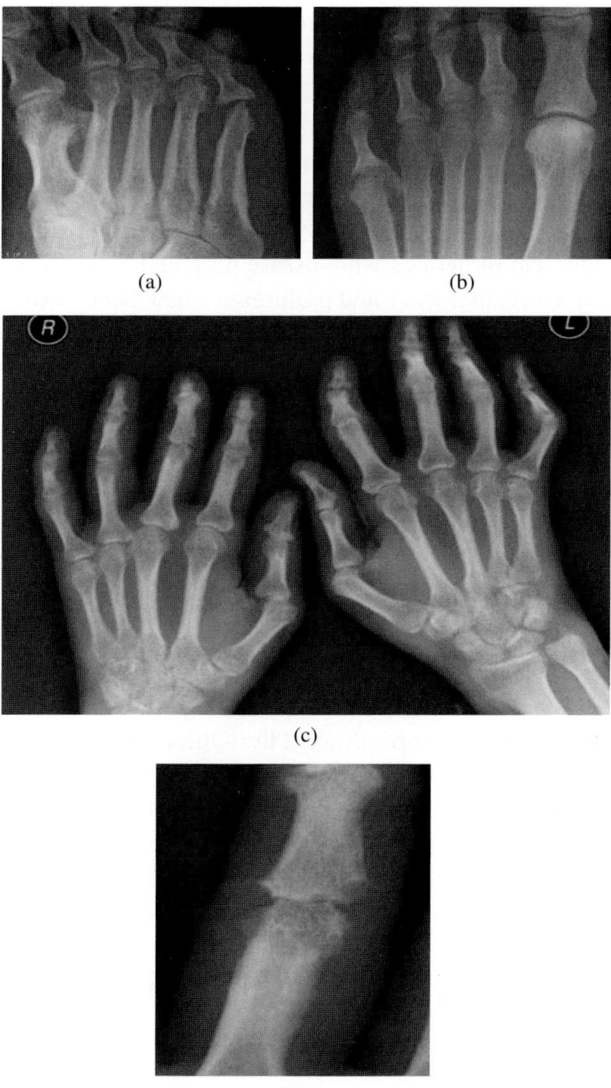

(a) (b) (c) (d)

Fig. 3.13. Radiological changes in psoriatic arthritis. (a) Psoriatic arthritis of the right 5th MTP joint with tapering of the metatarsal. These types of changes may progress to the classic 'pencil in cup' deformity. (b) Erosive arthritis affecting the left 5th MTP joint with erosions and periostitis of the fifth metatarsal in a patient with psoriasis. (c) Erosive arthritis of the PIP joints in a patient with psoriasis. (d) Magnified view of the periarticular erosions at the left middle finger PIP joint. Figures kindly provided by Dr Tom Marshall, Norfolk and Norwich Hospital.

resulting in the classic 'pencil in cup' deformity and in resorption of terminal phalanges. Bony proliferation is a feature with formation of spurs at sites of tendon insertions and ossification of spinal ligaments leading to ankylosis. US and MRI techniques have proved very useful in detecting early changes in PsA in the peripheral joints, peri-articular tissues and spine. Imaging appearances do differ from those seen in RA in that the joint involvement in PsA is often asymmetrical and involves the distal interphalangeal joints. The erosions seen in PsA may become irregular and ill defined with disease progression due to periosteal new bone formation. Gross osteolysis and proliferative new bone formation are characteristic of PsA whereas neither is usually seen in RA.

Management

A multidisciplinary approach

As in the case of other forms of inflammatory arthritis, management of PsA requires an integrated, multidisciplinary team approach. Patient education has a fundamental role to play in management. Improving patients' understanding of their disease can lead to better doctor–patient dialogue with positive effects on decision making, compliance, treatment outcomes and patient satisfaction. Involvement of a multidisciplinary team of health professionals will help to preserve patient function and independence. Physiotherapists can provide advice on joint protection and on tailored exercise programmes to promote muscle strength and improve range of movement at individual joints. Occupational therapists will be able to provide splints to rest joints where appropriate and can assess and support patients in a range of areas including personal self help. Provision of simple aids at home can often make a major difference to an individual's capacity to remain independent. Effective communication is required between rheumatologists and dermatologists and in some cases a referral to orthopaedic surgeons for arthroplasty or tendinoplasty may be indicated.

Pharmacological intervention

The major classes of drugs used in management of PsA are similar to those used in RA (see Table 3.6). The typical first-line drug therapy for mild to moderate PsA with no evidence of progressive joint damage is with NSAIDs. By reducing the level of inflammation, NSAIDs lead to an improvement in symptoms and joint mobility. The side effect profile of these drugs, especially their capacity to cause gastrointestinal irritation, needs to be considered and may restrict their use in a proportion of patients. Concomitant use of gastroprotective agents may be appropriate. There has been some concern that NSAIDs may aggravate the skin psoriasis and they should therefore be used with extra caution in these patients. Other therapies should be introduced when there is persistent inflammation and/or joint damage despite use of NSAIDS.

Corticosteroids

Oral and intramuscular (im) steroids can control the symptoms of PsA but their use is generally avoided because of the potential for steroid withdrawal to exacerbate the psoriatic skin disease. Intra-articular steroids may be useful, but care must be taken to avoid passing the needle through a psoriatic plaque as this may increase the risk of introducing infection into the joint.

DMARDs

There is evidence to show that certain DMARDs are effective in management of patients with PsA although, as yet, there is a paucity of good data showing that this group of drugs inhibits longer-term structural damage. Methotrexate is the most commonly prescribed DMARD for patients with PsA and has a positive effect on cutaneous as well as joint disease. Results of ongoing trials to assess the efficacy of methotrexate in reducing radiological progression are awaited. Leflunomide has been used to treat PsA with positive effects on both the skin and joints. Ciclosporin, at doses lower than those used for organ transplantation, has also been shown to be effective for both skin and joint disease. However, amongst other significant side effects such as hypertension, it is potentially nephrotoxic and its use is generally reserved for patients with severe and unresponsive disease. Several studies have demonstrated that sulphasalazine is effective in the treatment of peripheral arthritis in PsA although it has no proven effect on axial disease or cutaneous psoriasis and again there is no evidence that it inhibits joint destruction. Azathioprine or hydroxychloroquine are somtimes used in PsA although there has been some concern about the potential of the latter to exacerbate the skin lesions.

TNF-α antagonists

TNF-α antagonists have been shown to improve all facets of the disease. Importantly, there is evidence that these drugs reduce the extent of joint damage associated with PsA. These types of drugs are usually introduced where patients have failed to respond to conventional DMARDs and, in particular, where they are developing progressive joint damage. In contrast to their use in RA, studies suggest that TNF-α antagonists can be as effective in PsA when used as single therapy as when used in combination with DMARDs.

New agents

Other therapies are also being evaluated for use in PsA including alefacept, a recombinant fully human lymphocyte function antigen (LFA)3-IgG fusion protein that binds CD2 on T cells, thereby inhibiting T cell activation and allowing natural killer cell mediated T cell depletion. Early studies show evidence of benefit when the drug is used in association with methotrexate. Mycophenolate mofetil, Vitamin D3 and bromocriptine have all shown some positive effect in small numbers of patients with PsA. Further controlled trials of these and other agents are needed to confirm their efficacy.

3.4. Osteoarthritis

Osteoarthritis (OA) is the most common form of joint disease and is estimated to cost somewhere in the region of 1–1.5% of the gross domestic product of developed countries. The costs of the disease are those directly incurred from treating a chronic painful condition, as well as those associated with days off work through pain and disability. It is more prevalent in women and incidence increases with age. It is probably fair to say that this highly prevalent disease has suffered from academic neglect over recent decades; many clinicians still regard OA as simply a disease of 'wear and tear', even though the pathological processes appear to be a good deal more complex than this. In recent years, the identification of key degradative enzymes has opened the field up to potential new strategies for disease modification. Unfortunately, implementation into clinical trials is likely to be very slow as the tools for identifying early disease in patients remain poor and there are currently no good biomarkers for assessing disease development or progression. Synonyms for OA include 'osteoarthrosis' (this term reflects the typical lack of joint inflammation in the disease) or 'degenerative joint disease'.

Pathogenesis

In order to understand pathogenesis in OA it is first necessary to understand the structure of articular cartilage. Articular cartilage is the avascular and aneuronal tissue that overlies the ends of bone at synovial joints. It is principally composed of extracellular matrix (predominantly type II collagen and the proteoglycan aggrecan) in which are embedded a relatively small number (only 5–10% tissue volume) of cells called chondrocytes. The tissue is uniquely adapted to withstand mechanical stress; aggrecan is highly negatively charged, and so draws water into the tissue causing a swelling pressure, and type II collagen forms a highly robust scaffold in which the aggrecan and other minor components of the matrix are arranged.

The principal defect in OA is loss of articular cartilage which appears to occur initially at the articular surface, and which then spreads through the matrix (Fig. 3.14). Other changes that occur in the tissue include patchy loss of proteoglycan and clustering of articular chondrocytes. Within the joint there is also thickening, sometimes termed sclerosis, of the subchondral bone and episodic synovitis. It is possible that pain in disease arises from bone or synovial change, although other peri-articular structures, such as entheses, bursae

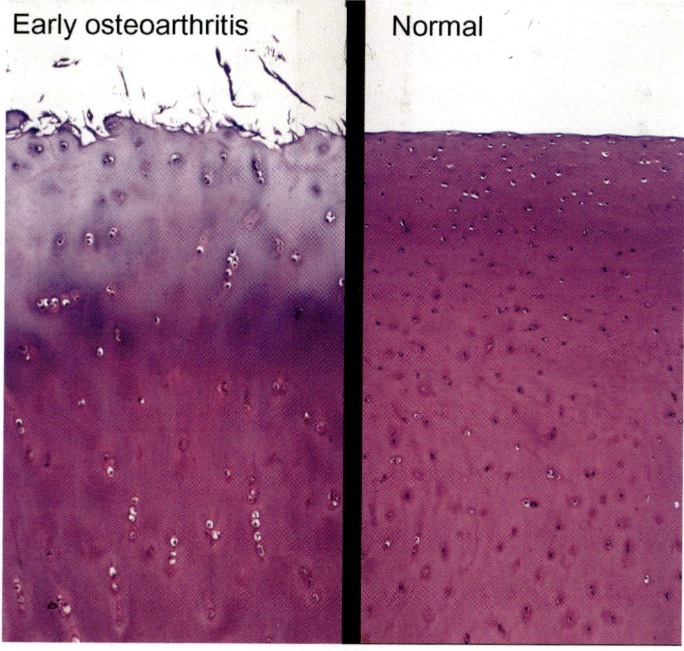

Fig. 3.14. Early osteoarthritic compared with normal human cartilage stained for proteoglycan (Toluidine blue). Courtesy of Professor Yasunori Okada.

Table 3.19. Historical theories of pathogenesis of OA over the past 50 years.

Decade	Theory
1960s	Failure of joint lubrication
1970s	Weakening of collagen network leading to over-hydration of cartilage
	Decreased compliance of the subchondral bone
1980s	Matrix degradation due to catabolic cytokines, e.g. IL-1
	Proteolysis by matrix metalloproteinases
1990s	Proteolysis by newly identified 'aggrecanases'

or tendons may be alternative sources. Persistence of pain, due to local sensitisation of nerve fibres and central nervous system changes, can also occur over time.

Theories of pathogenesis

A number of theories of pathogenesis have been proposed over the decades. These are listed in Table 3.19.

In the 1980s, the discovery of a family of matrix degrading enzymes, known as matrix metalloproteinases, substantially changed the face of OA research, and there evolved a new hypothesis, that cartilage damage was due to an imbalance between matrix degradation and synthesis. However, although fragments of aggrecan were identified in the joint fluid of patients with OA, they did not appear to have been generated by the action of known matrix metalloproteinases and it was determined that there must be an as yet undiscovered class of enzymes responsible for degradation in OA; these were termed 'aggrecanases'. It was not until 1999 that the first aggrecanase was purified and cloned. Soon after, a second homologous enzyme was discovered. Both of these are considered to be key aggrecanases in human articular cartilage and are the focus of much current OA research. Aggrecanases are classical inflammatory genes, which is to say that they are driven by inflammatory cytokines such as IL-1, suggesting inflammation may play a role in driving OA.

Risk factors

Epidemiological studies have suggested that many different factors predispose to the development of the abnormalities described above (Table 3.20).

Table 3.20. Risk factors in OA development.

Risk factors
Age
Obesity
Mechanical factors
Family history
Chondrodysplasias, e.g. defects in type II collagen
Other medical conditions, e.g. haemachromatosis
Joint damage due to other arthropathies

The role of age is controversial; it is likely that there is a reduction in new matrix synthesis, as well as an increase in activation of degradative pathways as we age, but how and whether these relate to mechanical 'wear' is unclear. Another complication is that mechanical stimulation of cartilage is also regarded as being anabolic for the tissue and may therefore help to protect against the development of OA.

The role of obesity in OA development is probably two-fold. Firstly, it increases the mechanical load on the joint, significantly contributing to 'mechanical wear'. Secondly, there is evidence that adipose tissue promotes inflammation and may contribute to OA pathogenesis through release of inflammatory cytokines that drive matrix degradation.

There is no doubt that mechanical factors are critically important during OA development; not only do we see markedly increased disease in individuals who have damaged their joints (either by destabilising the joint through meniscal and ligamentous injury or by direct trauma to the articular surface) but, in addition, disease is increased in those with joint malalignment, obesity and increasing age (Table 3.21).

From twin studies, hereditability in OA is calculated to be in the region of 60%. Much work has been conducted in recent years to determine the principal genes that contribute to this inherited risk. What has emerged from such studies is that OA is highly polygenic, in other words, disease is increased by polymorphisms in a number of different genes, although the relative risk attributable to each individual gene is small. Whole genome wide analysis is currently being carried out in OA to identify all polymorphic variants in this condition. Single-gene defects of major extracellular matrix components may give rise to developmental joint abnormalities which predispose to OA; these include the chondrodysplasias.

Table 3.21. Mechanical factors and osteoarthritis.

Evidence that mechanical factors contribute to osteoarthritis development
50% of individuals with mensical or cruciate ligament injuries develop osteoarthritis within 10–20 years
Intra-articular fracture increases the risk of osteoarthritis
Repetitive heavy use of a joint increases the risk of osteoarthritis, e.g 'foundry worker's elbow'
Malaligned joints develop osteoarthritis
Paralysed joints do not develop osteoarthritis

Clinical Features

OA is a syndrome characterised by joint pain and functional limitation. Typical radiographic changes are often absent in early disease, making accurate clinical assessment of the patient the key to diagnosis.

Symptoms and signs

OA may affect single, a few or multiple joints. Pain is typically worse with activity and there is usually a lack, or only a brief period (<30 minutes) of early morning stiffness. On examination an osteoarthritic joint is often tender and swollen. This swelling can be 'bony', reflecting bony expansion around the joint, or can be due to synovial or soft tissue inflammation. Figure 3.15 shows bony swelling or 'nodes' affecting the small joints of the hand. Restricted movement and joint crepitus (palpable 'crunching') may be evident on movement of the joint. Joint deformity can also be due to asymmetrical loss of articular cartilage. One such example is the varus knee deformity (bow legged) that occurs when cartilage is preferentially lost from the medial compartment of the joint. Careful clinical assessment usually allows the physician to discriminate between OA and RA (Table 3.22).

Joint distribution

OA can affect most synovial joints in the body. Commonly affected areas include the small joints of the hands and feet, the knee and the hip (Fig. 3.16). OA affecting these separate areas may represent subsets of the disease, with discrete genetic and environmental risk factors (see earlier). However, OA at one site increases an individual's risk of OA elsewhere, and some patients have 'generalised OA', i.e. OA affecting three or more sites.

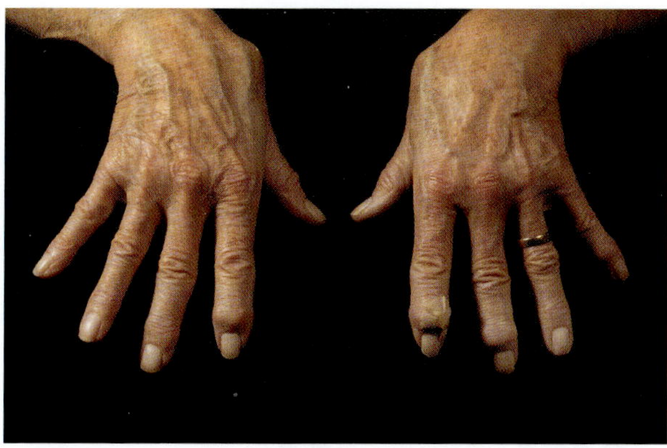

Fig. 3.15. Osteoarthritis of the hands affecting distal interphalangeal joints with development of Heberden's nodes, and the 1st carpometacarpal joints with 'squaring' at the base of the thumbs.

Table 3.22. Discriminating symptoms and signs in OA and RA.

Symptom/sign	OA	RA
Joint pain on activity	Worse	No difference/better
Metacarpophalangeal joint involvement	Rare	Frequent
Bony swelling of joint	Frequent	Not typical
Joint crepitus	Frequent	Not typical
Early morning stiffness	<30 min	>30 min
Lower back involvement	Frequent	Rare
Systemic involvement	No	Frequent
Number of joints affected	1+	Polyarticular

Hand

Hard swellings of the distal interphalangeal joints are referred to as 'Heberden's nodes' (Fig. 3.15), and swellings of the proximal interphalangeal joints are known as 'Bouchard's nodes'. These terms are only ever used in the context of OA. Patients with such 'nodes' are described as having nodal OA. The first carpometacarpal joint is also frequently affected by OA, and causes the appearance of 'squaring' of the base of the thumb (Fig. 3.15). The metacarpophalangeal joints are not typically involved in hand OA.

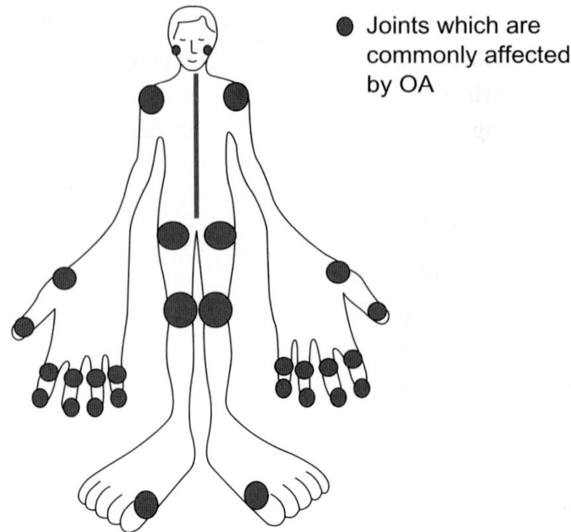

Fig. 3.16. Joint distribution in osteoarthritis. Metacarpophalangeal involvement is rare in osteoarthritis but common in rheumatoid arthritis. Conversely, distal interphalangeal joint involvement is common in osteoarthritis and is not a feature of rheumatoid arthritis.

Foot

Osteoarthritic changes in the metatarsophalangeal joints or interphalangeal joints can give rise to deformities such as hallux valgus, hallux rigidus (which can affect the 'toeing off' phase of gait) and hammer toe.

Knee

Typically the medial compartment is affected first in OA of the knee. The lateral compartment and patellofemoral compartment can also be affected, either in isolation or as part of 'tricompartmental' knee OA.

Hip

Congenital acetabular deformities predispose to hip OA. Obesity is also a potent risk factor.

Spine

The spine and sacroiliac joints can be affected by OA (in contrast to RA, where axial disease is unusual). Spinal OA is often associated with degenerative disc disease and ligamentous changes. Within this spectrum, diffuse idiopathic skeletal hyperostosis (often known by the acronym DISH) refers to florid ligamentous change and bony hypertrophy, which can cause a stiff back and fusion of vertebrae, sometimes causing diagnostic confusion with AS.

Other relevant patient history

A family history of OA should be sought because of the genetic predisposition to the disease. Occupational factors, a history of joint injury, deformity and joint surgery are also relevant. A history of diseases such as haemochromatosis and hyperparathyroidism which predispose to OA should be noted. Such cases would be considered as 'secondary OA'.

Investigations

Laboratory tests

These are normal in OA. Occasionally, patients with inflammatory symptoms and associated synovitis may have a modestly raised CRP. This can be associated with progressive 'erosive' OA seen in some patients. As yet, no biomarkers that might allow for reliable diagnosis and disease monitoring have been identified.

Imaging studies

Plain X-rays remain the most useful investigation, although may be normal in early disease. The classic features of radiographic OA are shown in Fig. 3.17 and include the following:

- Joint space narrowing
- Subchondral sclerosis
- Osteophytes
- Bone cysts

Not all of these four radiographic features must be present. Joint space narrowing on an X-ray reflects the progressive loss of volume of articular cartilage seen in the disease. Joint space narrowing is also seen in other arthropathies such as RA. In contrast, osteophytosis (formation of bony spurs around the joint) is quite specific to OA. Various grading systems, including the Kellgren–Lawrence scale allow for grading of severity of radiographic change in OA. It is now accepted practice that weight bearing X-rays must be taken of load-bearing joints such as

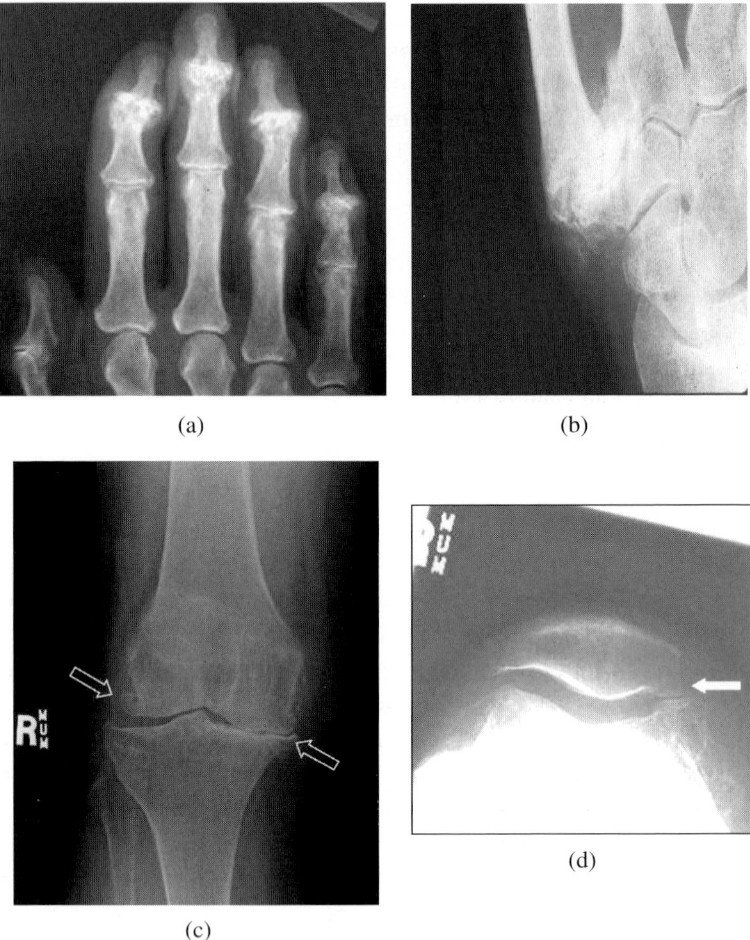

Fig. 3.17. X-Ray (a) interphalangeal joints (b) 1st carpometacarpal joint (c) AP standing knee (d) Skyline view of patellofemoral joint. X-Rays reveal all the classical features of osteoarthritis; reduction in joint space, subchondral sclerosis and osteophyte formation (open arrows). The skyline view of the knee demonstrates good preservation of the joint space except in the most medial aspect (filled arrow).

the knee, to accurately and reproducibly assess joint space narrowing. Sometimes calcification of the articular cartilage (chondrocalcinosis) due to secondary calcium pyrophosphate deposition may be seen on X-rays. This may give rise to episodic inflammatory symptoms.

Other imaging modalities, such as MRI and US, are not currently used for routine clinical assessment of OA but are being increasingly employed as research tools. MRI has a place in assessment of young patients who have isolated areas of cartilage loss amenable to surgical intervention, or those with symptoms suggestive of meniscal or ligamentous dysfunction.

Management

Despite the high prevalence of OA and its cost to society, there remains no medical therapy which can slow or reverse the disease process. The current management of patients can be thought of in three categories: supportive/lifestyle measures, medical and surgical therapies.

Supportive measures

Management should be tailored to the individual, who may have different needs at different stages of their disease. It should include an assessment of the effect of OA on their work, leisure activities, function and quality of life. Patients should be educated about the disease, and given access to appropriate information. All patients with OA should be encouraged to exercise. This may include specific manoeuvres, such as strengthening quadriceps exercises for the knee, but also regular aerobic exercise. A physiotherapist's involvement may be appropriate. If the patient is obese, weight loss should be a priority, as there is evidence that this will slow disease progression in all types of OA. Some patients may, in addition, benefit from supports and braces (particularly in the presence of deformity), specialist shoeware or wedges, and walking aids. Assessment by an occupational therapist may also be helpful, both in the patient's home and at their place of work.

Medical therapy

Not all patients will require oral analgesia. For those who do, paracetamol is the first line agent. Topical NSAID gel should be used in addition if necessary for symptomatic relief. Other drugs such as oral NSAIDs, cyclooxygenase (COX) II inhibitors or opioid drugs may be necessary. The potential risk of these therapies should always be considered in the elderly population. Topical capsaicin (an extract from chilli pepper) may also be pain-relieving when rubbed on an affected joint, although its irritant qualities are not tolerated by some patients. For flares affecting single joints, intra-articular steroid can improve symptoms for an average of six weeks. Such injections have no longer-term deleterious or joint-protecting effects in OA. Intra-articular synthetic hyaluronans and neutraceuticals such as glucosamine sulphate and chondroitin sulphate are not deemed to have a sufficient cost:benefit ratio to justify their widespread use in the treatment of large joint OA.

Surgery

For those patients who fail to respond to supportive and medical measures, surgical options should be considered (Table 3.23).

Ultimately, if the whole joint is affected and the patient is experiencing ongoing pain, stiffness, reduced function and reduced quality of life, which is refractory to non-surgical treatment, joint replacement (arthroplasty) should be considered. Arthroplasty is still a concern for active, younger patients who are likely to outlive the life of their prosthesis.

Concluding Comments

There is a huge unmet need to develop disease modifying OA drugs (DMOADs) for this highly prevalent condition. Future therapeutic strategies are likely to include specific inhibition of proteolytic activity in cartilage, e.g. aggrecanase inhibitors and promotion of intrinsic repair mechanisms. These

Table 3.23. Surgical interventions for OA.

Established procedures	Experimental procedures
Penetration of subchondral bone ('micro-fracture')	Autologous chondrocyte implantation
Cartilage plug/graft (for isolated defects)	Mesenchymal stem cell transplantation
Arthroscopy and debridement (for symptoms of true 'locking')	
Joint replacement (arthroplasty/unicompartmental/hemiarthroplasty)	
Joint fusion	
Osteotomy	
Soft tissue grafts (e.g. in carpometacarpal joint disease)	
Trapeziectomy (1st carpometacarpal joint disease)	

will necessarily require better tools for early diagnosis, determination of prognosis and disease monitoring.

3.5. Crystal Associated Disease

Crystals have a highly ordered, repetitive symmetrical molecular structure which often confers hardness and stability, making them well suited for strengthening skeletons. In humans, the hardness of bones and teeth results from compact deposition of basic calcium phosphates, predominantly partial carbonate-substituted hydroxyapatite. Such hard crystal formation in an otherwise soft body is necessarily under very tight control. Several factors influence crystal formation. Firstly, there must be a sufficient combined concentration of each of the individual chemical components (ionic product) to reach the saturation point at which crystallisation can occur. Whether crystals then form, however, critically depends on the balance of factors that either promote or inhibit crystal nucleation and growth. Many of our body tissues are supersaturated for various products but the presence of natural inhibitors prevents crystals from forming. A reduction in inhibitors and/or an increase in promoters may tip the balance in favour of crystallisation. Fibrous connective tissues seem to preferentially encourage crystal formation, possibly because highly structured collagen fibrils act as a template to encourage initial nucleation and ordered crystal growth. Crystallisation is a dynamic process and once formed, crystals can also dissolve, especially if the surrounding ionic product falls below the saturation point.

The most common crystals to deposit in and around joints are monosodium urate, calcium pyrophosphate dihydrate and basic calcium phosphate. Clinically, deposition of each of these crystals can associate with three common phenotypes:

- Asymptomatic deposition
- Acute, self limiting crystal-induced flares or attacks of florid inflammation
- Chronic damage

Crystals forming within cartilage or tendon are protected from interaction with inflammatory mediators. It is only when they escape from their site of origin ('crystal shedding') that they are exposed to inflammatory proteins and cells and cause acute flares of inflammation. Such flares often occur spontaneously, but recognised triggers to crystal shedding and acute crystal-induced inflammation include local trauma (shaking loose the crystals) and triggering of the acute phase response by inter-current illness or surgery. Mechanisms of acute crystal-induced inflammation include activation of the inflammasome, activation of soluble mediators (e.g. complement, Hageman factor) and cell membranolysis. Crystals may additionally cause tissue damage through mechanical effects. For example, large crystal concretions can cause pressure necrosis of joint tissues, and smaller deposits may act as abrasive wear particles at the cartilage surface.

3.5.1. *Gout*

Gout (from Latin *gutta*, 'a drop') is the most common inflammatory arthritis in men and older women. It is a true 'crystal deposition disease' caused by monosodium urate crystals forming in joints and other tissues. High uric acid levels are the main risk factor. Although identification of monosodium urate crystals is the gold standard for diagnosis, clinical presentation is often sufficiently distinctive to allow a confident diagnosis. Apart from septic arthritis, gout is the only arthritis in which one of the treatment aims is 'cure' — achieved by lowering uric acid levels to eliminate the crystals.

Pathogenesis and Risk Factors for Gout

In man uric acid is the end product of purine metabolism, formed by catalytic conversion by xanthine oxidase of hypoxanthine to xanthine and then xanthine to uric acid. Many animals possess the enzyme uricase (urate oxidase) which converts uric acid to highly soluble allantoin. However, in the Miocene era, humans and the great apes, as well as some birds and many reptiles lost the ability to produce uricase. In these animals the higher levels of uric acid may have conferred an evolutionary advantage because of the antioxidant properties of uric acid, but the disadvantage is that their uric acid levels may reach the saturation point for crystal formation. Humans are the only mammals to spontaneously develop gout because of the additional influence of lifestyle risk factors.

In humans approximately two-thirds of the body uric acid pool normally derives from breakdown of endogenous purines and one third from dietary intake (Fig. 3.18). About two-thirds is excreted by the kidneys, and one-third is secreted into the gut where it is converted to allantoin by colonic bacterial uricase. Renal elimination is mainly controlled by the urate transporter URAT1 (Fig. 3.19), which determines how much uric acid is reabsorbed in exchange for other ions (including lactate) following its filtration into the renal tubules.

The most important predisposing factor to gout is the degree of elevation of ionic product above the saturation point for monosodium urate crystallisation.

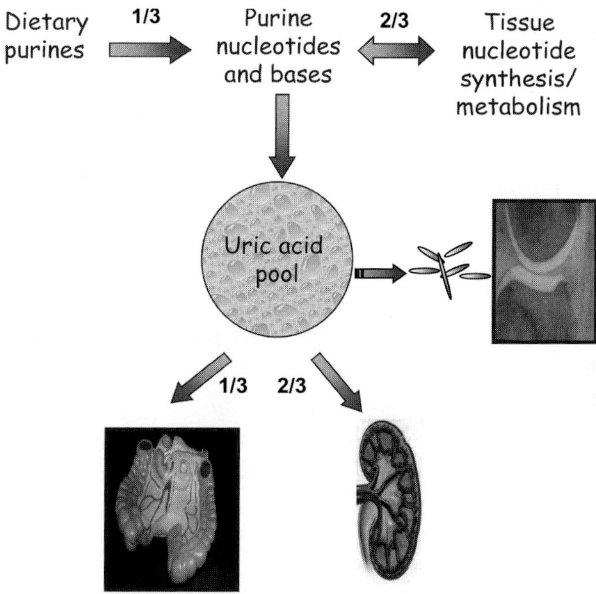

Fig. 3.18. Determinants of the uric acid pool.

Sodium concentration is tightly controlled, so uric acid is the main variable. Hyperuricaemia is defined traditionally in terms of serum uric acid levels more than two standard deviations above the mean for the population. However, the saturation point for monosodium urate crystal formation often lies within such a 'normal range', and for determination of gout risk it is best to consider the serum uric acid level that equates to the tissue saturation point, which is estimated at 360 μmol/l (or 6 mg/dl).

In addition to our shared evolutionary loss of uricase, a number of factors may result in elevation of serum uric acid.

Genetic factors

Gout shows high heritability, mainly due to an inherited renal defect in fractional uric acid excretion which impairs ability to increase excretion in response to a purine load ('under-excretors'). Certain polymorphisms of the gene encoding URAT1 have been incriminated, although the precise genetic mechanism in most 'under-excretors' remains unclear. Some gout patients are intrinsic 'overproducers' of uric acid through no identifiable cause. Inherited enzyme defects that cause

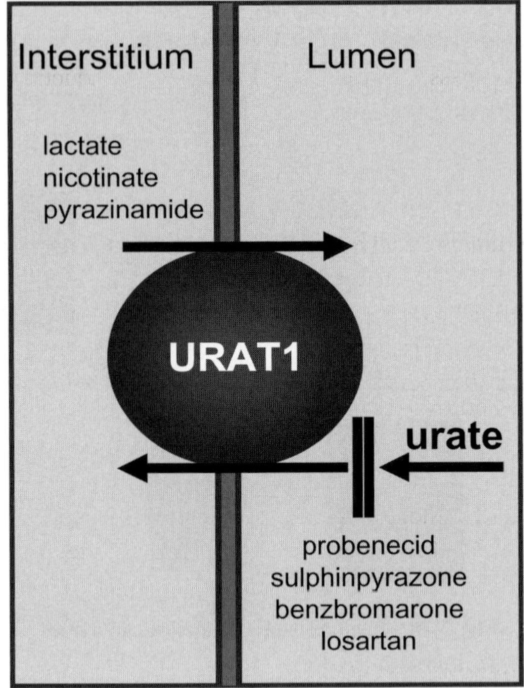

Fig. 3.19. The critical role of URAT1 in permitting re-absorption of urate in exchange for other ions such as lactate and certain drugs including pyrazinamide, following its filtration into the renal tubule lumen. Re-absorption of urate by this mechanism is blocked by 'uricosuric' drugs such as sulphinpyrazone.

uric acid overproduction are very rare, but should be suspected if gout develops under the age of 25 years, in patients presenting with uric acid renal stones, or if there is a strong family history of early onset gout.

Age and gender

Serum uric acid levels are higher in men than women at all ages. In men serum uric acid levels rise consistently from the third decade. Oestrogen increases renal uric acid excretion, so in women serum uric acid levels are low throughout reproductive years, but rise following the menopause, though not to levels seen in men. Apart from effects on serum uric acid, ageing may result in non-specific enhancement of crystal formation within fibrous connective tissues, through unknown mechanisms.

Obesity

The larger the body mass the higher the endogenous production of uric acid.

Specific dietary factors

High intakes of red meat, shellfish, fructose and alcohol are all independent risk factors for high serum uric acid and gout. In comparison, a diet high in dairy products is negatively associated with gout. With respect to alcohol, beer is the main risk for gout because of its high purine (guanosine) content. High spirit intake is also a risk but wine consumption is neutral. High intakes of coffee and vitamin C are negatively associated, due in part to their uricosuric effects mediated via URAT1.

Metabolic syndrome

Hyperuricaemia is an integral feature of metabolic syndrome. Hypertension, insulin resistance and hyperlipidaemia all independently reduce the efficiency of renal urate clearance.

Chronic renal impairment and drugs

Chronic renal impairment from any cause may reduce efficiency of renal urate clearance. Drugs that are either nephrotoxic or which act via URAT1 to reduce uric acid excretion may also elevate serum uric acid. The most important drugs in terms of attributable risk for gout are diuretics, specifically thiazides and loop diuretics (bumetanide causes less elevation of serum uric acid than furosemide). Ciclosporin, pyrazinamide and low (but not high) doses of aspirin may also cause modest elevation of serum uric acid. Gout that follows chronic renal disease or diuretic intake is a form of 'secondary gout'.

Osteoarthritis

Osteoarthritic cartilage encourages monosodium urate crystal formation via alteration in the balance of promotors and inhibitors of crystallisation. Interestingly there is a strong negative association between RA and gout, suggesting that it is OA rather than 'joint disease' that promotes crystallisation.

Epidemiology

The crude unadjusted prevalence of gout varies between populations but in the UK and Europe it occurs in 1.4% of adults, with a strong male predominance.

Prevalence increases with age, reaching a maximum of 7% in men aged over 75 years. Primary gout is more prevalent than secondary gout. Primary gout is extremely rare in pre-menopausal women because of their lower serum uric acid but after the menopause becomes more common with increasing age. In the past few decades there has been an increase in incidence and prevalence of primary gout in many countries including the UK and the United States. This increase has been mainly in men and in older age groups, and is attributed largely to (1) the increased prevalence of obesity and metabolic syndrome and (2) increasing longevity and an increased prevalence of OA.

Clinical Features

Acute gout

This usually affects a single distal joint. The first metatarsophalangeal joint is the first site affected in over 50% of cases of primary gout. Involvement of this joint is highly characteristic of gout and is called 'podagra' (literally 'seizing the foot') (Fig. 3.20). Other common sites are the mid-foot, ankle and knee, and then wrists,

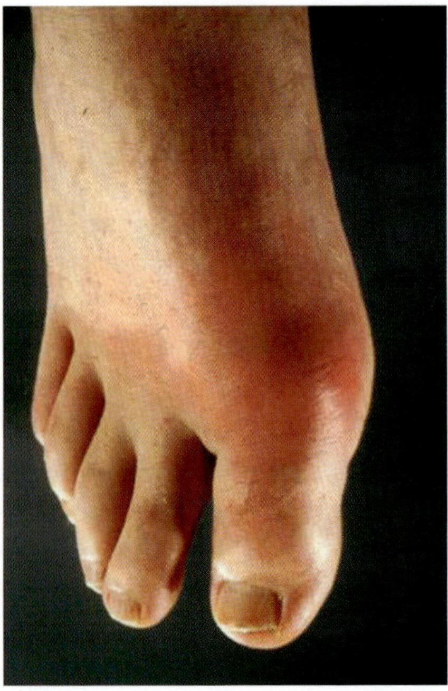

Fig. 3.20. An acute attack of gout involving the 1st metatarsophalangeal joint (podagra).

Table 3.24. Features of acute gout.

Clinical features of acute gout
Extremely rapid onset, reaching maximum severity within a few hours
Very severe pain, often described as the 'worst pain ever experienced'
Exquisite tenderness and hyperalgesia, the patient is unable to bear clothing or bed sheets touching the joint
Marked swelling, often with overlying red, shiny skin
Self limiting, with complete return to normality, usually over four to ten days but inevitably within two to three weeks

elbows and small joints of hands. Shoulders, hips and axial joints are hardly ever involved. The clinical presentation is usually characterised by rapid onset of severe pain, tenderness and swelling, with each episode of joint inflammation resolving spontaneously (Table 3.24).

Examination usually reveals signs of florid synovitis (capsular swelling, marked tenderness, increased local heat), adjacent peri-articular swelling and overlying erythema. As the attack subsides, the skin that was reddened often shows desquamation.

Attacks can affect two or more joints simultaneously, though polyarticular attacks are rare. When the knee or several joints are affected, especially in the elderly, the patient may be febrile and feel unwell or even confused.

Gout may also cause acute self-limiting bursitis, tenosynovitis or cellulitis. These have the same characteristics as joint flares, with very rapid onset, severe pain, florid inflammation and overlying erythema. Many patients also describe milder joint or peri-articular flares lasting only several hours.

The main differential diagnosis is synovitis due to another crystal (mainly calcium pyrophosphate dihydrate in the case of joints, basic calcium phosphate in the case of bursitis or peri-articular features) or acute bacterial arthritis or cellulitis. Septic arthritis is usually sub-acute and progresses in severity from day to day until treated. Sepsis and gout may coexist, so confirmation of gout does not exclude sepsis. Other causes of rapidly evolving inflammation are PsA (this can cause synovitis plus adjacent peri-articular inflammation, including dactylitis of the big toe), and palindromic rheumatism.

Recurrent and chronic tophaceous gout

After the first acute attack the patient is at risk of subsequent flares, although these may not occur for some months or years, and occasionally not at all (especially if presenting late in life). However, most people with primary gout suffer a second attack within one year, and subsequently the 'intercritical' periods between attacks get shorter. Apart from increased frequency, later attacks tend to be more severe and to involve new joints. The usual pattern of spread is to move from initial involvement of joints around the foot and ankle to the knee, and then to the upper limb with involvement of elbows, wrists and small hand joints.

Eventually, continuing monosodium urate crystal deposition may cause joint damage with more persistent pain, stiffness and impaired function. The time this takes to develop after the first attack is very variable but usually slow (one to two decades), but the higher the serum uric acid the more rapid and more extensive the monosodium urate deposits and tissue damage. Joints most commonly damaged are the same as those affected by acute attacks; the first metatarsophalangeal joint, mid-feet, ankles, finger joints, wrists and elbows. There may be additional chronic tenosynovitis and bursitis (most commonly olecranon bursitis). Examination may show joint restriction, crepitus, variable synovitis and sometimes severe deformity, especially of feet and hands (Figs. 3.21 and 3.22). Asymmetry of joint damage is characteristic.

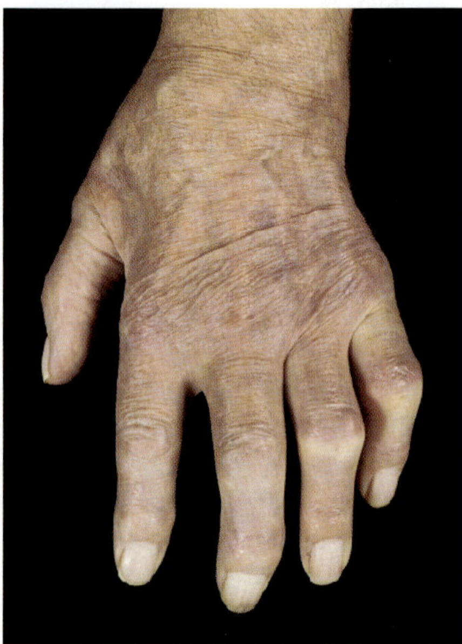

Fig. 3.21. Chronic gout with fixed flexion and radial deviation of interphalangeal joints, volar subluxation at the ring and little finger metacarpophalangeal joints, and crepitus and reduced movement of the radiocarpal joint.

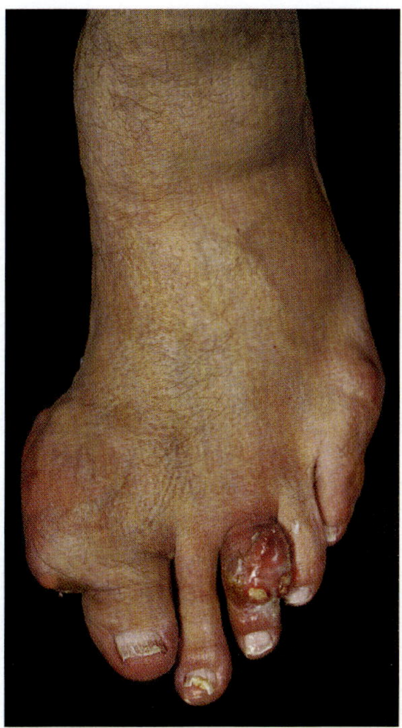

Fig. 3.22. Chronic gout with involvement of the ankle, mid-foot, and several metatarsophalangeal joints. There is synovial swelling at the ankle, loss of normal arches, and multiple eccentric tophi, including a very large tophus medial to the big toe and a discharging tophus over the middle toe.

Large concretions of monosodium urate crystals can produce irregular firm-hard nodules called 'tophi' (Latin for 'stones') (Figs. 3.22 and 3.23). These may be clinically evident at almost any site but particularly target the usual sites for nodules: extensor surfaces of fingers, hands, forearm, elbows and Achilles tendons. Occasionally the helix of the ear may be involved, although chondromalacia chronicus helicis is a more common cause of ear nodules. The whiteness of the monosodium urate crystals may be evident beneath the skin, allowing distinction from rheumatoid nodules. Tophi may ulcerate and discharge white, gritty toothpaste-like material with local inflammation. The term 'chronic tophaceous gout' is used when the patient has chronic symptoms and clinically evident tophi. However, imaging studies have confirmed common occurrence of subclinical 'microtophi' in many patients at initial presentation and in some hyperuricaemic people prior to any gout symptoms.

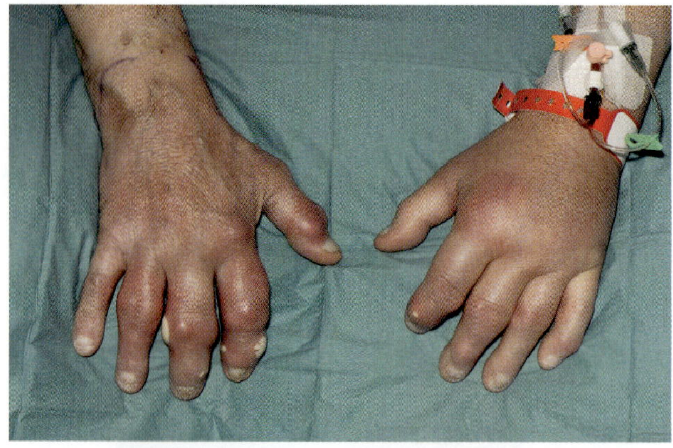

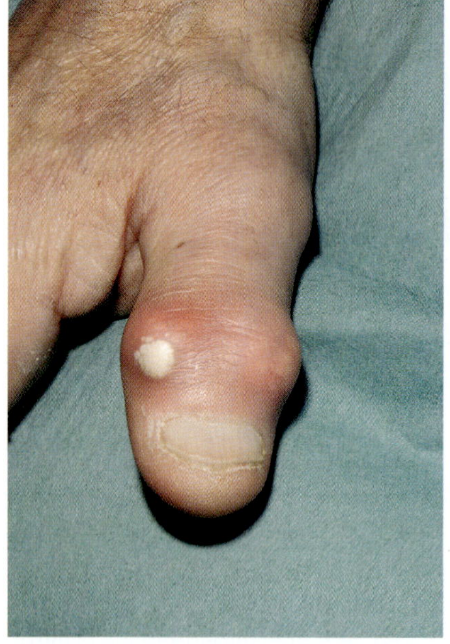

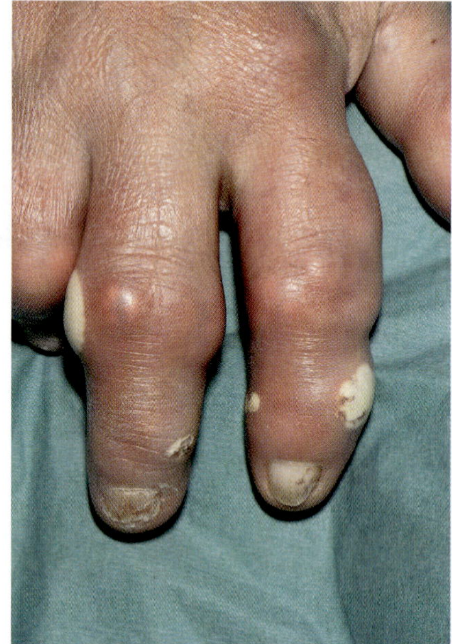

Fig. 3.23. Tophaceous gout. Severe inflammatory arthritis with multiple tophi in an individual with tophaceous gout.

Atypical presentations

Compared to the normal evolution of primary gout described above, some patients with secondary gout, and a minority with primary gout, may present with atypical features (Table 3.25).

Table 3.25. Presentation of atypical gout.

Atypical gout
Initial presentation with upper rather than lower limb symptoms
Presentation with chronic symptoms and tophi with no preceding acute attacks
Rapid development of tophi within months rather than years
Inflammatory distal arthritis with no features distinctive of crystals

One atypical phenotype is the older woman with nodal hand OA who develops painful, sometimes discharging tophi in their osteoarthritic finger joints as a result of chronic diuretic therapy. Because gout can present in protean ways, it is recommended that any patient with unexplained chronic inflammatory arthritis should undergo joint aspiration and examination for monosodium urate crystals.

Renal and urinary tract manifestations

About 10% of patients with primary gout suffer renal colic from nephrolithiasis. The incidence is higher in hot climates and is favoured by purine overproduction, uricosuric drugs, defects in tubular re-absorption of uric acid, dehydration and lowering of urine pH. Although gout patients are at increased risk of uric acid stones they predominantly develop the more usual calcium oxalate stones.

Patients with severe, untreated chronic tophaceous gout are at risk of progressive renal disease caused in part by deposition of monosodium urate crystals in the interstitium of the medulla and pyramids and consequent chronic inflammation with giant cell reaction, fibrosis and glomerulosclerosis. Secondary pyelonephritis is a common complicating factor.

Investigations

Laboratory tests

The 'gold standard' diagnosis of gout is demonstration of monosodium urate crystals in synovial fluid from a joint or bursa, or in a tophus aspirate. Synovial fluid during an acute attack has inflammatory characteristics; high volume, low viscosity and gross turbidity due to a very high cell count (>90% neutrophils). Synovial fluid from chronic gouty joints is variable but occasionally is white due to plentiful monosodium urate crystals. During intercritical periods aspiration of an asymptomatic first metatarsophalangeal joint or knee may still permit crystal identification, even if that joint has never suffered an acute attack. Under compensated

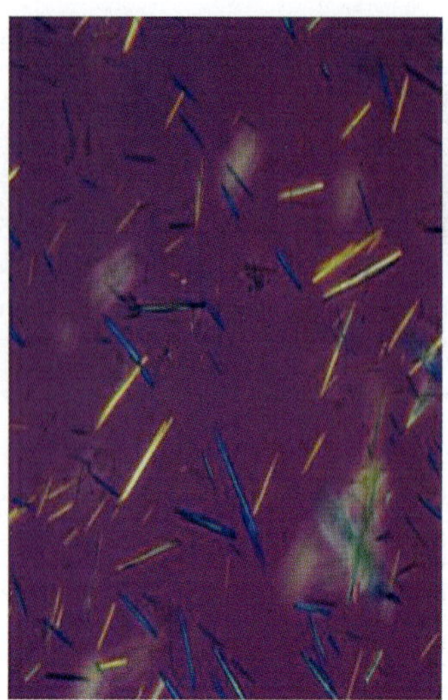

Fig. 3.24. Numerous needle-shaped monosodium urate crystals with bright birefringence (synovial fluid viewed under compensated polarised light microscopy with 400x magnification).

polarised light microscopy monosodium crystals are long and needle-shaped and show a strong light intensity and a negative sign of birefringence (Fig. 3.24).

High serum uric acid is usually present but does not confirm gout. Equally, a normal or low serum uric acid does not exclude gout, especially during an attack (serum uric acid falls as part of the acute phase reaction). Therefore serum uric acid is best assessed during the intercritical period, and at this time a urinary uric acid:creatinine ratio can be done to determine under-excretor or over-producer status. If over-production is suggested, a 24-hour urinary uric acid excretion should be done together with a FBC and ESR to screen for chronic myeloproliferative disease as a cause of hyperuricaemia and gout. Assessment of renal function and investigation for metabolic syndrome (hypertension, blood glucose, serum lipid profile) should be undertaken. During an attack a marked acute phase response (elevated CRP, neutrophilia) is usual, and the ESR and CRP are often modestly raised in chronic tophaceous gout.

Imaging studies

Radiographs of affected joints are often normal in early gout, but changes of OA (joint space narrowing, sclerosis, cysts, osteophyte) may develop in affected

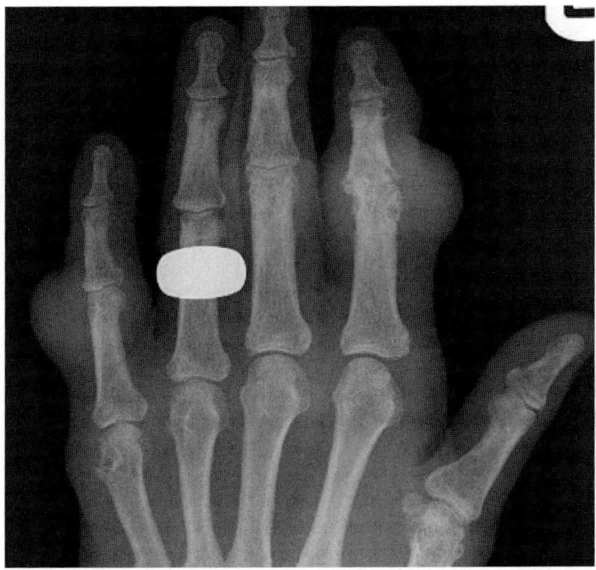

Fig. 3.25. Hand radiograph showing eccentric soft tissue swellings, "punched-out" cystic lesions (some extracapsular) and joint space narrowing in worst affected joints.

joints with time or be present as a predisposing factor. Cortical 'erosions', representing pressure defects caused by tophi, are a less common but more specific feature, appearing as para-articular 'punched-out' defects with well-defined borders and usually well-retained bone density. Eccentric soft tissue swellings from large tophi may also be evident (Figs. 3.25 and 3.26). In severe late tophaceous gout changes may be hard to distinguish from rheumatoid or other forms of inflammatory polyarthritis.

Management

Considerations relating to treatment of the acute attack can be separated from those that address modifiable risk factors and long-term urate-lowering therapy to effect "cure" (Table 3.26).

The acute attack

Application of an ice-pack is a simple, safe way of relieving pain that should be advised for every patient. A fast acting oral NSAID (e.g. naproxen, diclofenac,

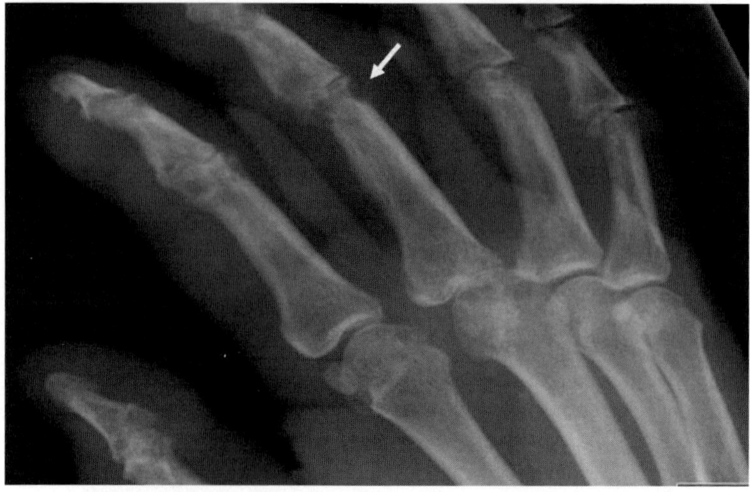

Fig. 3.26. Radiological appearances of gout. Para-articular erosions are evident particularly at the middle finger PIP joint (arrow).

Table 3.26. Drugs used in management of gout.

Drugs used in acute gout	Drugs used in long term management of gout
Non-steroidal anti-inflammatory drugs	Xanthine oxidase inhibitors (allopurinol, febuxostat)
Colchicine	Uricosuric agents (probenicid, sulphinpyrazone, benzbromarone)
Corticosteroids (intra-articular, intra-muscular, oral)	

indomethacin) or selective COX-2 inhibitor (e.g. etoricoxib) is the usual prescribed treatment; co-presciption of a proton pump inhibitor as prophylaxis against upper gastrointestinal toxicity is advised. These drugs are often contraindicated in older patients and in those with secondary gout due to renal impairment. Oral colchicine is an alternative agent that can give effective pain relief in acute attacks. It is an alkaloid derived from the autumn crocus and inhibits neutrophil activation. Dose regimens of 0.5 mg two or three times daily are generally recommended in order to avoid the severe gastrointestinal toxicity (diarrhoea, nausea) that often accompanies higher traditional doses. Where possible, joint aspiration gives instant relief by reducing the extreme intracapsular

Table 3.27. Indications for urate lowering therapy.

Indications for urate lowering therapy
Recurrent acute attacks
Presence of tophi
Radiographic evidence of bone or joint disease
Associated nephrolithiasis or renal disease
Gout with very high serum uric acid

pressure, and when combined with intra-articular steroid injection to prevent synovial fluid re-accumulation, is a very safe local treatment that often abbreviates the attack. Intramuscular corticosteroid is occasionally required for patients with severe upset from oligo- or polyarticuar attacks in whom both NSAIDs and colchicine are contraindicated.

Long-term management

As always, patient education concerning the nature of gout and treatment options are central to management. Modifiable risk factors should be addressed if possible. For example, weight reduction if overweight, reduction of excess beer consumption and stopping diuretics if possible. The patient should be advised to avoid high intake of specific dietary factors that elevate serum uric acid (e.g. seafood, red meat, offal) and to have a balanced diet with good intake of vitamin C, but there is no need for a highly restrictive or unpalatable diet.

In addition to lifestyle advice, many patients require urate lowering therapy. The indications for this are listed in Table 3.27.

The aim of urate lowering therapy is to reduce the serum uric acid well below the saturation point for monosodium urate crystal formation (360 μmol/l or 6 mg/dl), thereby preventing further crystal formation and encouraging dissolution of existing crystals. The lower the serum uric acid is below this point, the faster the tophus reduction and the elimination of existing crystals and the cessation of further flares. Because rapid lowering of serum uric acid may trigger acute attacks, the patient should be warned of this and told to continue treatment even if an attack occurs. In addition, flare prophylaxis with either low-dose colchicine (0.5 mg twice daily) or a NSAID is advisable for the first three to six months of urate lowering therapy. Once the therapeutic target is achieved, the serum uric acid should be checked infrequently to ensure that it is still sufficiently low. Urate lowering therapy is often continued indefinitely, unless successful modification of risk factors alone can sufficiently lower serum uric acid to maintain 'cure'.

The usual first line urate lowering therapy is allopurinol. This is a purine, non-specific inhibitor of xanthine oxidase that reduces conversion of xanthine and hypoxanthine to uric acid, thus reducing endogenous uric acid production. It is appropriate for both primary and secondary gout. The usual starting dose is 100 mg daily. This is then increased in 100 mg increments every two to four weeks, titrated against repeat serum uric acid levels, until the therapeutic target (<360 μmol/l) is achieved, up to a maximum dose of 900 mg daily. Such a slowly titrated regimen reduces the likelihood of triggering acute attacks and the requirement for flare prophylaxis. In patients with renal impairment, a lower starting dose (50 mg), smaller incremental increases (50 mg) and lower maximum dose are advised because the active metabolite of allopurinol (oxypurinol) is excreted via the kidney. Some people (<10%) are unable to tolerate allopurinol due to gastrointestinal upset or skin rash. Severe toxicity with fever, vasculitic rashes, hepatitis and multiple organ failure ('allopurinol hypersensitivity syndrome') is very rare and almost confined to patients with renal impairment within the first three months of treatment. Allopurinol has interactions with azathioprine, 6-mercaptopurine and warfarin.

Febuxostat is a new urate lowering therapy that is a non-purine, specific inhibitor of xanthine oxidase. It undergoes hepatic metabolism so does not require dose reduction in patients with renal impairment. It is given initially at 80 mg daily, increasing to 120 mg daily if required. Both doses are effective at reducing serum uric acid so require concomitant flare prophylaxis for six months. Febuxostat is recommended as second line urate lowering therapy in patients who cannot tolerate allopurinol or in whom allopurinol is contraindicated.

Probenecid and sulphinpyrazone are uricosuric drugs that increase renal uric acid excretion. Both are less efficient than the xanthine oxidase inhibitors at reducing serum uric acid. They require maintenance of a high urine flow to avoid uric acid crystallisation in renal tubules and are contraindicated in patients with renal impairment or urolithiasis, so are used only infrequently. In contrast, benzbromarone (50–200 mg daily) is highly efficient at reducing serum uric acid and is the only uricosuric that is effective and safe in patients with mild to moderate renal impairment. However, rarely benzbromarone may cause hepatotoxicity and has limited availability in most countries. The antihypertensive losartan and the lipid lowering agent fenofibrate both have uricosuric actions which can be an added advantage in gout patients requiring treatment for such comorbidity.

3.5.2. *Calcium Pyrophosphate Crystal Deposition*

Calcium pyrophosphate (CPP) crystal deposition (CPPD) is the usual cause of joint cartilage calcification or chondrocalcinosis. It may occur alone, or with

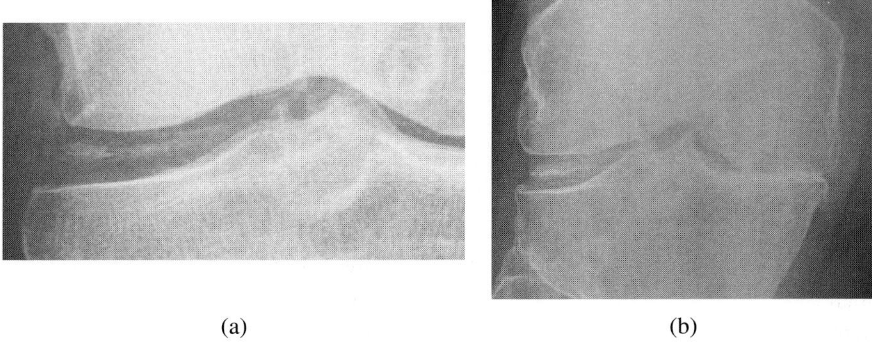

(a) (b)

Fig. 3.27. Radiographic chondrocalcinosis at the knee occurring (a) as an isolated finding or (b) in association with structural changes of osteoarthritis.

structural changes of OA (Fig. 3.27). Most cases are sporadic, but rare familial chondrocalcinosis and associations with diseases that increase pyrophosphate levels both occur. Radiographic chondrocalcinosis is rare below the age of 55 years, but the prevalence increases to 30–60% in those over the age of 85 years. Men and women are equally affected. The knee is the most common joint involved, followed by the wrist (triangular fibrocartilage) and pelvis (symphysis pubis). Although often asymptomatic, CPP crystals can cause acute self-limiting synovitis (acute CPP crystal arthritis previously termed 'pseudogout').

Pathogenesis

Inorganic pyrophosphate (PPi) is abundant in nucleoside triphosphates such as ATP and is produced in most biosynthetic reactions. PPi is not absorbed from the gut so all PPi is made endogenously. Most extracellular PPi is produced by breakdown of ATP by the ectoenzyme PC1 (plasma cell glycoprotein 1). PPi is then complexed with magnesium and broken down to orthophosphate by pyrophosphatases, principally alkaline phosphatase. PPi avidly adsorbs to the surface of basic calcium phosphate and has a key role in regulating calcification of bones and teeth, with lower PPi concentrations stimulating, but higher concentrations inhibiting, basic calcium phosphate crystal formation. PPi inhibits basic calcium phosphate crystallisation in urine and saliva as well as cartilage.

Calcium pyrophosphate crystals can form when the ionic product of calcium and PPi exceeds the saturation point for crystal formation. CPPD is

Table 3.28. Risk factors for calcium pyrophosphate crystal deposition.

Factors promoting crystal deposition
Ageing
Osteoarthritis
Genetic factors including mutations in ANKH gene
Metabolic diseases including haemochromatosis and hyperparathyroidism

almost confined to joint fibro- and hyaline cartilage, although shedding from cartilage can result in secondary uptake in synovium and joint capsule. The main risk factors for CPPD are shown in Table 3.28.

These factors affect levels of PPi and/or alter the balance of tissue promoters/ inhibitors of crystal formation.

Clinical Features

Acute CPP crystal arthritis (previously termed 'pseudogout')

This is a common cause of acute monoarthritis in older people. The knee is the most commonly affected joint, followed by the wrist, shoulder, ankle and elbow. It may be the first presentation of disease in that joint or occur on a background of chronic symptomatic OA. The typical attack closely resembles acute gout and develops very rapidly, with severe pain, stiffness and swelling, maximal within 6–24 hours of onset. Examination reveals a very tender joint with signs of synovitis and often overlying erythema. Especially with knee involvement, the patient may have a fever and appear confused and unwell. The attack is self-limiting but may take two to three weeks to resolve.

The main differential diagnosis is gout or sepsis. Gout is less likely in patients over the age of 65 without a prior history of primary gout or chronic diuretic therapy and seldom involves the knee in a first attack. Sepsis is usually sub-acute and progressive, but often needs to be considered, especially when the attack has been triggered by an intercurrent infection or surgery. As with gout, pseudogout can coexist with sepsis.

Osteoarthritis with CPPD

Most patients with OA and CPPD are older women. The knee is the commonest joint to be affected, followed by wrists, shoulders, elbows, hips and midtarsals. The second and third metacarpophalangeal joints are often targeted in the hand. Symptoms are similar to OA, with 'mechanical' pain (worse on use, relieved by rest, variable or intermittent), only mild early morning and inactivity stiffness, and functional restriction. Acute attacks may be superimposed on these chronic symptoms. Examination may reveal signs of OA, specifically bony swelling, crepitus, restriction and deformity. Effusion and synovial thickening are variable and usually most evident at knees and wrists. Examination may reveal more widespread signs of generalised OA.

Although inflammatory features are occasionally sufficient to suggest RA ('chronic CPP crystal inflammatory arthritis') OA with CPPD targets large rather than small and medium-sized joints and tenosynovitis and extra-articular involvement are absent. Rarely, severe damage and instability of knees or shoulders may suggest a neuropathic joint, but this can be excluded by a normal neurological examination.

Incidental finding

As with OA, asymptomatic X-ray features of chondrocalcinosis are a common incidental finding in older people. Only a thorough history and examination can determine the relevance of such findings to symptom causation.

Investigations

As with acute gout, aspirated synovial fluid in acute CPP crystal arthritis is inflammatory and occasionally uniformly blood-stained. The gold standard for diagnosis is demonstration of synovial fluid CPP crystals by compensated polarised light microscopy. CPP crystals are smaller, rhomboid or rod-shaped, and usually less numerous than monosodium urate crystals, and have weak light intensity and positive birefringence (Fig. 3.28). Gram stain and culture of synovial fluid will exclude sepsis. CPP crystals are also identified in the less inflamed fluids aspirated from OA with CPPD.

Radiographs may show chondrocalcinosis in fibro-cartilage and/or hyaline cartilage with or without associated structural changes of OA (Fig. 3.27). Chondrocalcinosis is not always evident, especially in joints with cartilage loss, and absence of chondrocalcinosis does not exclude the diagnosis. Synovial and capsular calcification are occasional accompaniments.

Screening for metabolic predisposition (serum ferritin, calcium, alkaline phosphatase, magnesium) should be undertaken if patients are under the age of

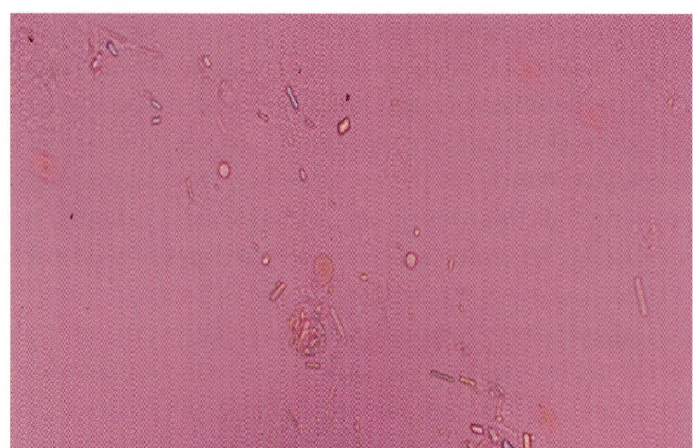

Fig. 3.28. Rhomboid, rod-shaped calcium pyrophosphate crystals showing weak birefringence (synovial fluid viewed under compensated polarised light microscopy with 400x magnification).

55 years, have florid polyarticular chondrocalcinosis or have additional clinical or radiographic features of predisposing disease.

Management

Treatment options for acute CPP crystal arthritis are the same as for acute gout, but because of the late age of presentation, ice packs plus aspiration and injection of corticosteroid are the usual preferred treatments. Early active mobilisation is also important in this age group. For chronic arthritis (OA with CPPD or chronic CPP crystal inflammatory arthritis) the management is the same as for OA.

3.5.3. *Basic Calcium Phosphate Deposition*

Basic calcium phosphate (apatite) deposition is the usual cause of metastatic calcification in which a high ionic product of calcium and orthophosphate results in calcification in normal tissues (e.g. chronic renal dialysis, hyperparathyroidism, vitamin D intoxication). Basic calcium phosphate deposition is also the usual cause of dystrophic calcification which results from alterations in tissue promotors and inhibitors of calcification, usually secondary to chronic inflammation and fibrosis (e.g. in fibrotic lung parenchyma, scarred lymph nodes, atherosclerotic blood vessels). Dystrophic calcification may also occur in musculoskeletal tissues, for example tendons (calcific periarthritis), hyaline cartilage (in association with OA) and in subcutaneous tissue and muscle (calcinosis due mainly to connective tissue diseases). In most situations such calcification is of no consequence, but basic calcium phosphate crystals have inflammatory potential and in some situations may associate with clinical problems. The crystals are too small to be viewed by light microscopy although their aggregated spherulites can be seen using non-specific calcium stains. For clinical purposes presumptive diagnosis is often based on radiographic calcification alone.

Calcific Periarthritis

Population screening has shown that up to 7% of adults aged 20–40 years have radiographic calcification of one or both supraspinatus tendons. This mainly occurs proximal to the humeral attachment where the tendon is compromised by low oxygen tension and most commonly develops degenerative change. Such calcification remains occult provided the basic calcium phosphate crystals remain within the tendon. However, crystal shedding from the tendon can trigger severe acute inflammation of the subacromial and subdeltoid bursa. The acute episode may occur spontaneously or follow local trauma. Within just a few hours, shoulder pain and tenderness are extreme and the area appears swollen and hot. Pain severity usually plateaus within the first 48 hours and then resolves spontaneously over one to three weeks.

At the start of the attack the calcification is usually evident on radiographs, but this may disperse and disappear over several weeks if crystal shedding is complete. Aspiration of the subacromial or subdeltoid bursa may reveal inflammatory, often white, fluid containing many calcium-staining aggregates (only seen with a calcium stain such as alizarin red). Calcific periarthritis may associate with renal failure, hyperparathyroidism or hypophosphatasia, but serum creatinine, calcium and alkaline phosphatase are normal in most cases. The CRP is often elevated during the episode.

Oral analgesics, NSAIDs or colchicine may give some pain relief but aspiration and injection of corticosteroid provide greater benefit and often abbreviate the attack. Exceptionally large deposits may cause chronic mechanical blocking and painful impingement on abduction and require surgical removal. Calcific periarthritis may also affect other periarticular sites, such as the greater trochanter of the hip, or around the wrists, hands and feet. Clinical features, investigation and management are the same as for the shoulder.

Osteoarthritis and Basic Calcium Phosphate Crystal Deposition

If specifically sought, basic calcium phosphate aggregates are often identified in synovial fluid from knees with OA, either alone or with CPP crystals ('mixed crystal deposition'). Whether they cause inflammation or contribute to joint damage is unclear. However, very high synovial fluid concentrations of basic calcium phosphate have been associated with an uncommon OA phenotype called 'apatite-associated destructive OA', representing the worst end of the spectrum of OA (Table 3.29 and Fig. 3.29).

Table 3.29. Apatite-associated destructive osteoarthritis.

Features of apatite-associated destructive osteoarthritis
Age >75 years
Involvement of hips, knees or shoulders
Rapid clinical and radiological progression over few months
Development of instability and large cool effusions of knees and shoulders
Markedly atrophic radiographic changes with severe attrition of cartilage and bone but minimal osteophytosis

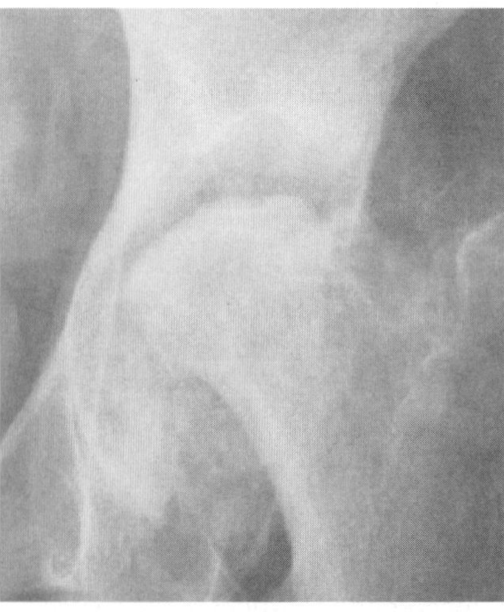

Fig. 3.29. Hip radiograph showing marked loss of bone with no osteophytes. Although the joint space is widened in this supine view there is complete loss of cartilage and a weight-bearing view showed 'bone on bone'.

The differential diagnosis of such rapidly destructive arthropathy is end-stage avascular necrosis, chronic sepsis or neuropathic joint. Treatment is the same as for OA, but most patients quickly come to joint replacement. It is thought that the basic calcium phosphate aggregates, rather than being causal pathogenic agents, are a marker of the speed of joint damage and originate largely from sub-chondral bone damage.

3.6. Bacterial Infection and Arthritis

3.6.1. *Septic Arthritis*

Septic arthritis is an important diagnosis to consider in the assessment of an individual with arthritis. Acute bacterial infection can rapidly destroy articular cartilage and cause significant morbidity and even mortality. Irreversible loss of joint function may develop in up to half of all patients if management is delayed. The incidence of bacterial arthritis has been reported as up to 10 per 100,000 per annum in the normal population. This is at least three times as high in patients with RA and joint prostheses. Despite the development of anti-microbial agents the mortality rate has not changed, with poor outcome being associated with age over 65 years, diabetes mellitus, delayed diagnosis, open surgical drainage and a Gram-positive infection other than *Staphylococcus aureus*.

Prosthetic implants are now frequently used by orthopaedic surgeons. Despite improvements in surgical techniques and routine prophylactic antibiotics, prosthetic joint implantation and replacement has remained the single most common cause of joint infections. The prevalence of infection after total knee or hip arthroplasty is estimated to be approximately 1–2%.

Aetiological Agents

The bacterial pathogens in joint and bone infections depend on the type and route of infection and host factors. The infection may be acute or chronic, haematogenous or contiguous and may vary in locality. The important host factors are the age of the patient, presence of co-morbid disease and immunosuppressive therapies.

S. aureus is the most common pathogen and accounts for 40–70% of all cases. After *S. aureus*, *Streptococcus* species are the next most commonly isolated bacteria from adult patients with septic arthritis. Gram negative bacilli are found in intravenous drug users and at the extremes of age. Anaerobic bacteria are usually the pathogens in diabetic patients and patients with joint prostheses.

Historically, *Haemophilus influenzae* was a common pathogen in septic arthritis in children. However, in response to the *H. influenzae* type b vaccination its incidence is falling. Many other micro-organisms are found in orthopaedic infections. In the context of immunocompromised patients, *Mycoplasma* species, *Ureaplasma* species and *Mycobacteria* species are opportunistic pathogens of septic arthritis.

The predominant pathogens involved in prosthetic joint infections are low-virulence bacteria (e.g. coagulase-negative staphylococci). Such bacteria produce a biofilm that protects them from anti-microbial agents as well as the humoral and cellular immune systems of the host. Antibiotic resistance found in prosthetic joint infections with methicillin-resistant *S. aureus* (MRSA), coagulase-negative staphylococci and *Enterococcus faecium* creates additional challenges in joint infection management.

Pathogenesis

In order to develop septic arthritis, bacteria must reach the synovial membrane. There are several mechanisms for this (Fig. 3.30). Haematogenous seeding, involving bacteria travelling to the synovium from a distant site of infection (e.g. abscesses, dental infections, skin wounds, respiratory tract and urinary infections and rarely endocarditis) is the most common route of infection. Whatever the route, bacteria reach the well-vascularised synovial membrane which is particularly susceptible to microbial invasion. An inflammatory reaction begins. A pro-inflammatory response is created by migrating leukocytes. Synovial membrane proliferation ensues and blood flow increases. Bacteria, inflammatory cells and proteins move into the joint cavity. There, phagocytes may try to engulf and kill the bacteria. The joint becomes swollen and the joint pressure rises and can cause cartilage damage. The enzymes elastase and collagenase are released from polymorphonuclear and synovial cells and degrade the cartilage. A potent inflammatory response may also arise from bacterial superantigens that behave in a similar manner to the staphylococcal toxins in toxic shock syndrome. The tissue changes can cause irreversible joint damage within a few days.

There is an increased risk of developing septic arthritis in patients at the extremes of age and in pre-existing arthritis, particularly RA, but also OA and gout. Systemic diseases and medications that cause immunosuppression are important risk factors. These include diabetes mellitus, alcohol and intravenous drug abuse, liver cirrhosis, chronic haemodialysis, cancer and corticosteroids.

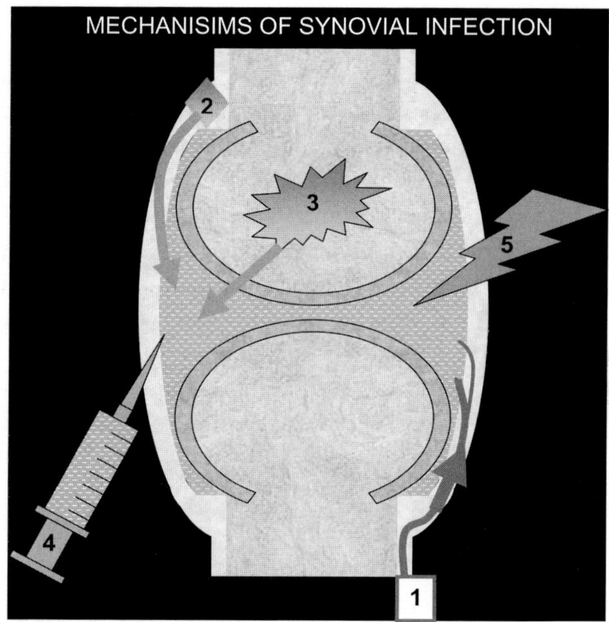

Fig. 3.30. Mechanisms of synovial infection. Pathogens may enter the joint (1) via the blood stream (2) from local infection via lymphatics (3) from osteomyelitic bone (4) by iatrogenic means or (5) from penetrating trauma or surgery.

Clinical Features

Patients with septic arthritis have different clinical features depending on their age. Infants have a predominance of systemic illness over local arthritis. As children increase in age they behave more like adults and develop more local signs. Adult patients with bacterial arthritis typically present with a short history of a hot, swollen and tender joint(s) with restriction of movement. The pain is often severe and the patient may not be able to weight bear. The joint may be erythematous and hot with an effusion. The lower limb joints are most frequently involved with the knee accounting for more than half of cases. Ankles, wrists and hips are also commonly infected.

Investigations

Any patient who presents with acute monoarticular arthritis, especially in the context of underlying joint disease, should be suspected of having a bacterial arthritis and investigated accordingly.

Laboratory tests

Blood cultures are positive in half of all cases and should be obtained in any patient with suspected bacterial arthritis. Synovial fluid should be viewed under direct microscopy with Gram staining and cultured prior to starting antibiotics. Multiple joint aspirations increase the sensitivity and specificity of diagnosing septic arthritis. The diagnosis of septic arthritis must still be considered even in the absence of identifying a microorganism on Gram stain or synovial fluid culture. In this situation patients with probable septic arthritis should be treated empirically to avoid the morbidity and mortality associated with treatment delay.

Elevation of white cell count, CRP and ESR are common but not specific to septic arthritis. They are useful for monitoring response to treatment. Renal and hepatic functions should also be assessed as multiple organ failure carries a poor prognosis in septic arthritis.

Imaging studies

Plain radiography should be requested initially. Changes on plain radiographs suggest that an infection has been present for more than two weeks. Ultrasonography assists in identifying fluid collections in a joint or in the extra-articular soft tissues. CT scanning can identify adjacent lesions such as a sequestrum and MRI can also be used to help rule out a secondary osteomyelitis.

Echocardiography

Bacterial arthritis may be the first sign of infective endocarditis. Endocarditis should be suspected in septic arthritis cases caused by *S. aureus*, enterococci or streptococci in patients without an obvious predisposing cause. Echocardiography should be used to identify cardiac valve vegetations.

Management

In order to successfully treat acute septic arthritis, the identification of the pathogen with corresponding antibiotic sensitivities is important. The antibiotic drug selected should have sufficient tissue penetration to the affected joint. There is no clear evidence to suggest the optimal duration of intravenous or oral antibiotic therapy. Conventionally, antibiotics are given for up to two weeks intravenously or until signs improve. Thereafter a four-week course of oral antibiotics is given. Stopping antibiotics should be based on symptoms, signs and acute phase responses. The successful treatment of acute septic arthritis also requires the removal of pus. Medical needle aspiration or surgical aspiration via arthroscopy can be used.

The choice of antibiotic in empirical therapy should be based upon the patient's risk group. If the patient has no risk factors for atypical organisms, intravenous flucloxacillin at two grams four times a day (with gentamicin if advised by local policy) should cover the most likely staphylococcal and streptococcal pathogens. Clindamycin or second and third generation cephalosporins are alternatives in patients with penicillin allergy. If Gram-negative sepsis is likely (patients who are elderly, have recurrent urinary tract infections or had recent abdominal surgery) a second or third generation cephalosporin should be used. For possible MRSA septic arthritis in patients from a nursing home or those at risk, vancomycin with a second or third generation cephalosporin should be used. If there is any uncertainty a microbiological opinion should be sought.

3.6.2. *Gonococcal Arthritis*

Neisseria gonorrhoea is a Gram-negative coccus that typically forms in pairs or diplococci. It usually infects young sexually active people via mucosal surfaces. This organism then disseminates via the blood and causes gonococcal arthritis by replicating in the synovium and provoking an immune response from cells in the synovium. Antibiotic resistance determines efficacy of therapy and awareness of local sensitivities is important because resistance to beta-lactam, tetracycline and quinolone antibiotics has developed.

Epidemiology and Risk Factors

Gonococcal arthritis used to be a common cause of septic arthritis. However, public health programmes have reduced the incidence of this arthritis in developed countries and developing countries have the highest incidence of this infection. Risk factors for disseminated gonococcal infection include lower socioeconomic status, promiscuity, early sexual activity, homosexuality, previous gonococcal infection and intravenous drug use. Asymptomatic carriage increases the prevalence of this condition.

Clinical Features

The symptoms of disseminated gonococcal infection may occur between one day and three months after primary infection. Gonococcal arthritis can develop as a localised septic monoarthritis with a positive synovial fluid culture. However, it can also develop as an arthritis-dermatitis syndrome with bacteraemia, fever, dermatitis and migratory polyarthralgia. The dermatitis is typically manifest as multiple tiny small painless papules, vesicles or pustules which usually disappear promptly after treatment is commenced. Erythema nodosum and multiforme may also be seen. The migratory polyarthralgias may resolve without treatment or may develop into a septic mono- or polyarthritis. This typically involves the knee, ankle, elbow or wrist joints in an asymmetric fashion. It is unusual to develop a destructive gonococcal arthritis but this has been observed with concomitant HIV infection. Disseminated gonococcal infection can involve meningitis and clinical sepsis. Endocarditis may be a feature and is associated with marked fever and embolic phenomenon in the viscera. Pericarditis and myocarditis may also occur. The Fitz-Hugh–Curtis syndrome or gonococcal perihepatitis may present like acute cholecystitis and be associated with derangement of liver function tests.

Investigations

Gonococcal aetiology should be suspected in young, sexually active patients with acute arthritis and dermatitis. Microbiological investigation is an essential step in investigation. A classic synovial fluid Gram stain may infrequently identify Gram-negative intracellular and extracellular cocci; however, 50% of synovial fluid cultures are positive. In order to improve the culture rate further, samples from all sexual mucous membranes should be taken and transferred promptly to a microbiology laboratory for accurate testing. Polymerase chain reaction techniques may identify the causative organism when the cultures are negative.

Radiographs will only identify evidence of soft tissue swelling and effusions and are therefore not diagnostic.

Management

Gonococcal arthritis is predominantly managed with judicious use of antibiotics. In view of resistance patterns, im ceftriaxone at 1 g per day is the recommended initial treatment for eradication of the primary infection and arthritis. However, microbiological antibiotic sensitivities are essential for management. Surgical drainage is only needed if the joint does not respond to medical treatment.

Patients should be screened and treated for other sexually transmitted diseases including HIV and contact tracing should be performed by a sexual health clinic. Finally, patient education to prevent further dissemination of the bacterium should be offered.

3.6.3. *Syphilitic Arthritis*

Articular manifestations can develop in different stages of syphilis but most typically occur in secondary syphilis. These manifestations include arthralgia and a polyarthritis that symmetrically affects the knees, ankles and occasionally the shoulders. The patient will also usually have a maculopapular rash involving the palms of the hands and soles of the feet. There may be non-tender general lymphadenopathy. Patients in the developed world rarely progress to develop Charcot joints (painless destruction of joints due to sensory neuropathy referred to as 'Tabes dorsalis'). Syphilis is identified by a positive VDRL (indirect treponemal screening test) result and then a fluorescent treponemal antibody (direct treponemal screening test) performed on samples of venous blood. In contrast, analysis of synovial fluid or biopsy rarely identifies the pathogens. Secondary syphilis is treated with three doses of weekly intramuscular penicillin G.

3.6.4. *Lyme Arthritis*

The spirochete *Borrelia burgdorferi* causes Lyme arthritis. Following inoculation by a tick bite the majority of patients develop the clinical hallmark of erythema migrans at the site of the bite creating a ring like appearance. There is usually intermittent arthralgia and myalgia within the first few weeks. Half of the patients who are untreated go on to develop monoarthritis or oligoarthritis involving the knee and/or other large joints. These symptoms can wax and wane for many months. A small percentage of affected individuals develop a chronic inflammatory synovitis. Diagnostic testing is performed by measuring IgG antibodies to *B. burgdorferi.* The test is positive in 90% of patients with Lyme arthritis. Lyme arthritis generally responds well to therapy with oral doxycycline for 30 days or parenteral ceftriaxone for four weeks.

3.6.5. *Mycobacterial Arthritis*

Only 1% of cases of tuberculosis develop tuberculous arthritis. This most typically presents as a chronic monoarthritis. Classically it involves the large weight bearing joints, in particular the hips, knees and ankles. A progressive monoarticular swelling and pain develop over months to years. Systemic symptoms are only seen in half of these cases. The arthritis occurs as part of a disseminated primary infection or through late reactivation. The latter may occur in the context of HIV infection and serological investigations for this should be done. Diagnosis can sometimes be made using samples of synovial fluid although biopsies of synovial membrane will give a higher yield. Ziehl–Neelson staining is used for detection of acid–alcohol fast bacilli and samples should also be cultured in a specialist medium to detect mycobacterium. Anti-tuberculous medication is the same as for the treatment of pulmonary disease and ideally should be guided by the organism's sensitivities.

3.7. Viral Infection and Arthritis

Viral induced arthritides are usually acute and self-limiting diseases. They commonly occur with fever, dermatological manifestations, haematological abnormalities and other clinical features. Parvovirus, rubella, alphaviruses, hepatitis B and hepatitis C are some of the commonest viral pathogens to cause arthritis and arthralgia. Mumps, enteroviruses and herpes viruses cause joint symptoms less frequently.

Pathogenesis

The mechanism by which a virus induces arthritis and the clinical expression of this depends on host and viral factors. The host factors include age, sex, genetic background and immune response. Viral factors include the route of entry into the host, the tissues infected by the virus, the cytopathological effects of the virus, the ability to establish a chronic infection and viral expression of host-like antigens. Joint inflammation and damage may be mediated via several different routes (Table 3.30).

Direct infection of synovial cells may mediate joint tissue damage through two mechanisms. Viral infection may directly cause cell destruction or initiate programmed cell death (apoptosis) or the processed viral antigens expressed on the infected cell surfaces may stimulate immune-mediated cell destruction.

Table 3.30. Viral arthritogenic mechanisms.

Pathological basis for arthritis induced by virus infection
Direct infection of synovial cells resulting in cell damage
Direct infection of synovial cells stimulating immune-mediated destruction
Immune complex formation
Molecular mimicry
Modulation of gene expression in host cells

Immune complexes may form when the humoral immune system produces antibodies that bind viral antigens. These immune complexes may be deposited in the joints and skin causing a typical clinical picture of rash and arthralgia or arthritis. This is classically seen in hepatitis B and C, parvovirus and alphavirus infections. Alternatively, where there is molecular similarity between host antigens and viral antigens, the antibodies may cross react with host antigens, leading to an autoimmune response. This is referred to as molecular mimicry. Finally, viral infection of host cells may result in modulation of gene expression and stimulation of production of pro-inflammatory molecules that initiate inflammation and synovial hyperplasia.

Clinical Features

Viral arthritis typically presents with abrupt onset of arthralgia or arthritis. This is often polyarticular and symmetrical and a concurrent fever and rash may be noted. Viral arthralgia and arthritis is typically self-limiting although persistent and recurrent symptoms have been infrequently noted with rubella, parvovirus and alphaviruses. Viral arthritis does not cause erosive damage to joints.

Investigations

Diagnosis of viral arthritis may be difficult and depends on a high degree of clinical suspicion along with the support of suggestive viral serology. Identification of an acute IgM antibody response followed by IgG antibody production to a specific virus confirms acute viral infection. Notably, identification of a stable level of IgG does not distinguish a previous from current infection. Therefore an acute serum sample should be obtained as soon as possible to optimise the chances of identifying the acute IgM response and a convalescent serology sample should be repeated at two to three weeks for comparison. The virus specific antibodies are identified by immunoassay and selection of specific viral immunoassays should be based on clinical and epidemiological data.

Synovial fluid analysis is usually of limited use in diagnosing viral arthritis, particularly given that few viruses actually invade the joint. However, if achievable, virus isolation from synovial fluid or synovium formally confirms the diagnosis of viral arthritis. Polymerase chain reaction can identify viral nucleic acid although high rates of detection are found in asymptomatic patients which limit its clinical usefulness. Synovial fluid should be cultured for the important differential of bacterial arthritis.

Management

Viral arthritis should be treated by symptom control. This includes addressing pain with NSAIDs and transient functional impairment with occupational therapy and physiotherapy input if required.

3.7.1. *Parvovirus B19*

Parvovirus B19 is a single-stranded DNA virus that is a member of the family Parvoviridae. Parvovirus infection is common with transmission via nasopharyngeal secretions. Many parvovirus B19 infections in the community remain asymptomatic or are undiagnosed. Epidemics are frequent in children in school and hence teachers and professionals with exposure to children are at increased risk. Following infection there is an incubation period of seven to 18 days. In children parvovirus B19 cause erythema infectiosum and transient aplastic crisis. The most typical features of parvovirus B19 infection in adults include a sudden-onset, peripheral polyarthralgia, myalgia, fever and evanescent rash. Arthralgia and arthritis are usually symmetrical and occur mainly in the wrists, hands, knees and ankles, often with a distribution similar to that found in RA. The features are usually self-limiting but infrequently persist and may mimic RA with synovitis, morning stiffness and low to moderate RF and ANA titres. However, joint erosions and rheumatoid nodules do not occur. This condition should be diagnosed with serological identification of anti-parvovirus B19 IgM and should be treated symptomatically with NSAIDs.

3.7.2. *Rubella Infection*

Rubella is a single-stranded RNA virus that is a member of the Togaviridae family. It is transmitted via nasopharyngeal secretions and infection is most common in winter and spring. A characteristic morbilliform facial rash that descends to the body occurs two to three weeks after infection. In association, affected individuals develop flu-like symptoms and post-auricular and occipital lymphadenopathy. The development of arthralgia and arthritis is more common in women. Typically half of women display arthralgia and a fraction of them suffer arthritis within a week of the characteristic rash. The arthritis is symmetrical and involves inflammation of the metacarpophalangeal and proximal interphalangeal joints, wrists, knees and elbows. It usually resolves within two weeks. Similar features may arise after live rubella vaccination. Rubella infection can be diagnosed by demonstration of a typical humoral immune response with early anti-rubella IgM and subsequent anti-rubella IgG antibodies. The virus can also be isolated from synovial fluids. Treatment is symptomatic with NSAIDs being beneficial for the arthritis.

3.7.3. *Arthropod-Borne Alphaviruses*

Arthritogenic alphaviruses are mosquito-borne RNA viruses. They typically cause epidemics of polyarthritis and arthralgia in Africa, South East Asia and South America. These can affect thousands of people and increasingly frequent cases are being reported in travellers.

Ross River virus is found in Australia and the Pacific Islands. The O'nyong-nyong group causes epidemics in Central and East Africa and the Chikungunya group is found mainly in South and East Asia and Africa. Two rarer groups include the Sindbis virus group which occurs in Africa and Asia and the Mayaro virus group which is found mainly in South America.

These alphaviruses are transmitted in a continuous cycle between mammals and birds by mosquitoes. Bites from infected mosquitoes can lead to infection in humans. This is most commonly seen following increased rain fall when mosquito numbers are high. Unlike other arthritogenic viruses, the alphaviruses are distinguished by the fact that almost all symptomatic infections in adults result in joint symptoms.

The incubation period lasts from several days to three weeks. The infection is typically associated with a triad of fever, arthritis and rash. However, the diagnosis is made difficult by frequently missing features of the triad. The onset in Chikungunya and O'nyong-nyong viruses is abrupt with fever and polyarthritis which can be severe in nature. The other alphaviruses are associated with a more gradual onset of fever and non-specific constitutional symptoms prior to joint involvement.

Alphaviruses typically cause polyarthralgias usually involving the feet, ankles, knees, lower back, fingers, wrists, elbows, shoulders, and neck. The rash is short-lived and involves the face and trunk. It normally occurs shortly after the onset of joint symptoms. It is usual for a progressive resolution of symptoms to take place over three to six months. The diagnosis of alphavirus infection is made by serology. Treatment is based around symptom control with NSAIDs.

3.7.4. *Hepatitis B Virus*

This is a member of the Hepadnaviridae family and is a DNA virus. It is most common in Asia and the Middle East. Transmission is haematogenous or sexual.

Following primary infection there is usually a two to four month incubation period before hepatitis ensues. It is during this interval that a prodromal illness with flu-like symptoms, urticaria and arthritis may occur. Joint involvement typically manifests as a symmetrical arthritis of the hands, wrists, ankles, elbows and shoulders and may persist for weeks.

Viral antigens will stimulate a host immune response which may clear the virus from the host and confer lasting immunity. Infrequently the host is unable to clear the infection and a chronic infection ensues during which it remains possible to detect viral antigens in serum. Recurrent polyarthralgia and polyarthritis may be a feature of chronic infection but joint damage does not occur.

The presence of an urticarial rash and biochemical hepatitis should raise suspicion of hepatitis B infection. This can be confirmed by serological identification of viral antigens. Arthralgias should be treated symptomatically but patients with persistent infection should be referred to a liver unit for longer-term follow-up.

3.7.5. *Hepatitis C Virus*

Hepatitis C virus is an RNA virus of the Flaviviridae family. Its prevalence in Africa and Japan is higher than in Europe. It can be transmitted haematogenously or sexually and may cause an acute or chronic hepatitis. The virus can sustain a chronic infection by frequent mutations of envelope proteins which facilitate the evasion of the adaptive immune response. The virus infects lymphocytes and bone marrow cells leading to extra-hepatic disease and the production of cryoglobulins. Up to one fifth of infected patients have an associated arthropathy. This is often similar to RA with symmetrical involvement of multiple small joints, shoulders and knees. However, in contrast to RA, it is a non-deforming and non-erosive arthropathy. Hepatitis C-induced arthritis should be investigated by serological testing for anti-hepatitis C virus antibodies with immunoassays and a confirmatory immunoblot. Arthralgias may be treated symptomatically in the first instance. Anecdotal evidence suggests that use of disease modifying agents such as methotrexate may be of benefit in managing joint symptoms in some patients. All patients should be referred to a liver unit for consideration of anti-viral and pegylated IFN alpha treatment.

The sections of this chapter were contributed by Peter Taylor (rheumatoid arthritis), Bina Menon and Andrew Keat (spondyloarthropathies), Elena Nikiphorou and Sonya Abraham (psoriatic arthritis), Fiona Watt and Tonia Vincent (osteoarthritis), Michael Doherty (crystal associated disease), Andrew Barr and Sonya Abraham (infection and arthritis). Figures were provided by Leena Patel.

Chapter 4

Connective Tissue Disease and Vasculitis

Editor: Frances Hall

Shweta Bhagat, Amel Ginawi, Frances Hall, Pippa Watson, Richard Watts

4.1. Connective Tissue Disease

4.1.1. *Systemic Lupus Erythematosus*

Systemic lupus erythematosus (SLE) is a systemic autoimmune disease characterised by production of a range of autoantibodies, including hallmark antibodies specific for nuclear components.

Pathogenesis

SLE arises as a result of genetic susceptibility and one or more environmental triggers. It is a highly heterogeneous disease and current understanding of the pathogenesis suggests that the nature of the genetic predisposition and the identity of triggers vary between patients. SLE may more appropriately be viewed as a syndrome in which a variety of different immunopathological pathways lead to clinical features recognized as typical of SLE.

Genetic factors

The genetic contribution to SLE is evident from the familial clustering of cases. A number of genetic loci have been associated with SLE, at least in certain populations. These include genes involved in both innate and adaptive immune responses. Genetically encoded variation in innate pathways controlling apoptosis, type I interferon (IFN) production, complement activation and opsonisation may each be important in subgroups of patients. For example, polymorphisms (or mutations) affecting production of C-reactive protein (CRP), mannose-binding lectin and complement component C4 influence complement activation and, directly or indirectly, opsonisation and clearance of microbes or cell debris. Genetic variants leading to over-expression of type I IFNs produce a persistent state of impaired cellular gene expression and natural killer (NK) cell activation (producing chronic 'flu-like' symptoms in patients). Certain human leukocyte antigen (HLA) DR alleles and polymorphism in genes encoding co-stimulatory molecules, cytokines, chemokines and intracellular signalling pathways influence the adaptive immune response in patients with SLE, having effects on antigen presentation and lymphocyte activation, differentiation and survival.

The greater susceptibility to SLE of women is presumed to relate to the female hormonal milieu but the mechanisms remain to be clarified.

Environmental factors

A variety of environmental influences appear to modify the risk of developing or severity of SLE. Suggested infectious triggers include Epstein–Barr virus (EBV), cytomegalovirus (CMV) and Hepatitis C virus (HCV). Non-microbial triggers or promoters include smoking, ultraviolet light (well-recognised as a trigger of cutaneous lupus it probably also activates systemic disease) and stress. Exogenous sex hormones may modify risk of lupus, or flares in patients with established disease although this remains controversial. Moderate levels of alcohol, vitamin D and antioxidants may be protective but these observations are also contentious.

Aberrant immune responses

A number of aberrant immune responses flow from the interplay of the genetic and environmental factors discussed above. These are summarised schematically in Fig. 4.1. Autoantibodies may directly cause cell death, leading to anaemia, leukopenia (frequently lymphopenia) and thrombocytopenia. Autoantibody binding may also affect a plethora of pathways, causing molecular and cellular dysfunction. Thus, antibody-mediated signals may contribute to renal, neural, gastrointestinal and endocrine dysfunction. Autoantibodies may form immune complexes which are deposited in the microcirculation and activate complement and leukocytes to cause small vessel vasculitis. Well-established examples of

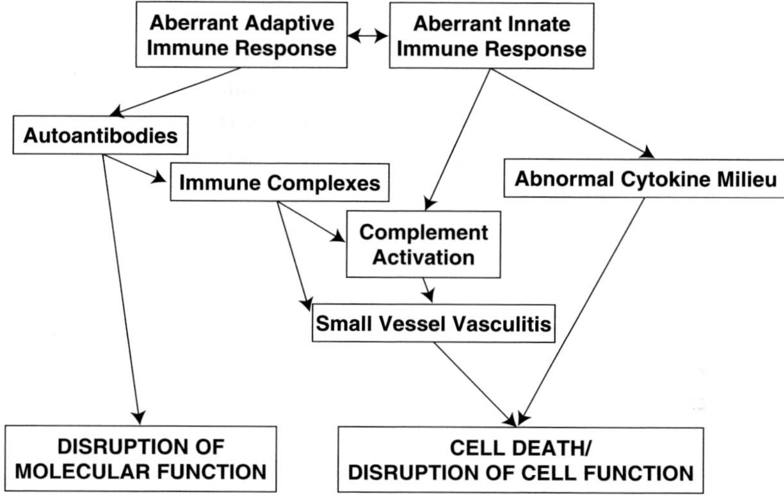

Fig. 4.1. Schematic summary of the immunopathogenesis of systemic lupus erythematosus.

immune-complex-mediated pathology occur in lupus nephritis, lupus synovitis, lupus rashes and in the vegetations of Libman–Sacks endocarditis.

Endothelial cell damage

Endothelial damage and dysfunction is caused not only by autoantibodies and immune complexes but also by a myriad of circulating cytokines and innate mediators and probably also by lipoproteins oxidised in the chronic inflammatory environment. Endothelial damage is likely to occur throughout the circulation and this contributes to macrovascular as well as microvascular disease.

Drugs

Several drugs are known to trigger a lupus-like disease in susceptible individuals (Table 4.1). This is a distinct entity from SLE and has been designated 'drug-related lupus'.

Anti-tumour necrosis factor (TNF)-α agents also may induce a lupus-like syndrome with production of anti-nuclear antibodies (ANA) and sometimes clinical features of SLE. This may occur because TNF-α blockade leads to dereg-ulated type I IFN production.

Table 4.1. Drugs implicated in drug-related lupus.

Definite	Probable	
Hydralazine	Allopurinol	Sulphasalazine
Isoniazid	Atenolol	IFN-alpha
Minocycline	Enalapril	Ibuprofen
Methyldopa	Propanolol	Sulindac
Procainamide	Penicillin	Statins
Quinidine	Nitrofurantoin	Quinine
Chlorpromazine	Tetracycline	Phenytoin
	Griseofulvin	

Epidemiology

The ratio of females to males with SLE is ~10:1, with onset most commonly occurring in the second and third decades. The incidence of SLE is higher in individuals with African or Asian ancestry.

Clinical Features

The clinical manifestations of SLE are diverse and a series of classification criteria have been published by the American College of Rheumatology (ACR), most recently in 1997 (Table 4.2). The classification criteria were designed for use in clinical trials but provide a useful guideline in clinical practice. A patient needs to fulfil four or more criteria for a diagnosis of SLE to be made. It is important to be aware that several clinical features that occur commonly in SLE such as Raynaud's phenomenon and diffuse alopecia are not included in the criteria. Other features that are included, such as mouth ulcers, are not very specific for the condition. Clinical features may occur over several years or decades and, for example, an episode of unexplained pleurisy or nephritis several years previously can contribute to the diagnosis.

It is important to listen carefully to the patient. The protean manifestations of lupus will often lead to unusual symptoms which may be dismissed as functional; the thoughtful clinician may make a link with lupus pathogenesis. Conversely, one has to be careful about applying a label of SLE inappropriately; it is important to consider whether there may be alternative explanations for any of the clinical features.

In making an assessment of the patient consider whether the features reflect currently active disease, damage from previously active disease, co-morbidity or an entirely different clinical condition. The use of validated disease activity

Table 4.2. ACR 1997 revised criteria for the classification of SLE.

Criterion	Comments
1. Malar Rash	
2. Discoid Rash	
3. Photosensitivity	
4. Oral ulcers	Oral or nasopharyngeal
5. Arthritis	Objective synovitis
6. Serositis	Pleurisy
	Pericarditis
	Peritonitis*
7. Renal disorder	Renal histology indicating immune-complex-mediated glomerulonephritis*
	Persistent proteinuria >0.5 g/24 hours or 3+
	Cellular casts
8. Neuropsychiatric disorder	Central or peripheral nervous system involvement or psychiatric condition
9. Haematological disorder	Haemolytic anaemia
	Leukopenia: <4000/μl on ≥ two occasions
	Lymphopenia: <1500/μl on ≥ two occasions
	Thrombocytopenia: <100 000/μl
10. Immunological disorder	Anti-double-stranded DNA antibody
	Anti-Sm antibody
	Anti-phospholipid antibodies (either elevated anti-cardiolipin IgM or IgG or a positive lupus anticoagulant test)
	False positive serologic test for syphilis, positive for at least six months
	Positive LE preparation
	Low levels of complement C3/C4*
11. Antinuclear Antibody	Raised titre

LE lupus erythematosus.
*Additional criteria proposed (and widely used) since 1982 publication.

scores such as the British Isles Lupus Assessment Group (BILAG) score or SLE disease activity index (SLEDAI) can be helpful.

Constitutional symptoms

Patients commonly experience fatigue, fever, night sweats, weight loss and lymphadenopathy.

Joint and muscle symptoms

Polyarthralgia occurs in the majority of patients, often with early morning stiffness. Arthritis with objective synovitis occurs in ~10% (Fig. 4.2). Jaccoud's arthropathy, a reducible deformity without radiological erosions, is usually due to tenosynovitis. Myalgia is present in the majority but myositis occurs in only ~5%.

Cutaneous features

A malar (butterfly) rash (see Fig. 4.2) is a well-recognised feature of disease, and cutaneous photosensitivity and diffuse alopecia are also common. Palpable purpura may occur and reflects a small vessel vasculitis. Livedo reticularis occurs particularly in individuals with an associated anti-phospholipid antibody syndrome (APLS). Raynaud's phenomenon often develops early during the course of

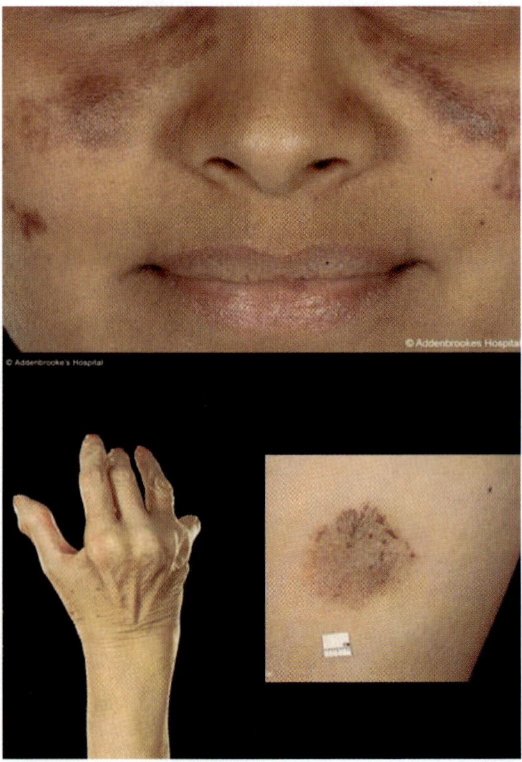

Fig. 4.2. Malar rash, arthritis and discoid rash in systemic lupus erythematosus.

SLE. Discoid rashes are a feature of discoid lupus erythematosus rather than SLE and may form scars.

Pulmonary disease

Inflammatory disease affecting the pleura commonly causes pleurisy and pleural effusions (Fig. 4.3a). Insterstitial lung disease, which affects the lung tissue itself, is less often seen (Fig. 4.3b). Pulmonary embolus is associated with anti-phospholipid antibodies or nephrotic syndrome.

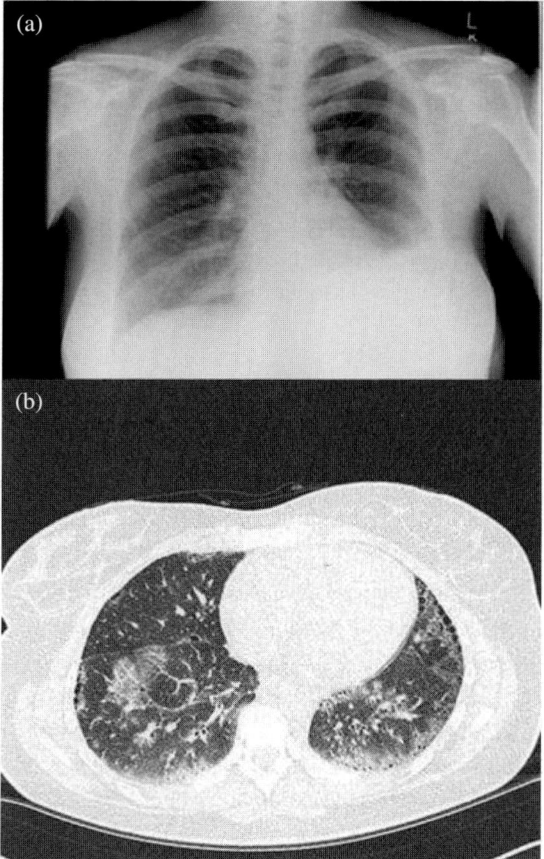

Fig. 4.3. Radiographic manifestations of pulmonary disease in systemic lupus erythematosus. (a) In the upper panel, a chest X-ray reveals a left pleural effusion. (b) In the lower panel, a high-resolution chest CT scan demonstrates interstitial lung disease.

Cardiovascular disease

The pericardium is most commonly involved and patients usually present with pericarditis or a pericardial effusion. Endocardial lesions are associated with antiphospholipid antibodies (Libman–Sacks endocarditis). In the longer term the incidence of ischaemic heart disease and stroke is increased between three- to ten-fold.

Renal dysfunction

Glomerular disease may manifest as a nephritic or a nephrotic syndrome. The former presents as acute renal failure with hypertension, active renal sediment (haematuria, cellular casts) and proteinuria and is usually associated with proliferative glomerulonephritis. Nephrotic syndrome presents with peripheral oedema, hypoalbuminaemia, hyperlipidaemia and nephrotic range proteinuria $\geq$ 3.0 g/day and is usually associated with membranous glomerular changes. All patients should have their blood pressure and urinalysis checked at every visit to ensure that glomerulonephritis is detected early. Tubulointerstitial nephritis can also be a feature of SLE. It may present with sterile pyuria and may rarely cause renal tubular acidosis type 1 or nephrogenic diabetes insipidus. Renal vein thrombosis may rarely occur in association with APLS or nephrotic syndrome.

Neuropsychatric syndromes

SLE may involve both the central and peripheral nervous systems, with a plethora of clinical presentations (Table 4.3).

Haematological disorders

Anaemia is present in the majority of cases and is often normochromic normocytic, reflecting an anaemia of chronic disease. Autoimmune haemolytic or microangiopathic haemolytic anaemia may also occur. Lymphopenia is common and may correlate with disease activity. Neutropenia is uncommon but may reflect drug toxicity. Thrombocytopenia, if present, is usually only modest ($50–100 \times 10^9$/1) and serious bleeding is uncommon.

Reticulo-endothelial involvement

Lymphadenopathy is common in SLE but the possibility of co-existing lymphoma should be considered. Hepato- and/or splenomegaly may occur but rarely cause serious problems. Functional hyposplenism with the associated increased risk of infection with encapsulated bacteria is well reported.

Table 4.3. Manifestations of neuropsychiatric systemic lupus erythematosus.

Central nervous system	Peripheral nervous system
Cerebrovascular disease (common)	Mononeuropathy
Headache	Polyneuropathy
Demyelinating syndrome	Cranial neuropathy
Seizures	Plexopathy
Movement disorder	Autonomic neuropathy
Myelopathy	Guillain–Barré syndrome
Cognitive dysfunction	Myasthenia gravis
Acute confusional state	
Aseptic meningitis	
Mood disorder	
Psychosis	

Gastrointestinal disease

Mouth ulcers are common and episodic abdominal pain, bloating, constipation and diarrhoea are frequently reported. Autoimmune hepatitis, malabsorption, colitis, mesenteric vasculitis and mesenteric or hepatic vessel thrombosis are all rare but more serious.

Associated conditions

Patients with SLE may have an associated APLS. Sjögren's syndrome (SS) also commonly occurs in association with SLE. Thyroid disease, predominantly hypothyroidism, is a feature in ~6% of SLE patients, compared with ~1% of the general population. Approximately 25% of patients with SLE have osteoporosis and ~10% suffer fractures. The risk of infections is increased by SLE (relative risk of ~1.6 compared with controls overall). Urinary tract infections and pneumonia are the commonest types of infection. Infective endocarditis may occur, especially where pre-existing endocardial lesions are present. Central nervous system infections are uncommon in SLE (Table 4.4).

Drug-related lupus

Drug-related lupus may be considered as a separate entity from SLE. Typical features include constitutional symptoms, arthralgias/arthritis, myalgia, rashes and serositis with a raised erythrocyte sedimentation rate (ESR) and a positive ANA

Table 4.4. Checklist for clinical assessment of patients with SLE.

Common features of active SLE	Commonly associated conditions
Constitutional symptoms with malaise, fevers, sweats	Anti-phospholipid syndrome
Joint pain and swelling	Sjögren's syndrome
Skin rashes: malar, sun-sensitive, purpura	Thyroid disease
Raynaud's phenomenon	Cardiovascular disease
Mouth ulcers	Osteoporosis
Hair fall	Infections
Lymphadenopathy	
Chest pains with evidence of pleurisy or pericarditis	
Headaches, fits or other neurological features	
Hypertension	
Abnormal urinalysis with haematuria and proteinuria	

with elevated anti-histone antibodies. The condition usually develops within weeks to months of introduction of the triggering medication. Note that anti-double stranded DNA (dsDNA) antibodies suggest SLE rather than drug-related lupus.

Investigations

Investigations will contribute to making a diagnosis, assessing overall disease activity, evaluating involvement of specific organs and monitoring for development of co-morbidities (Table 4.5).

Immunological abnormalities are key in investigation of SLE and form part of the ACR diagnostic criteria. The ANA is positive in ~95% of SLE patients. The presence of anti-dsDNA or anti-Sm is more specific although less sensitive for making the diagnosis. Levels of anti-dsDNA antibodies may reflect disease activity in some patients. Patients may also have antibodies to other extractable nuclear antigens (ENA) including Ro and La. Levels of complement C4 are usually low and levels of complement C3 may also be low in active disease. Some patients will have anti-phospholipid antibodies (anti-cardiolipin antibodies) or a positive lupus anticoagulant test indicating the possibility of an associated APLS. Anti-histone antibodies should be checked if drug-induced lupus is suspected.

Table 4.5. Investigation of patients with SLE.

Purpose	Specific investigation
Tests that contribute to ACR diagnostic criteria	ANA, dsDNA antibodies Complement C3 and C4 levels FBC U&Es, urinalysis, urine microscopy, renal biopsy
Markers that may fluctuate with disease activity	dsDNA Complement C3 and C4 levels ESR (with normal CRP)
Investigation of specific organ involvement	Lungs: CXR, pulmonary function tests, CT scan (high resolution) Heart: ECG, echocardiogram Kidneys: U&Es, urinalysis and microscopy, renal biopsy Liver: LFTs, US scan, liver biopsy (rarely) Gastrointestinal disease: endoscopy Nervous system: MRI, LP to assess CSF, neurophysiological studies Muscle: CK, EMG, MRI scan, biopsy
Monitoring for associated conditions	APLS: anti-cardiolipin antibodies and lupus anticoagulant Sjögren's syndrome: Schirmer's test, salivary flow, anti-Ro/La antibodies Thyroid disease: thyroid function tests Cardiovascular disease: lipid profile, doppler studies Poor bone health: Bone density scan, vitamin D Infection risk: Anti-*S. pneumoniae* and anti-*H. influenzae* antibodies

ANA anti-nuclear antibody, APLS anti-phospholipid syndrome, CK creatine kinase, CRP C-reactive protein, CSF cerebrospinal fluid, CT computed tomography, CXR chest X-ray, ECG electrocardiogram, EMG electromyogram, ESR erythrocyte sedimentation rate, FBC full blood count, LFT liver function tests, LP lumbar puncture, MRI magnetic resonance imaging, U&E urea and electrolytes, US ultrasound.

Haematological disorders are also included within the ACR diagnostic criteria and a full blood count (FBC) should be performed in all patients to detect anaemia, thrombocytopenia and leukopenia, particularly lymphopenia. Renal function should be assessed, both with urinalysis to detect microscopic haematuria/proteinuria and with a blood test. Abnormal urinalysis should prompt a request for microscopy to look for red cells and cellular casts. A renal biopsy may be required if there is an active urinary sediment and/or proteinuria >1 g/24 hours and/or raised creatinine.

The ESR will be elevated but the CRP is often normal in active SLE; when considered together these tests can be helpful in distinguishing between active SLE and infection in an individual with SLE.

Further investigations will depend on the clinical presentation. Chest X-ray (CXR) and echocardiogram will be helpful in detecting pleural and pericardial effusions respectively. Pulmonary function tests, including assessment of lung volumes and transfer factor, may be indicated. A parallel decrease in lung volumes and transfer factor is usually indicative of interstitial lung disease, a disproportionate decrease in transfer factor raises suspicion of pulmonary arterial hypertension. Liver function tests (LFTs) should be requested; these may be abnormal due to lupus hepatitis but are more commonly disturbed by drugs such as non-steroidal anti-inflammatory drugs (NSAIDs). Endoscopic studies may identify gastrointestinal pathology, often due to use of NSAIDs rather than a primary manifestation of SLE. A magnetic resonance imaging (MRI) scan of the brain and a lumbar puncture to obtain cerebrospinal fluid for analysis can be helpful in investigation of cerebral SLE. The creatine kinase (CK) value is usually elevated in patients with myositis and abnormalities may be seen on electromyography (EMG). MRI will help to localise involved muscle which can then be biopsied.

Monitoring for development of associated conditions should be performed annually. Thyroid function tests will detect associated hypothyroidism. A lipid profile will help in evaluation of longer-term cardiovascular risk. Vitamin D levels should be checked and a bone density scan may be appropriate particularly if patients are taking corticosteroids. Serological tests for antibodies specific for *Streptococcus pneumoniae* and *Haemophilus influenzae* may be helpful in evaluation of risk of infection, particularly where there is prolonged hypocomplementaemia or functional hyposplenism.

Management

There are three major strands to management of patients with SLE. Firstly, disease activity needs to be controlled. Secondly, attention should be paid to minimising symptoms that relate to damage caused by previously active disease. Thirdly, it is important to prevent and manage associated co-morbidities. As with all chronic conditions, patient education is key to a successful outcome.

Control of SLE disease activity

This should be achieved using the minimal immunosuppressive regime to reduce risk of adverse effects. Topical or local (e.g. intra-articular) immunosuppression is preferable to systemic immunosuppression if disease activity is truly localised to a single area. A short burst of moderate dose corticosteroids is better than progressive escalation from a small starting dose and is likely to result in a lower cumulative corticosteroid dose. The most serious organ involvement should always be considered and treatment tailored to that; the lesser manifestations of disease activity will likely also then be adequately controlled. Disease activity should be monitored objectively, both by clinical assessment and by blood tests, to determine whether treatment is effective.

Corticosteroids

Prednisolone at doses of >20 mg once a day (od), depomedrone 80–120 mg intramuscularly (im) or methylprednisolone 500–1000 mg intravenously (iv) daily for up to three days, are useful for gaining rapid control of activity but their long-term use should be minimised. Topical corticosteroids should be used in preference to systemic corticosteroids where possible.

Hydroxychloroquine

Hydroxychloroquine use is associated with fewer disease flares and reduced long-term damage and should be used in the majority of patients; patients need to arrange annual eye checks with their optician in view of the possible association with maculopathy.

Anti-metabolites

Agents such as azathioprine, mycophenolate mofetil or methotrexate may all be used to control chronic SLE activity. All require regular blood tests to monitor for possible toxicity.

Cyclophosphamide

Cyclophosphamide has traditionally been used, together with high-dose corticosteroids, to treat severe, organ-threatening SLE activity, classically lupus-related proliferative glomerulonephritis. However, cyclophosphamide is a toxic drug with adverse effects including bone marrow suppression, infertility and an increased risk of malignancy. It is still widely used but recent studies suggest that it may be superseded by mycophenolate mofetil and/or B cell depletion therapy.

B cell depletion therapy

Rituximab, a monoclonal antibody specific for CD20, can be used to induce B cell depletion and may be effective in management of some manifestations of SLE. Clinical trials are ongoing. Several weeks usually elapse before clinical benefit occurs.

Anti-TNF-α agents

TNF-α antagonists should generally be avoided due to the risk of lupus exacerbation.

Minimising symptoms related to tissue damage

Many symptoms arise as a result of previous tissue damage; immunosuppression is then inappropriate and ineffective and management strategies should largely be aimed at relieving symptoms. Examples include:

- Neuropathic pain: may be relieved by amitriptyline, gabapentin, pregabalin or carbemazepine.
- Skin hyper- or hypopigmentation: refer for appropriate cosmetic advice via dermatologists.
- Joint damage: simple analgesia and physiotherapy may be sufficient in mild cases but joint replacement may be required if severe hip or knee arthritis has occurred.
- Chronic renal impairment: control of hypertension, prevention of renal osteodystrophy with phosphate binders and alphacalcidol, dialysis if required.

Prevention and management of associated morbidity

Specific measures may be required if patients suffer from APLS, SS or hypothyroidism. Depression is common and may require pharmacological treatment. Patients with SLE are at increased risk of cardiovascular disease, osteoporosis, infection and depression (Table 4.6).

Drug-related lupus

For patients with drug-related lupus, the suspected triggering medication should be withdrawn. In general, symptoms improve within days or a few weeks. The positive ANA and anti-histone antibodies may persist for months to years.

Table 4.6. Management of co-morbidities associated with SLE.

Comorbidity	Management
Anti-phospholipid antibodies or syndrome	Consider low dose aspirin or hydroxychloroquine if antibodies present but no history of thrombosis. Anti-coagulate with warfarin if history of thrombosis.
Sjögren's syndrome	Tear replacement and advice about oral hygiene.
Hypothyroidism	Thyroxine replacement.
Cardiovascular disease	Advise smoking cessation and reduction of body mass index to <25. Manage hypertension and hyperlipidaemia.
Osteoporosis	Minimise corticosteroid use. Consider prescription of calcium/vitamin D and bisphosphonates for patients taking corticosteroids for >three months or for patients with osteoporosis (T score <−2.5)
Infection risk	Vaccinate against influenza, pneumococcus and *Haemophilus influenzae* and check antibody titres to ensure adequate response. Treat intercurrent infections promptly.
Depression	Consider treatment with selective serotonin re-uptake inhibitors (e.g citalopram or fluoxetine). Amitriptyline may be useful in patients with coexisting fibromyalgia.

4.1.2. *Anti-Phospholipid Antibody Syndrome*

Anti-phospholipid antibody syndrome (sometimes known as Hughes' Syndrome) is an autoimmune disease in which antibodies against phospholipids and associated proteins cause an acquired thrombophilia or tendency to inappropriate blood clotting. This gives rise to thromboses, spontaneous abortion and premature births.

Pathogenesis

The development of anti-phospholipid antibodies (APLA) reflects a breakdown of tolerance. APLA frequently recognise a phospholipid/protein combination; the most important protein co-factors are beta-2-glycoprotein I and pro-thrombin. Both genetic susceptibility and an environmental trigger (e.g. infection or certain drugs) are probably required. The APLA cause prolongation of the activated partial thromboplastin time (APTT) *in vitro* probably by forming complexes with certain clotting factors which are required for the *in vitro* coagulation assay. However, *in vivo*, the effect of APLA is to promote rather than to retard clotting. This reflects the activating effects of APLA on endothelial cells (promoting a pro-coagulant environment) and platelets, acquired protein C resistance and possibly also impairment of fibrinolysis.

APLA are believed to interfere with placental development due to ischaemia arising from thrombosis in placental vessels, defective maturation of trophoblast cells and activation of complement by bound APLA.

Clinical Features

Making a diagnosis of APLS is complicated by the diversity of clinical manifestations, the high prevalence of some features, such as miscarriage, in the normal population and the presence of anti-cardiolipin antibodies and/or lupus anti-coagulant in 1–2% of the population. The 2006 international consensus criteria are generally used for making a diagnosis of definite APLS (Table 4.7). A diagnosis

Table 4.7. 2006 International consensus criteria for diagnosis of APLS.

Diagnosis of APLS
Clinical criteria
1. Vascular thrombosis.
Arterial, venous or small vessel thrombosis in any tissue or organ (excluding superficial venous thrombosis) confirmed by appropriate imaging or histopathology
2. Pregnancy morbidity involving at least one of the following:
a) One or more unexplained deaths of a morphologically normal foetus at or beyond tenth week of gestation
b) One or more premature births of a morphologically normal neonate before thirty-fourth week of gestation due to eclampsia or severe pre-eclampsia or placental insufficiency
c) Three or more unexplained consecutive spontaneous abortions before tenth week of gestation, with hormonal, chromosomal or maternal anatomic causes excluded
Laboratory criteria
1. Lupus anti-coagulant
2. Anti-cardiolipin antibody of IgG and/or IgM isotype
3. Anti-beta-2-glycoprotein-I antibody of IgG and/or IgM isotype in medium/high titre

Laboratory criteria must be present on two or more occasions at least 12 weeks apart and must be measured according to the appropriate guidelines. Definite APLS is present if at least one clinical criterion and one laboratory criterion are satisfied.

of possible or probable APLS may be given to a patient who fulfils some of these criteria.

The main clinical feature is thrombosis which may occur at any level in the vascular tree, leading to stenosis or occlusion in the affected vessels (Table 4.8). The diagnosis of APLS should, for example, be considered in individuals who present with strokes or myocardial infarctions at a young age. The condition may present less obviously with hypertension (due to renal artery stenosis), proteinuria (as part of the nephrotic syndrome) or relatively non-specific neurological features such as headaches, hearing loss or cognitive dysfunction. A prominent livedo reticularis rash may be a helpful pointer. It is important to enquire about oral and genital ulceration in order to exclude the differential diagnosis of Behçet's disease which may also present with thrombosis. Likewise weight loss might point to a malignancy as an alternative explanation for thrombosis.

Patients with APLS are at risk of pregnancy loss, which may occur in the first, second or third trimester; APLS is currently the commonest cause of avoidable foetal loss.

The third common feature of disease, which is not included in the consensus criteria, is a mild thrombocytopenia.

The anti-phospholipid syndrome is often found in association with SLE and/or SS and features of these diseases may therefore be present.

Distinct syndromes within the diagnostic label of APLS have been identified as follows:

- Catastrophic APLS: life threatening condition in which three different organ systems become objectively involved within weeks.
- Sneddon's syndrome: clinical triad of stroke, hypertension and livedo reticularis.
- Libman–Sacks endocarditis: sterile vegetation on heart valves.

Table 4.8. Thrombosis in APLS.

Arterial	Venous	Thrombotic microangiopathy
Stroke syndromes	Deep vein thrombosis +/– pulmonary embolus	Livedo reticularis
Myocardial infarction	Budd–Chiari syndrome (hepatic vein thrombosis)	Splinter haemorrhages
Renal artery stenosis	Retinal vein thrombosis	Nephrotic syndrome
Digital gangrene	Renal vein thrombosis	Avascular necrosis
Mesenteric ischaemia	Saggital sinus thrombosis	Neurological features*

* Including headache, seizures, cognitive dysfunction, depression, psychosis, sensorineural hearing loss, parkinsonism, Guillain–Barré syndrome, amaurosis fugax, optic neuropathy, intracranial hypertension.

Investigations

The diagnosis of APLS requires the detection of at least one of three abnormalities:

- Presence of anti-cardiolipin antibodies detected by enzyme linked immunosorbent assay (ELISA). IgG anti-cardiolipin antibodies are more significant than IgM or IgA antibodies.
- Presence of anti-beta-2-glycoprotein I antibodies detected by ELISA.
- Presence of a lupus anti-coagulant. This may be detected using a variety of tests, each of which demonstrate that a phospholipid-dependent clotting assay is prolonged *in vitro* due to the presence of an inhibitor which is generic to all phospholipid-dependent steps and not specific to a single clotting factor.

A thrombophilia screen to exclude abnormalities of protein S, protein C and antithrombin as a cause for thrombosis is also usually appropriate. A FBC may demonstrate a mild thrombocytopenia. ANA, dsDNA and ENAs may be positive if the APLS is associated with a connective tissue disease such as SLE. Further tests including imaging studies may be required depending on the clinical manifestations.

Management

The objectives of management are to prevent thromboembolic episodes and maximise the chance of a successful pregnancy. The evidence base for the management of definite or probable APLS is poor and the criteria determining use and degree of anticoagulation are controversial. Therapeutic strategies are generally tailored to the degree of perceived risk (as outlined below) but there is considerable variation in protocols used by different units (Table 4.9).

Prevention of thromboembolic episodes

Patients should be advised to avoid smoking, use of oral contraceptives and prolonged periods of immobility. Where there is no history of thrombosis but there is a persistently positive anti-phospholipid test then some units suggest use of low dose aspirin or hydroxychloroquine, particularly in patients with SLE. Where thrombosis has occurred then life-long anti-coagulation is recommended and consideration should also be given to use of hydroxychloroquine. The target international normalised ratio (INR) should be 2.0–3.0 where a single venous thrombosis has occurred and 3.0–4.0 where recurrent venous thromboses or an arterial thrombosis has occurred. Heparin may be used and/or an anti-platelet

Table 4.9. Management of APLS.

History	Non-pregnant patient	Pregnant patient
APLA	Consider aspirin +/– hydroxychloroquine	Consider post-partum aspirin or LMWH
APLA + thrombosis	Warfarin +/– hydroxychloroquine	LMWH + aspirin
APLA + foetal loss	Consider aspirin +/– hydroxychloroquine	LMWH

APLA anti-phospholipid antibody, LMWH low molecular weight heparin.

agent may be added if patients continue to experience thrombosis despite anticoagulation to achieve an INR of 3.0–4.0.

Maximising chance of successful pregnancy

The principles here are to minimise the risks of thromboembolism (and hence placental insufficiency) and of maternal or foetal adverse effects from medication. Patients should be advised not to smoke. They should have regular ultrasound scans to monitor foetal growth. Doppler studies of uterine and umbilical artery blood flows may be helpful during the second trimester.

Where a patient has a persistently positive anti-phospholipid test but no history of thromboembolic events or pregnancy loss, no specific treatment is required during pregnancy although consideration should be given to the use of aspirin or low molecular weight heparin (LMWH) in the post-partum period. Where there has been a prior thromboembolic event the patient should stop warfarin and take aspirin and LMWH during pregnancy, switching back to warfarin in the post-partum period. Where there has been prior pregnancy loss the patient should be given LMWH during pregnancy and in the post-partum period.

Calcium and vitamin D supplements should be given to women receiving LMWH during pregnancy although there is no clear evidence that this has any effect on the risk or severity of heparin-induced osteoporosis.

Calcium channel antagonists are usually used to manage hypertension and early delivery may be necessary in response to pre-eclampsia and placental insufficiency.

With careful pregnancy management, the probability of a live birth in a patient with APLS is ~80%.

4.1.3. *Sjögren's Syndrome*

Primary Sjögren's syndrome (pSS) is an autoimmune disease, primarily of exocrine glands, especially salivary and lacrimal glands. Secondary Sjögren's syndrome (sSS) occurs in the context of another autoimmune disease.

Pathogenesis

SS is characterised by T and B lymphocytic infiltration and destruction of salivary and lacrimal glands and systemic evidence of aberrant B cell activation in the form of hypergammaglobulinaemia, autoantibodies (typically anti-Ro and anti-La but also rheumatoid factor (RF), antibodies to the M3 receptor on epithelial cells and antibodies specific for proteins implicated in apoptosis). Immune complex deposition and complement fixation in the microvasculature sometimes occur, giving rise to small vessel vasculitis. Aberrant B cell proliferation and survival underlies the increased risk of lymphoma in patients with SS.

Both environmental and genetic factors have been implicated in the development of SS. HLA DR3 is associated with presence of anti-Ro and anti-La antibodies. EBV has been proposed as an infectious trigger. Both androgen deficiency and microchimerism (commonly arising during pregnancy) have also been suggested as triggers or promoters for the development of pSS. Human immunodeficiency virus (HIV) and HCV infection are associated with sicca symptoms and are generally considered as exclusion criteria for a diagnosis of pSS to be made.

Epidemiology

The prevalence of SS is approximately 1%, with a female:male ratio of 9:1. Onset is most common between 45–55 years. Lymphoma develops in about 5% of patients; risk factors for lymphoma are presence of autoantibodies, low complement C4, monoclonal gammopathy, CD4+ T lymphopenia, decrease in immunoglobulins (Igs), presence of cryoglobulins, immune complex-mediated vasculitis, lymphoid or glandular swellings.

Clinical Features

The most widely-used classification criteria for pSS are those from the American–European consensus group (Table 4.10).

Table 4.10. American–European consensus group criteria for the diagnosis of SS.

Criteria	Details
I Ocular symptoms	1. Have you had daily, persistent, troublesome dry eyes for more than three months? 2. Do you have a recurrent sensation of sand or gravel in the eyes? 3. Do you use a tear substitute more than three times a day?
II Oral symptoms	1. Have you had a daily feeling of dry mouth for more than three months? 2. Have you had recurrently or persistently swollen salivary glands as an adult? 3. Do you frequently drink liquids to aid in swallowing dry foods?
III Objectively dry eyes	Positive Schirmer's Test (≤5 mm in 5 min) or Rose Bengal score
IV Histopathology	Minor salivary gland (lower lip) biopsy reveals focus score of ≥1
V Objectively dry mouth	1. Unstimulated whole salivary flow ≤1.5 ml in 15 min 2. Parotid sialography showing diffuse sialectasis without major duct obstruction 3. Salivary scintigraphy showing delayed uptake of tracer
VI Serology	Anti-Ro, anti-La antibodies, or both

Exclusions: previous head and neck radiation, hepatitis C infection, acquired immunodeficiency syndrome (AIDS), graft-versus-host disease, pre-existing lymphoma, sarcoidosis, use of anti-cholinergic drugs.

Diagnosis requires either:

- the presence of four of six criteria, including either histopathology (IV), or serology (VI), or
- the presence of three of four objective criteria (III, IV, V, VI)

The diagnosis of sSS is based on the presence of symptoms of dry eyes or dry mouth (I or II) plus two other criteria from III, IV and V, occurring in a patient with a well-defined connective tissue disease.

Other causes of the ocular and oral symptoms, including HIV or HCV, use of anti-cholinergic drugs, prior head/neck radiation or pre-existing lymphoma or sarcoidosis should be considered.

Glandular involvement

The most obvious features in pSS usually arise from glandular involvement. Patients experience a sensation of dryness or grittiness affecting the eyes (keratoconjunctivitis sicca). An objective test for tear secretion, the Schirmer's test, involves placing a standard strip of filter paper in the inferior conjunctival sac and instructing the patient to close their eyes. Normally at least 10 mm wetting of the paper strip will occur in five minutes. The test is regarded as definitely positive if <5 mm wetting occurs in five minutes. Rose Bengal is an aniline dye that stains exposed epithelium; abnormal uptake is best seen by slit lamp examination performed by an ophthalmologist.

Patients may also complain of dryness affecting their mouth (xerostomia) and the need to take frequent sips of water. Saliva secretion over five to fifteen minutes may be measured by asking the patient to spit all saliva secreted over this time into a container. A secretion rate of <0.1 ml/min is abnormal. The lack of saliva leads to an increased tendency to dental caries.

The parotid or other salivary glands may become swollen, reflecting lymphocytic infiltration (Fig. 4.4). Vaginal dryness may lead to dyspareunia. Abnormal pancreatic function may occasionally lead to malabsorption.

Extra-glandular features

Fatigue occurs in the majority of patients and is often the major presenting feature. Lymphadenopathy is common both as a feature of SS and as a sign of developing lymphoma. Interstitial lung disease, usually of the lymphocytic pneumonia subtype, occurs in ~30% of cases but is usually subclinical (Fig. 4.5). Raynaud's phenomenon, arthralgias and myalgias are well-recognised features

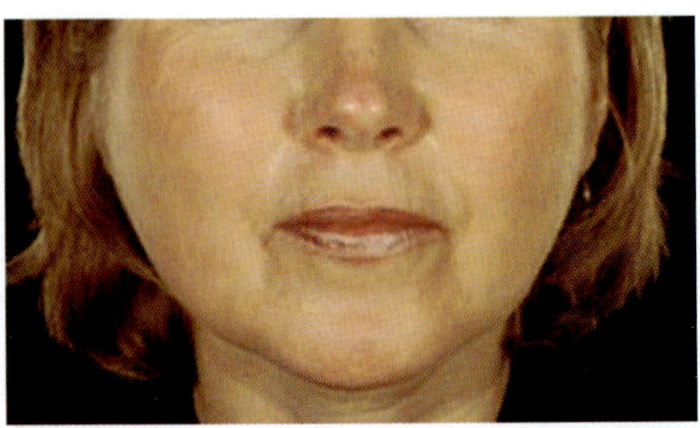

Fig. 4.4. Right parotid salivary gland swelling in primary Sjögren's syndrome.

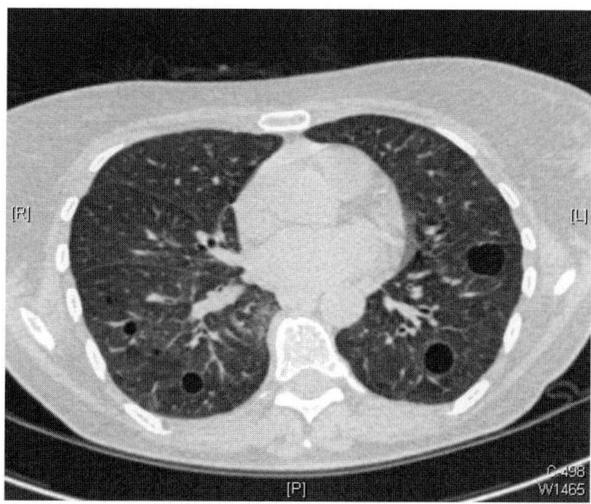

Fig. 4.5. Lymphocytic interstitial pneumonia in primary Sjögren's syndrome. CT scan showing areas of ground glass attenuation, thickening of bronchovascular bundles and cystic airspaces.

of disease although joint swelling or myositis is rare. Palpable purpura or urticaria may indicate small vessel vasculitis affecting the skin. A mononeuritis multiplex likewise may reflect vasculitis affecting peripheral nerves. Immune complex mediated glomerulonephritis is a rare manifestation of disease. An interstitial nephritis may cause biochemical abnormalities including acidosis, hypokalaemia and nephrogenic diabetes insipidus. Interstitial cystitis may occur leading to urinary symptoms such as frequency, dysuria, urgency and nocturia. Approximately 30% of patients with pSS also have hypothyroidism and 20% fulfil diagnostic criteria for fibromyalgia. A smaller number develop primary biliary cirrhosis.

Investigations

Laboratory tests

Immunological abnormalities form part of the diagnostic criteria; an ANA should be requested and tests for antibodies to Ro and La done if the ANA is positive. In some patients the RF is positive at high titre. Complement C3 and C4 proteins may be reduced. There is usually a marked hypergammaglobulinaemia which is generally polyclonal. A fall in the level of Igs or development of a monoclonal band or cryoglobulin is associated with an increased risk of lymphoma development. FBC may show lymphopenia and renal function tests may show hypokalaemia and low bicarbonate. Thyroid function should be checked in all patients because of the high frequency of associated hypothyroidism. Abnormal LFTs and a positive anti-mitochondrial antibody may point to the development of primary biliary cirrhosis. The lactate dehydrogenase (LDH) should be checked if lymphoma is suspected. Serological tests for HCV and HIV should be done where appropriate to exclude these as differential diagnoses.

Imaging and other studies

A lip biopsy may show evidence of involvement of the minor salivary glands, one of the criteria that contribute to diagnosis. Salivary gland imaging with ultrasound, MRI or scintigraphy may demonstrate enlargement. Lung function tests may reveal decreasing lung volumes (e.g. forced vital capacity) and transfer factor if there is respiratory involvement. A high resolution computed tomography (CT) scan of the chest may show changes of interstitial lung disease (Fig. 4.5). Biopsy of skin or peripheral nerve tissue may show evidence of vasculitis. Renal biopsy may occasionally be required to investigate for glomerulonephritis or interstitial nephritis. Excision biopsies of enlarged lymph nodes may be required for diagnosis of an associated lymphoma.

Management

Patients require education about eye and mouth care. They should avoid dry environments and protect their eyes when performing dirty/dusty tasks and should be shown how to apply topical treatments to their eyes. They need to see their dentist regularly for check-ups. Very importantly they should be advised to report salivary gland or lymph node swelling to their doctor in view of the increased risk of lymphoma associated with SS.

Topical treatments

Artificial tear drops such as hypromellose should be applied frequently. Ophthalmic ointments such as lacrilube may be applied at night. Lacrimal duct plugging or cauterization may be considered in more severe cases. Patients should take regular sips of water or may find that chewing gum or using an artificial saliva spray such as glandosane is helpful. Skin emollients and vaginal lubricants can be beneficial.

Systemic treatments

If there is some residual gland function then pilocarpine will promote secretions; its use is often limited by side effects including flushing, sweating, diarrhoea and urinary urgency. Prednisolone may be useful in patients with more severe disease, particularly where there is lymphadenopathy or salivary gland enlargement. Hydroxychloroquine has a role in managing the joint manifestations of SS but does not relieve the sicca symptoms. Where there is clear synovitis and particularly if erosive disease develops then patients should be treated as for rheumatoid arthritis (RA), using methotrexate as first line therapy. Major organ involvement such as interstitial lung disease may require treatment with immunosuppressive agents such as mycophenolate mofetil or cyclophosphamide. Rituximab may come to play a role in management of both glandular and extraglandular disease; results of clinical trials are awaited.

4.1.4. *Systemic Sclerosis*

Systemic sclerosis (SSc) is a rare multisystem autoimmune disease of unknown aetiology. It is characterised by an abnormal immune response, widespread microvascular disease and excessive fibrosis.

Pathogenesis

Aberrant immune responses

Autoreactivity is a feature of disease with the presence of autoantibodies such as ANA, anti-centromere or anti-Scl-70 antibodies and the occurrence of a chronic inflammatory response within some tissues. Florid cutaneous inflammation is often evident in the early stages of SSc, with an infiltrate containing T cells (mainly CD4+), macrophages, mast cells and occasional B cells. The CD4+ T cells in the tissues predominantly exhibit T helper (Th)2 or Th17 activity. Th2 cells secrete interleukin (IL)-4 and transforming growth factor (TGF)-beta, both of which promote synthesis of the matrix constituents collagen, proteoglycans and fibronectin and inhibit production of matrix metalloproteinases. IL-17, the signature Th17 cytokine, promotes proliferation of fibroblasts, and activation of both endothelial cells and macrophages. Other pro-fibrotic cytokines, which are elevated in affected tissues, include connective tissue growth factor and platelet-derived growth factor. With time, the overtly inflammatory phase usually gives way to cutaneous fibrosis, causing the characteristic skin thickening, tightening and tethering, known as scleroderma. However, chronic inflammation may continue in some tissues and underlies interstitial lung disease and perhaps also gastrointestinal dysfunction.

An interesting hypothesis regarding the aetiology of SSc has been proposed, suggesting that microchimerism (persistence of small numbers of lymphocytes from a different donor of the same species) may result in a chronic graft-versus-host immune response leading to the clinical features recognised as SSc. Microchimerism may be established in women after pregnancy, during which foetal cells cross the placenta to the maternal circulation; conversely, maternal cells may cross into the foetal circulation.

Microvascular disease

Raynaud's phenomenon occurs in >90% of patients with SSc, often years before the onset of other symptoms. The pathogenesis of Raynaud's phenomenon in SSc is incompletely understood but may reflect intrinsic abnormalities of endothelial cells or vascular smooth muscle cells, increased concentrations of paracrine or endocrine vasoconstrictors and, possibly, aberrant autonomic control. The potent pressor peptide secreted by endothelial cells, endothelin-1, is increased in SSc. Gradually, the intermittent vasoconstriction is accompanied by proliferation of vascular smooth muscle cells and deposition of excessive extracellular matrix in vessel walls, processes in which endothelin-1 is also involved. This leads to narrowing and, ultimately, occlusion of small arteries (Fig. 4.6). The resulting tissue ischaemia and infarction leads to tissue re-absorption,

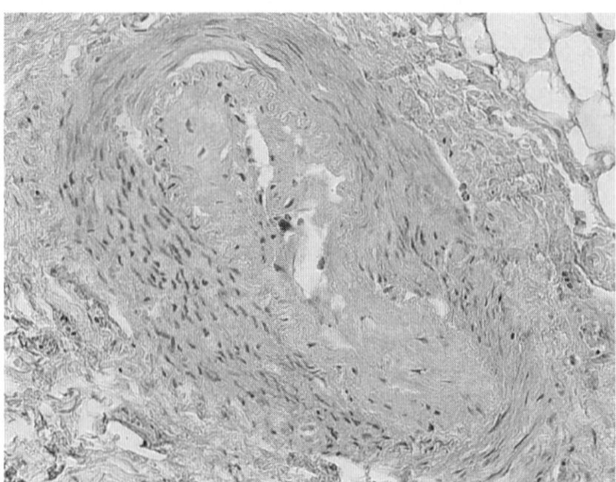

Fig. 4.6. Cross-section of a digital artery from a patient with systemic sclerosis showing wall thickening and luminal narrowing. From Herrick AL, Pathogenesis of Raynaud's phenomenon. *Rheumatology* 2005 **44**: 587–596 by permission of Oxford University Press and Professor A Freemont.

ulceration and scarring. These processes are most obvious in the digits but occur in other tissues, including lung, kidney and gut, and are responsible for many of the clinical features of SSc.

Fibrosis

The nature of the aberrant immune response in SSc may itself drive excessive matrix deposition. However, in some populations/cases, a predisposition to fibrotic disease *per se* may contribute to the clinical picture. Association with polymorphisms in genes encoding type I collagen alpha 2 chains (COL1A2), fibrillin 1 (FBN1) and the pro-fibrotic cytokine, TGF-β, have been described in different populations.

Epidemiology

SSc occurs with a UK prevalence of approximately 120 per million, a female:male ratio of 3:1 and a peak age of onset ~30–50 years. Genetic predisposition is important and a positive family history is the strongest risk factor for the development of SSc, although the absolute risk for a first-degree relative of an index case is still low (<1%). Certain genetically isolated populations exhibit higher risk, e.g. the Choctaw American Indians.

Many environmental agents have been suggested as triggers for SSc including silica, organic chemicals and drugs including appetite suppressants, bleomycin, hydroxytryptophan and cocaine. The possibility that silicone breast implants may increase the risk of SSc has received a great deal of coverage but recent meta-analyses and a large case-control study do not support an association.

Clinical Features

SSc is a multi-system disease and clinical assessment must therefore cover all organ systems.

Raynaud's phenomenon

Raynaud's phenomenon is the manifestation of transient vasospasm, usually most evident in the fingers. It is the initial symptom in more than 90% of SSc cases. Abnormal widening of capillary loops within the nail beds helps to distinguish

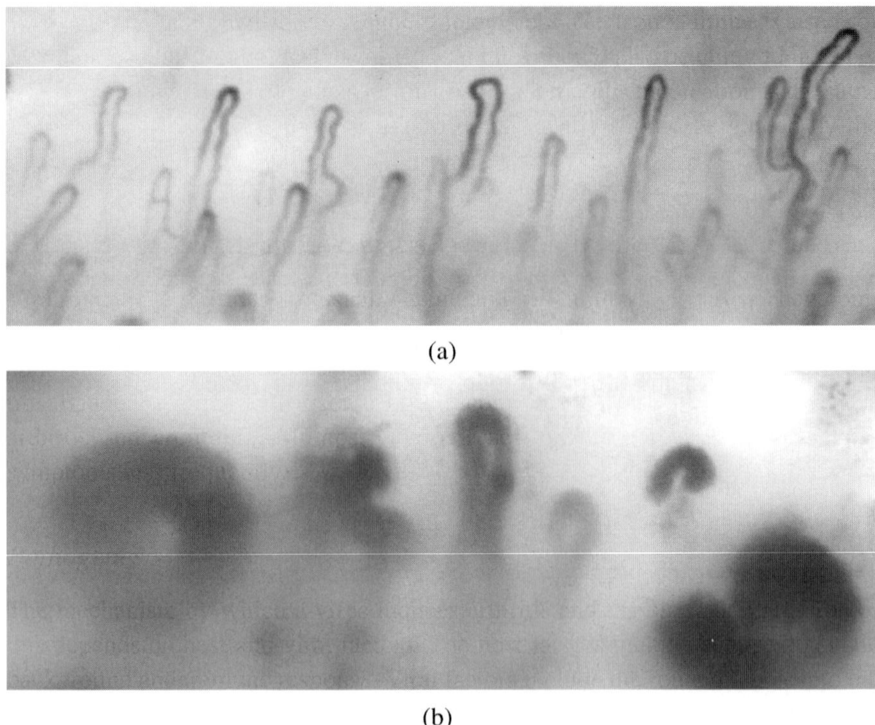

(a)

(b)

Fig. 4.7. Nailfold capillaries from (a) healthy control subject and (b) patient with systemic sclerosis showing abnormal widened capillary loops. From Herrick AL, Pathogenesis of Raynaud's phenomenon, *Rheumatology* 2005, **44**: 587–596, by permission of Oxford University Press and Dr A Herrick.

the Raynaud's phenomenon in connective tissue disease from primary Raynaud's phenomenon. Nailfold capillaroscopy, performed with an opthalmoscope using oil or gel as a magnifying lens, allows better visualisation of the nail bed capillary loops (Fig. 4.7). Severe Raynaud's phenomenon may lead to ulceration, gangrene and loss of fingertips (Figs. 4.8 and 4.9). Acroosteolysis describes the resorption of bone of the terminal phalanges that may occur with severe Raynaud's phenomenon or more generally in SScl (Fig. 4.10).

Skin disease

The term 'scleroderma' is derived from the Greek *skleros* (hard) and *derma* (skin) and describes characteristic skin changes in SSc, in which skin becomes thickened, shiny, smooth and tethered to underlying tissues. Sclerodactyly

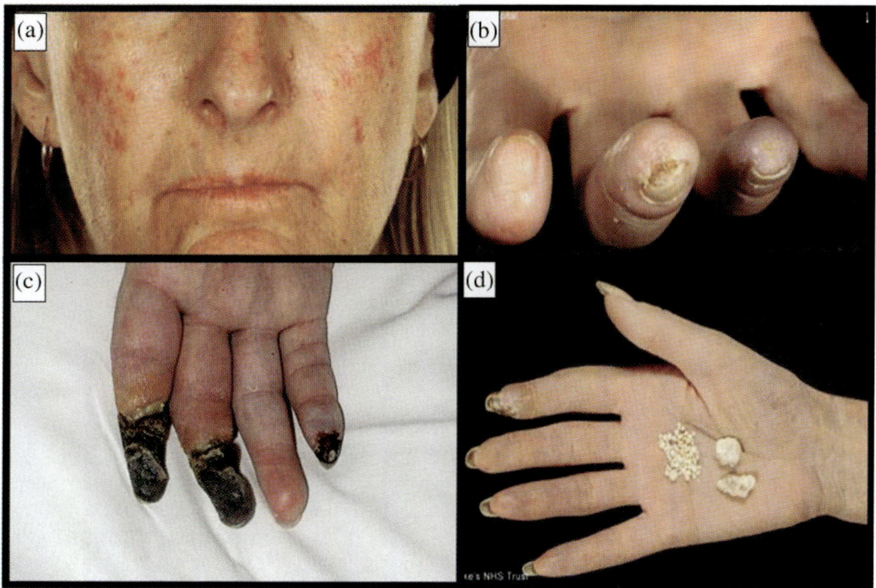

Fig. 4.8. Clinical features of systemic sclerosis. (a) Facial telangectasia and drawstring mouth. (b) Digital ischaemia. (c) Sclerodactyly with digital ulcers. (d) Calcinotic extrusions collected by a single patient.

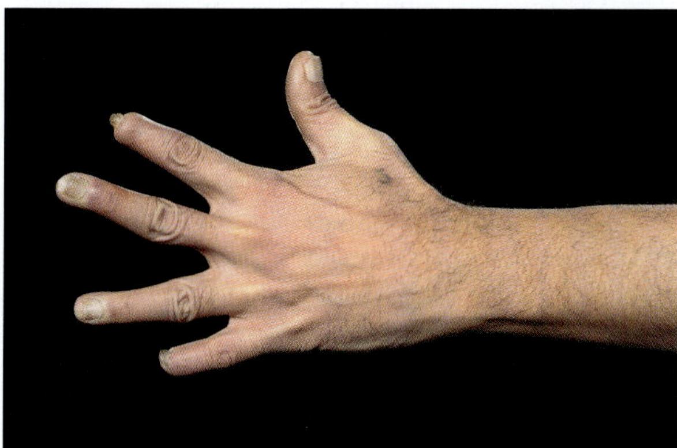

Fig. 4.9. Loss of distal tissue affecting the left index and little finger in a patient with limited cutaneous systemic sclerosis and severe Raynaud's phenomenon.

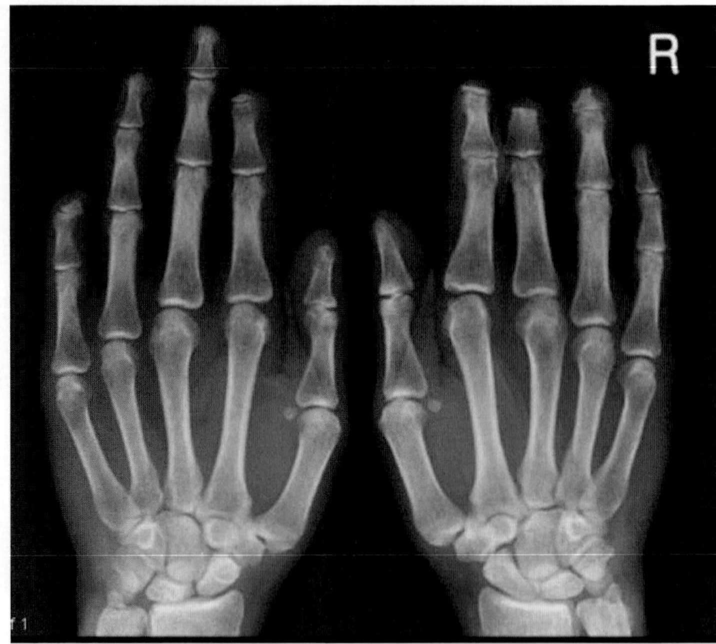

Fig. 4.10. Acroosteolysis in systemic sclerosis. Resorption of the terminal phalanges affecting the left index and little fingers and the right index, middle and ring fingers.

occurs when scleroderma affects the digits, resulting in joint contracture and loss of function (see Fig. 4.8). Circumoral scleroderma causes microstomia and the impaired mouth-opening leads to difficulties with dental work and even eating (see Fig. 4.8). Patients may develop prominent telangiectasiae which are dilated capillaries and arterioles that occur mainly on the face and upper trunk but also develop in the gut, where they can cause occult bleeding (see Fig. 4.8). Calcium deposits termed 'calcinosis' may form in the skin and subcutaneous tissue and often extrude through the skin causing an ulcer (see Fig. 4.8).

Lung disease

Interstitial lung disease occurs in the majority of SSc patients but is clinically significant in ~40% of patients. It is usually a non-specific interstitial pneumonitis (Fig. 4.11). Pulmonary artery hypertension occurs in ~12% of patients with limited cutaneous SSc and is the most common cause of death in this group.

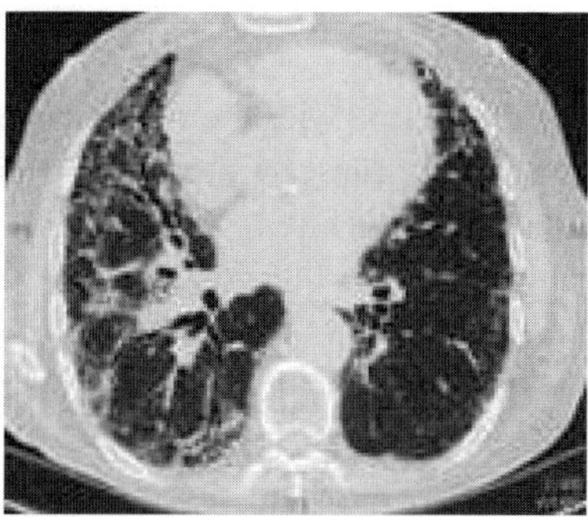

Fig. 4.11. High resolution CT image of non-specific interstitial pneumonitis in a patient with systemic sclerosis.

Hidebound chest results from sclerodermatous involvement of the chest wall and may result in a restrictive lung defect.

Gastrointestinal disease

Oesophageal dysmotility occurs in the majority of patients with SSc. This may be associated with aspiration pneumonia. Bowel dysmotility is common; stasis facilitates bacterial overgrowth and hence may lead to malabsorption.

Kidney disease

Scleroderma renal crisis is characterised by hyperreninaemia with rapidly increasing blood pressure and rising creatinine. Patients may present with hypertensive encephalopathy and often have an associated microangiopathic haemolytic anaemia. Although the use of angiotensin converting enzyme (ACE) inhibitors to manage hypertension in patients with SSc has decreased the incidence of renal crisis, it is still an important cause of mortality and end-stage renal failure.

Cardiac disease

Myocardial fibrosis may cause arrhythmias and/or conduction disturbances. Right heart failure may complicate interstitial lung disease or pulmonary artery hypertension.

Joint disease

Polyarthralgia is common, arthritis occasional but erosive disease unusual.

Associated medical conditions

Carpal tunnel syndrome is associated with the inflammatory early stages of scleroderma. An associated SS may cause dry eyes and mouth. Hypothyroidism occurs in approximately 40% of patients.

Subsets of SSc

The heterogeneity of SSc has resulted in a number of suggested classification systems. The most widely used scheme was initially developed by Le Roy *et al.* in 1988 (Table 4.11). It is based on the extent of skin involvement and allows

Table 4.11. Le Roy classification scheme for systemic sclerosis.

Subsets of systemic sclerosis
Limited cutaneous systemic sclerosis
Skin involvement restricted to hands, forearms (distal to elbow), face, and feet
Raynaud's phenomenon is usually the presenting feature
Telangectasiae
Calcinosis
Oesophageal dysmotility
Pulmonary artery hypertension occurs in ~10% of patients
Interstitial lung disease
Associated with anti-centromere antibody
Diffuse cutaneous systemic sclerosis
Skin involvement extending proximal to the elbow and involving the trunk
Raynaud's phenomonen often develops later in the course of the disease
Constitutional symptoms
Internal organ involvement involving kidneys, lungs, heart, gastrointestinal tract
Associated with anti-Scl-70, anti-RNA polymerase I/III antibodies
Pre-scleroderma
No skin involvement
Raynaud's phenomenon
Associated with anti-centromere, anti-Scl 70, anti-RNA polymerase I/III antibodies
Systemic sclerosis sine scleroderma
No skin involvement
Raynaud's phenomenon
Internal organ involvement involving kidneys, lungs, heart, gastrointestinal tract
Associated with anti-Scl 70, anti-RNA polymerase I/III antibodies

classification into four subsets of disease with relatively distinct clinical and immunological features. The designation of a 'limited cutaneous' category of SSc should not distract the clinician from the very 'systemic' nature of the disease which was previously best known as 'CREST' (calcinosis, Raynaud's phenomenon, oesophageal dysmotility, sclerodactyly and telangiectasia); many students still find this acronym a useful aide-memoire.

Investigations

Investigations may be performed to assist with the diagnosis of SSc or to monitor and investigate new clinical features in patients with known disease.

Whilst the diagnosis is predominantly a clinical one, serological studies can be very helpful. The majority of patients are ANA positive. Approximately 75% of patients with the limited cutaneous form of disease have anti-centromere antibodies and around 55% of patients with the diffuse cutaneous form of disease have anti-Scl 70 antibodies (directed at topoisomerase) or anti-RNA polymerase antibodies. A small proportion of patients have anti-U3RNP antibodies. Patients with the SSc without scleroderma variant also tend to have antibodies specific for Scl70 or RNA polymerase. Any of the antibodies may be present in patients with pre-scleroderma. Patients with overlap syndromes with sclerodermatous features may have other autoantibodies including anti-PM/SCL, anti-cyclic citrullinated peptide (CCP) antibodies and RF (Table 4.12).

Further tests need to be performed at least annually to look for common complications of the disease. Blood tests including FBC, ESR, urea and electrolytes (U&E), LFT and CK will provide information about disease activity and possible kidney, liver or muscle involvement with immune-mediated disease. Abnormalities of renal or liver function may also reflect drug toxicity. Low levels of vitamin D, ferritin, folate and vitamin B12 may reflect malabsorption due

Table 4.12. Serological tests to aid diagnosis in SSc.

Test	Association
Anti-nuclear antibody	Positive in ~95% of SSc patients
Anti-centromere antibody	Associated with limited cutaneous SSc
Anti-Scl 70 antibody	Associated with diffuse cutaneous SSc
Anti-RNA polymerase I/III	Associated with diffuse cutaneous SSc
Anti-U3RNP (fibrillarin)	Associated with diffuse cutaneous SSc

to gastrointestinal involvement. As with other autoimmune diseases it is wise to check thyroid function because of the frequency of co-existence of hypothyroidism and to measure a lipid profile to ensure that cardiovascular risk is managed appropriately. An electrocardiogram (ECG) and echocardiogram should be performed annually to detect conduction or rhythm abnormalities and development of pulmonary hypertension. Likewise, pulmonary function tests should be performed on a yearly basis; lung volumes and transfer factor decrease proportionately in interstitial lung disease whereas an isolated fall in transfer factor suggests pulmonary hypertension. A high resolution CT scan of the chest is useful for further investigation of patients with possible interstitial lung disease and right heart catheterisation studies are required to more fully investigate patients with pulmonary hypertension. Barium swallow, upper gastrointestinal tract endoscopy and colonoscopy may be helpful in investigation of oesophageal dysmotility or lower gastrointestinal tract disease.

Management

The treatment of scleroderma is difficult and challenging. Therapies are directed towards modifying the progress of microvascular disease, suppressing abnormal inflammatory responses and managing symptoms and associated co-morbidities. Patient education is important and a multidisciplinary approach is essential, with referral to appropriate specialties for the management of complications.

Patient education

This should include advice about protecting fingers and keeping them warm, regular hand exercises to maintain mobility, stopping smoking, raising the head of the bed to reduce nocturnal gastric reflux, taking gentle aerobic exercise and maintaining good dental hygiene. Patients should be aware that they need to seek medical advice if they develop shortness of breath or digital ulcers.

Managing microvascular disease

Raynaud's phenomenon

Drugs that alter behaviour of the vasculature can be beneficial in management of patients with Raynaud's phenomenon, pulmonary artery hypertension or scleroderma renal crisis.

Raynaud's phenomenon may be symptomatically improved by calcium channel antagonists such as nifedipine or angiotensin receptor antagonists such as losartan.

Bosentan, an endothelin receptor antagonist, has recently been licensed for use in SSc patients with digital ulceration, following publication of evidence indicating that it reduces the incidence of new ulcers. Intravenous iloprost, a synthetic analogue of prostacyclin, is often used as salvage therapy for patients with digital ulceration. Phosphodiesterase V inhibitors (e.g. sildenafil) and selective serotonin re-uptake inhibitors (e.g. fluoxetine) are also used to treat Raynaud's phenomenon.

Pulmonary artery hypertension

Bosentan and sitaxsentan, a selective endothelin receptor A antagonist, have demonstrated efficacy for management of pulmonary artery hypertension in SSc. Continuous intravenous epoprostenol (prostacyclin) is used in patients who deteriorate despite treatment. Sildenafil is also sometimes helpful. Anti-coagulants are generally used in patients with pulmonary hypertension but careful consideration must be given to the risk of bleeding from the gastrointestinal tract.

Scleroderma renal crisis

Although formal clinical trials have not been conducted, historical comparison suggests that ACE inhibitors have significantly reduced the incidence and improved the outcome of scleroderma renal crisis. Unfortunately, ACE inhibitors have yet to be shown to improve other manifestations of microvascular disease in SSc. Glucocorticoids should be avoided, especially in patients with diffuse cutaneous SSc, since moderate to high doses may precipitate scleroderma renal crisis.

Immunosuppressive treatment

A variety of immunosuppressive agents are used in SSc patients with overt inflammatory disease, particularly those with interstitial lung disease. A large trial has recently demonstrated that cyclophosphamide has a significant albeit modest efficacy in SSc-associated interstitial lung disease. Smaller studies suggest that mycophenolate mofetil may be effective. Methotrexate, azathioprine and D-penicillamine appear to be ineffective.

Haematopoietic stem cell transplantation is currently being evaluated in two controlled trials in Europe and the USA; preliminary data suggest that skin and microvascular disease may be improved. There is currently only anecdotal evidence for the use of biologic agents including anti-TNF-α agents and B cell depleting agents but these and the use of tyrosine kinase inhibitors (which inhibit platelet-derived growth factor signalling) need further study.

Managing symptoms and co-morbidity

Arthralgias and arthritis may merit treatment with analgesics or NSAIDs and, occasionally, intra-articular corticosteroid injection. It is sometimes possible to resect calcinotic lesions although skin healing is poor in this group of patients. Proton pump inhibitors and metoclopramide will improve symptoms associated with oesophageal dysmotility. Supplementation with vitamin D, iron, vitamin B12 and folate may be required where small bowel involvement results in malabsorption; it is occasionally necessary to use parenteral nutrition. Bacterial overgrowth will respond to a course of antibiotics. Diarrhoea and constipation may be treated simply with loperamide and agents such as lactulose and fybogel respectively. Patients with interstitial lung disease should receive vaccinations against influenza, pneumococcus and *H. influenzae*. Associated conditions such as hypothyroidism and osteoporosis require management in the usual way.

4.1.5. *Inflammatory Myopathies*

This group of conditions includes polymyositis (PMy), dermatomyositis (DMy) and inclusion body myositis (IBM). Juvenile DMy is considered in Chapter 7 (Paediatric Rheumatology). Both PMy and DMy are autoimmune myopathies that predominantly involve proximal muscles; patients with DMy also have a characteristic skin rash. IBM is characterised by inflammatory and degenerative changes that affect both proximal and distal musculature.

Pathogenesis

Both PMy and DMy are thought to arise in genetically predisposed individuals following exposure to an environmental trigger. Several infective triggers have been proposed including coxsackie virus, influenza, parvovirus, CMV and toxoplasma but have not been substantiated. PMy and DMy are both considered to be immune-mediated diseases; ANA is positive in ~80% of patients although the specificity of the autoantibodies differs between the two conditions. Histological studies also suggest the pathophysiology of PMy and DMy is distinct. In PMy, cytotoxic CD8+ T cells surround HLA class I-expressing myofibres and utilise perforin and granzyme to induce muscle necrosis. In contrast, in DMy, humoral mechanisms are more prominent. A perivascular CD4+ T cell and B cell infiltrate is evident. Immune complex-mediated small vessel vasculitis, often with evidence of complement activation, occurs in muscle, skin and other locations. Up-regulation of HLA class I molecules and increased production of cytokines, such as TNF-α, are both manifestations of aberrant autoimmune activity in PMy and DMy.

The aetiology of IBM is unknown but familial forms and HLA associations have been documented. Ageing appears to be an important factor in the pathogenesis. IBM is characterised by both inflammation and degeneration of myocytes but it is unclear which of these is the primary defect. Many histological features of IBM are shared with PMy. The presence of vacuoles and amyloid-like deposits is distinct; ubiquitin-positive inclusions are thought to be significant since ubiquitin is a molecular marker for proteins which are destined for degradation.

Epidemiology

The annual incidence of PMy and DMy combined is approximately ten per million with the disease most commonly presenting at 40–50 years. IBM is the most common inflammatory myopathy in the over 50s with a prevalence of five to ten per million although this may be an underestimate due to under diagnosis.

Clinical Features

Muscle weakness

Both PMy and DMy are characterised by muscle weakness which is usually insidious in onset, symmetrical, mainly proximal and usually painless (myalgia in ~30% of patients but rarely severe). Patients have difficulty with activities such as climbing stairs, brushing hair or standing up from sitting. They may be unable to hold their head up well if the neck musculature is involved. Pharyngeal and respiratory muscle weakness leading to dysphagia and respiratory failure can occur and may be life-threatening. Myocardial involvement is rare but serious.

IBM differs from PMy and DMy in that it characteristically involves both the proximal and distal musculature; patients often describe falls due to quadriceps weakness and difficulty manipulating keys and pens reflecting loss of manual dexterity due to distal muscle weakness. The disease is usually gradual in onset and tends to occur in individuals over 50 years old.

Skin rash

Dermatomyositis is also characterised by a heliotrope (violaceous) rash that occurs over eyelids, Gottron's patches or papules which describe purple/dusky red lichenoid patches over the metacarpophalangeal (MCP) and proximal interphalangeal (PIP) joints (Fig. 4.12), and an erythematous rash over the face, neck and anterior chest (V sign) or over the back and shoulders (shawl sign).

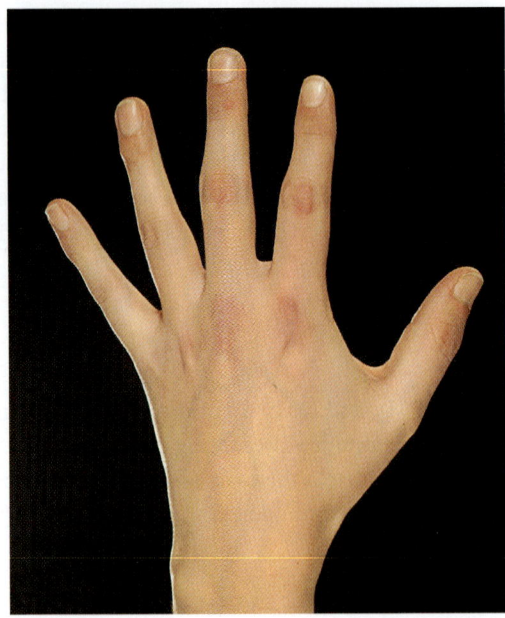

Fig. 4.12. Gottron's papules in a patient with dermatomyositis.

Systemic features

Fever, fatigue, anorexia and arthralgias are common in both DMy and PMy. Interstitial lung disease occurs in ~30% of patients and usually presents with cough and breathlessness. The combination of DMy, interstitial lung disease and polyarthritis is often associated with presence of antibodies specific for aminoacyl transfer RNA synthetases and is referred to as 'anti-synthetase syndrome'. A small vessel vasculitis is sometimes a feature of DMy.

Malignancy

Both PMy and DMy are associated with malignancy; the association is most clear for DMy with estimates suggesting that 25% of patients over 45 years old develop cancer. The malignancy may emerge before or after the diagnosis of inflammatory myositis, the most common tumours being ovarian, lung, pancreatic, stomach, colorectal and lymphoma. It is important to perform a full systems enquiry and examination to detect any localising symptoms or signs that point to the development of a cancer. Continued vigilance is necessary as malignancies may present up to two years after the initial presentation with myositis.

Differential diagnoses

The differential diagnosis of muscle disease is wide and inflammatory myositis only accounts for a small proportion of myopathies. Alternative diagnoses need to be considered. A family history may indicate an inherited muscular dystrophy. Pigmented urine after exercise points to a metabolic myopathy. Involvement of facial or external ocular muscles suggests myasthenia gravis. Muscle fasciculation suggests motor neurone disease. Features of hypo- or hyperthyroidism or of acromegaly suggest an endocrine cause for the myopathy.

Diagnostic criteria

There are no universally accepted diagnostic criteria for the inflammatory myopathies. The Bohan and Peter criteria for diagnosis of PMy and DMy are widely used (Table 4.13) although they have been criticised for lack of specificity.

Diagnostic criteria for IBM have been developed by Griggs (Table 4.14). The histological appearances are the most specific. Therefore, if all characteristic features are evident in the biopsy, no other criteria are required. However, if the histology is inconclusive, clinical and laboratory criteria are utilised.

Investigations

Diagnosis rests on demonstrating elevated muscle enzymes, characteristic abnormalities on EMG and hallmark histopathological features on muscle biopsy.

Table 4.13. Bohan and Peter diagnostic criteria for inflammatory myopathies.

Criteria for diagnosis of PMy and DMy
1. Symmetrical proximal muscle weakness with or without dysphagia and respiratory muscle weakness
2. Elevation of serum muscle enzymes especially CK
3. Electromyographic evidence of myositis
4. Muscle biopsy reveals degeneration, regeneration, necrosis, phagocytosis and interstitial mononuclear infiltrate
5. Pathognomic rash of dermatomyositis (heliotrope, Gottron's patches)

CK creatine kinase.

PMy is 'definite' in the presence of criteria 1–4, 'probable' with three of the first four criteria and 'possible' with two of the first four criteria. DMy is classified as 'definite' if all five criteria are met.

Table 4.14. Griggs 1995 diagnostic criteria for IBM.

Diagnostic criteria for IBM
Clinical Features
Duration of illness >6 months.
Age at onset >30 years.
Slowly progressive muscle weakness of arms and legs, including finger flexors, wrist flexors or quadriceps
Laboratory Features
Creatine kinase <12× upper limit reference range.
Electromyogram showing myopathic or missed pattern +/– short and long duration motor unit potentials
Muscle biopsy
Inflammatory infiltrates, rimmed vacuoles and abnormal protein deposits

Definite IBM: Satisfies all muscle biopsy criteria
Possible IBM: Equivocal muscle biopsy + clinical features + laboratory features

The CK is nearly always high in active PMy and DMy, often 50-fold higher than the upper limit of the reference range. The CK may be used to track activity of the disease as it is treated. Other muscle enzymes including transaminases and LDH are less sensitive than CK but are often also high. In IBM, the CK may be normal or mildly elevated, usually within 10-fold of upper limit of reference range. The γ-glutamyl transferase is a specific liver marker and, unlike transaminases, will not be raised by myositis.

Electromyography will usually show low-amplitude, short duration, polyphasic units on voluntary activation and increased spontaneous activity. It does not distinguish between PMy, DMy or IBM but is useful for excluding other conditions such as neurogenic disorders.

MRI using fat-suppressed T2 weighted and short T1 inversion recovery (STIR) images is highly sensitive for muscle inflammation and oedema. It is sometimes used to determine the optimal biopsy site and may, in future, have a role in monitoring disease.

Muscle biopsy is usually taken from the quadriceps provided the MRI has confirmed local involvement. The hallmark of PMy is endomysial infiltration of CD8+ T cells, which surround morphologically normal myocytes expressing HLA class I molecules. In DMy, the inflammatory infiltrate consists mainly of CD4+ T cells and B cells. Immune complexes and deposition of complement components C5–9 can be detected and myofibre necrosis and regeneration is typical. In IBM, the histology reveals the classical triad of inflammatory infiltrates, rimmed vacuoles and abnormal protein deposits (amyloid and filamentous inclusions).

Serological tests are not included in diagnostic criteria for the inflammatory myopathies. However, the ANA is positive in the majority of patients with DMy or PMy with specific patterns of reactivity. Anti-aminoacyl transfer RNA synthetase antibodies, particularly anti-Jo-1 antibodies, occur in association with DMy and are a hallmark feature of the 'anti-synthetase syndrome'. Anti-signal recognition peptide (SRP) antibodies occur in association with PMy. Anti-Mi2 antibodies occur in both groups but more commonly with DMy than with PMy.

A malignancy screen should be considered in patients with DMy or PMy over the age of 45 years and will usually involve CT scans of chest, abdomen and pelvis. Pulmonary function tests and high-resolution CT scan of the chest may be indicated if respiratory symptoms develop, to assess for respiratory muscle involvement or interstitial lung disease. ECG and echocardiogram will be required if involvement of myocardium is suspected.

Management

The prime aim of treatment of DMy and PMy is to control muscle inflammation and thereby prevent muscle loss. Glucocorticoids are the mainstay of treatment. Prednisolone at a dose of 1 mg/kg per day is typically used for approximately four weeks and then, provided the symptoms and acute phase response have improved, is tapered to the minimum maintenance dose (usually 5–15 mg od). Pulses of intravenous methylprednisolone are often used at disease onset or during flares of activity. Concomitant treatment with bisphosphonates, calcium, vitamin D and a proton pump inhibitor should be given to reduce the risk of side effects.

Methotrexate and azathioprine are second line agents that can be used for their steroid sparing effects. Ciclosporin, tacrolimus, mycophenolate and cyclophosphamide are sometimes used as alternatives. Intravenous Ig can be used in refractory cases. Rituximab, an anti-CD20 antibody, has also been reported to be effective in refractory disease in case reports and small case series. Anti-TNF-α agents have been variably reported to improve or exacerbate myositis. Early referral to physiotherapy helps to prevent development of contractures and to improve muscle function. Referral to a speech therapist is required for patients who develop dysphagia with its associated risk of aspiration.

Management of IBM differs in that there is no evidence that immunosuppression affects the course of the disease. However, an initial trial of high-dose corticosteroid may be performed to assess whether there is any steroid responsiveness in a given individual. Patients should be referred for physiotherapy and to an appliances department as orthoses to improve stability at the knee and ankle can be helpful.

4.1.6. *Sarcoidosis*

Sarcoidosis is a chronic multisystem granulomatous disorder of unknown cause. The term is derived from the Greek: *sarco* — flesh, *eidos* — like, *osis* — condition.

Pathogenesis

Both genetic susceptibility and an environmental trigger appear to be important in the pathogenesis of sarcoidosis. Data from monozygotic twins and siblings who live in different environments indicate a polygenic genetic component to susceptibility. Candidate genes include HLA class I (HLA B7 in African-Americans and HLA B8 in most racial groups), HLA class II (mainly HLA DR5 and HLA DR3) and polymorphisms in the TNF-α promoter, vitamin D receptor, natural resistance associated macrophage protein (NRAMP)-1 and ACE.

The environmental trigger for sarcoidosis is likely to be an agent which produces persistent and poorly degradable particles, which are ingested by macrophages. Intracellular microbes such as mycobacteria and non-infective particles including pine pollen, talc and beryllium have all been explored as potential aetiological agents but, as yet, the triggering agent(s) remain unknown.

Sarcoidosis is defined by the presence of non-caseating granulomas. These are formed during an adaptive immune response, starting with presentation of antigen, presumably from the microbial or other particulate trigger, by antigen-presenting cells to CD4+ T cells. Cytokines and chemokines released by the antigen-presenting cell and T cells cause local proliferation and the recruitment of further monocytes and T cells to the lesion. Some monocytes differentiate into epithelioid cells (Fig. 4.13) which form layers around the granuloma; others form multinucleated giant cells, probably by fusion (Figs. 4.13 and 4.14). In sarcoidosis, a dominant Th1 response appears to drive this process, since Th1 cytokines IFN-γ, IL-12 and IL-18 have all been found to be up-regulated in affected tissues. In patients with acute sarcoidosis (Löfgren's syndrome), circulating immune complexes are present, indicating that a humoral response is also important, at least in this form of the disease. In some patients with chronic

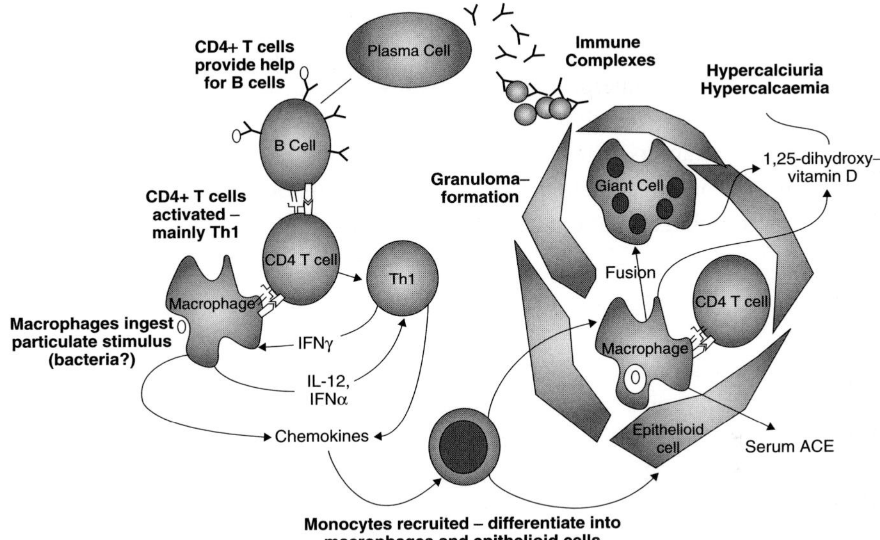

Fig. 4.13. Schematic representation of the pathogenesis of sarcoidosis.

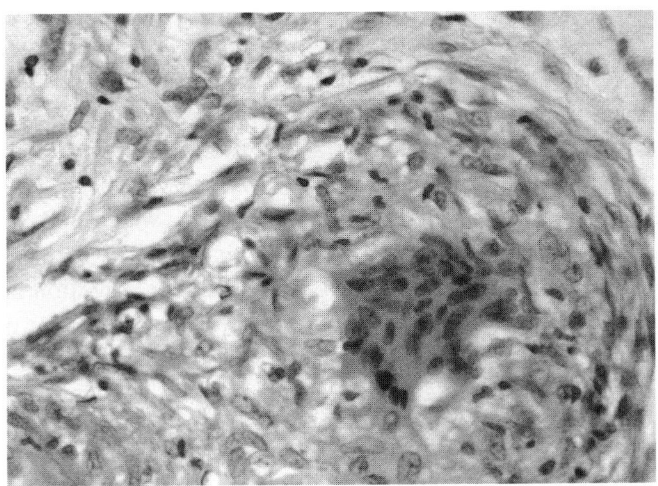

Fig. 4.14. A multinucleated giant cell in a sarcoidosis granuloma.

sarcoidosis, fibrosis is an important cause of tissue damage and the cytokine TGF-β has been implicated in this response.

Activated macrophages in granulomatous lesions may exert systemic metabolic effects. Increased activity of 1-alpha hydroxylase increases the conversion of 25-hydroxyvitamin D to 1,25-dihydroxyvitamin D. This causes hypercalcaemia in 10% and hypercalciuria in 40% of patients. ACE is also produced by activated macrophages and epithelioid cells.

Epidemiology

Sarcoidosis is relatively common, with an incidence of 1–64 per 100,000 worldwide. It usually presents between the ages of 20 and 40 years and there is a female predominance. The prevalence is highest in White Scandinavians and African-Americans and the clinical presentation and severity also vary with race and ethnicity. Disease in Caucasians tends to be less severe with erythema nodosum being a common manifestation; disease in Japanese is characterised by cardiac involvement; disease in African Americans is often severe.

Clinical Features

Acute sarcoidosis (Löfgren's syndrome)

Acute sarcoidosis classically presents as a triad of arthritis, erythema nodosum and hilar lymphadenopathy. Constitutional features (malaise and/or fever) are present in the majority of cases. Careful examination will show that the arthritis is actually a periarthritis and joint movements are usually full. It most commonly involves ankles but may include knees, wrists and small joints of hand. Erythema nodosum may be absent particularly in male patients. Acute uveitis occurs in a small minority of cases. The condition needs to be distinguished from other causes of inflammatory mono- or oligoarthritis, particularly reactive arthritis or psoriatic arthritis, and of lymphadenopathy with erythema nodosum, particularly lymphoma and infections such as with *Mycobacterium tuberculosis*. Acute sarcoidosis is almost always self-limiting (Table 4.15).

Chronic sarcoidosis

Chronic sarcoidosis is a multisystem disease. As in acute sarcoidosis, arthritis, erythema nodosum and hilar lymphadenopathy may be features. Patients also

Table 4.15. Acute sarcoidosis.

Features of acute sarcoidosis	Differential diagnoses
Periarthritis	Reactive arthritis
Erythema nodosum	Tuberculosis
Hilar lymphadenopathy	Lymphoma
	Systemic lupus erythematosus

Table 4.16. Chronic sarcoidosis.

Features of chronic sarcoidosis	Differential diagnoses
Pulmonary infiltrates and fibrosis	Sjögren's syndrome
Intrathoracic lymphadenopathy	Behçet's disease
Lupus pernio, erythema nodosum, nodular rashes	Psoriatic arthritis
Arthritis, dactylitis, tenosynovitis	Reactive arthritis
Parotid swelling	Tuberculosis
Cranial (VIIth) and peripheral neuropathies	Lymphoma
Uveitis	Berylliosis
Sicca syndrome	Systemic lupus erythematosus
Cardiac arrythmias, conduction defects and failure	

develop other manifestations of disease which can affect virtually every organ. Chronic sarcoidosis needs to be distinguished from other forms of multisystem disease, particularly SS and Behçet's disease and from infectious disease such as tuberculosis (Table 4.16).

Pulmonary disease

Interstitial lung disease with development of pulmonary infiltrates and fibrosis is a common feature of chronic sarcoidosis (Fig. 4.15). Pulmonary disease may be asymptomatic or may present with cough, dyspnoea or wheeze. The clinical course is heterogeneous with spontaneous remissions occurring in nearly two thirds of patients.

Lymphadenopathy

Intrathoracic lymphadenopathy may be striking with obvious bilateral hilar lymph nodes seen on plain CXR.

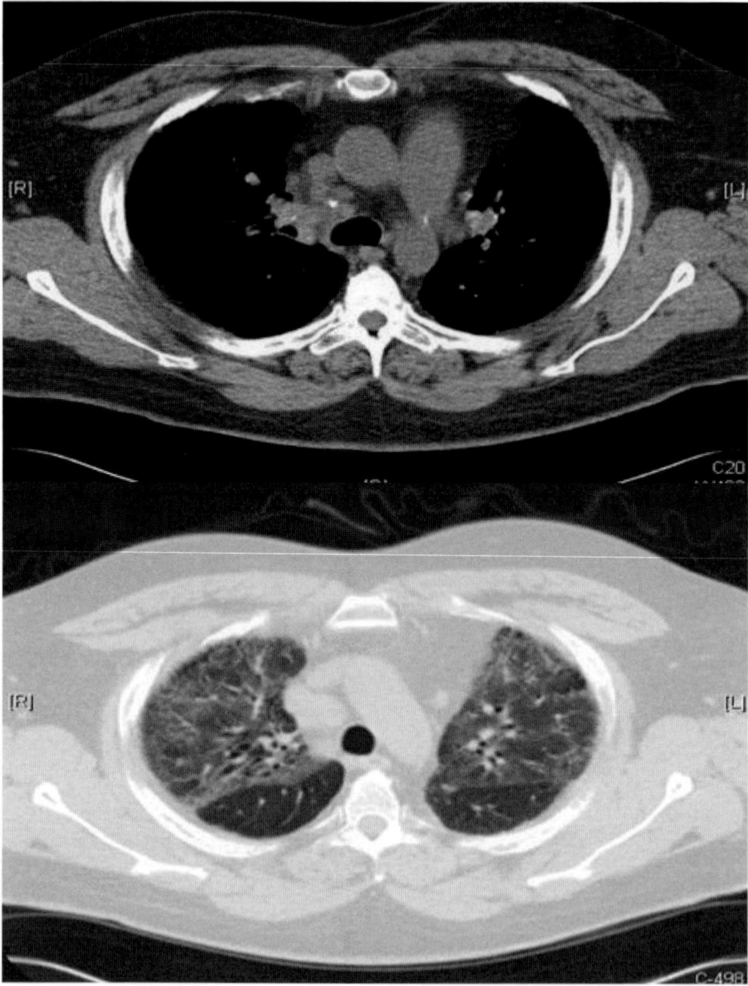

Fig. 4.15. Chest CT scan in a patient with pulmonary sarcoidosis. The upper panel demonstrates hilar lymphadenopathy and the lower panel shows interstitial fibrosis.

Cutaneous disease

Skin involvement occurs in ~30% of cases and may take many forms. A maculopapular eruption usually involves the nose, lips, eyelids, forehead, back of neck and scars or tattoos. Waxy pink nodular lesions may develop on the face, trunk and extensor surfaces of extremities. Erythema nodosum classically occurs on the lower legs. Lupus pernio describes violet discolouration of nose, cheeks, chin and ears.

Parotid involvement

Unilateral or bilateral parotid swelling may occur.

Musculoskeletal

Patients may experience a chronic polyarthritis, tenosynovitis or dactylitis. Rarely, bone cysts, particularly affecting the middle and proximal phalanges, occur.

Neurological

Cranial neuropathies, most classically a unilateral lower motor neuron seventh nerve palsy, may occur. Peripheral neuropathies, aseptic meningitis and granulomatous space occupying lesions in the central nervous system are also features in some patients.

Ocular

Both anterior and posterior uveitis can occur. Lacrimal gland involvement usually presents as painless, bilateral, palpable swellings and may be a cause of dry eyes (sicca symptoms).

Cardiac

Arrythmias, conduction disturbances, cardiac failure and sudden death are all well described; cardiac disease accounts for ~25% of sarcoidosis-associated mortality.

Investigations

Acute sarcoidosis

Positive findings include a neutrophilia, elevated CRP and ESR and presence of bilateral hilar lymphadenopathy on CXR (Stage I; see Table 4.17). Serum ACE and calcium are elevated in only a minority of cases and reflect macrophage hyperactivity. It may be appropriate to check the LDH, ANA, anti-neutrophil cytoplasmic antibody (ANCA), RF, anti-CCP antibodies and carry out an enzyme linked immunosorbent spot (ELISPOT) assay for *M. tuberculosis* to exclude other diagnoses as far as possible. Lymph node biopsy is rarely required if the presentation is classical.

Table 4.17. Staging of pulmonary involvement in sarcoidosis.

Stage	CXR features
Stage 0	Normal chest X-ray
Stage I	Bilateral hilar lymphadenopathy without pulmonary infiltrates
Stage II	Bilateral hilar lymphadenopathy with pulmonary infiltrates
Stage III	Pulmonary infiltrates without hilar adenopathy
Stage IV	End-stage fibrosis, bullae, honeycombing and cavities

Chronic sarcoidosis

Blood tests may be abnormal with an elevated CRP and ESR. Serum ACE and calcium are more commonly elevated than in patients with acute sarcoidosis. An ECG may show conduction abnormalities or arrythmias. The CXR is abnormal in ~95% of cases and is usually described using a staging system (Table 4.17). Further investigation of pulmonary disease with pulmonary function tests, CT scan and bronchoscopy and lavage may be required.

Definitive diagnosis in chronic sarcoidosis is usually made on the basis of biopsy of an affected tissue. This will show non-caseating granulomata, with negative stains for fungus and mycobacteria.

Management

Acute sarcoidosis

Acute sarcoidosis is self-limiting and typically no treatment is required. Arthritis is generally responsive to NSAIDs or a short course of corticosteroids in more severe cases.

Chronic sarcoidosis

Treatment required will depend on the extent and severity of disease. In mild disease no treatment is necessary. Corticosteroids will be effective in more severe disease. The use of other agents such as methotrexate, azathioprine and mycophenolate has not been extensively studied although there is some evidence that these drugs may be effective in arthritis, cardiac and cutaneous disease. There have been case reports of the successful use of anti-TNF agents, especially infliximab, for refractory pulmonary and ocular disease.

Table 4.18. Classification of vasculitis.

Dominant vessel	Primary	Secondary
Large arteries	Takayasu's arteritis Giant cell arteritis	Infection (e.g. syphilis, tuberculosis) Rheumatoid arthritis
Medium arteries	Classic polyarteritis nodosa Kawasaki disease	Hepatitis B associated polyarteritis nodosa
Medium arteries and small vessels	Wegener's granulomatosis* Churg–Strauss syndrome* Microscopic polyangiitis*	Rheumatoid arthritis Systemic lupus erythematosus Sjögren's syndrome, Infection (e.g. HIV) Drugs
Small vessels	Henoch–Schönlein purpura Cryoglobulinaemia Cutaneous leukocytoclastic angiitis	Infection (e.g. HCV) Drugs

* Diseases most commonly associated with anti-neutrophil cytoplasmic antibodies and a significant risk of renal involvement, and most responsive to immunosuppression with cyclophosphamide.
HIV human immunodeficiency virus, HCV hepatitis C virus.

4.2. Vasculitis

The heterogeneity of the systemic vasculitides has resulted in a number of different classification schemes being proposed. Most are based on a division of vasculitis into primary and secondary forms with further subdivision according to the size of vessels involved (Table 4.18). A subset of primary vasculitides involving medium arteries and small vessels are associated with the presence of ANCA. The majority of secondary forms of vasculitis occur in the context of infection, drugs or connective tissue disease.

4.2.1. *Takayasu's Arteritis*

Takayasu's arteritis (TA) is a rare, large vessel vasculitis of unknown cause. The Chapel Hill Consensus Conference defined TA as 'granulomatous inflammation of the aorta and its major branches that usually occurs in patients younger than 50'.

Aetiopathogenesis

The aetiology of TA is unknown. It has been linked to infection but no clear organism has yet been identified. There are weak associations with the HLA molecules HLA B52 and HLA DR4. Anti-endothelial antibodies may be detected in some patients. Pro-inflammatory cytokines IL-12, TNF-α, IL-6 and IL-1 are elevated in the serum and may promote granuloma formation. However, the extent to which the abnormal antibody and cytokine profiles are primary or secondary is unclear.

The pathological changes are a granulomatous necrotising vasculitis (inflammation with cell death) affecting large vessels. There is adventitial thickening, cellular infiltration of the tunica media and local destruction of the vascular smooth muscle. The intima becomes fibrosed which leads to stenosis.

Clinical Features

The clinical features of TA are predominantly a consequence of ischaemia due to narrowing of the lumen of the aorta or its major branches. Patients commonly experience claudication of their arms or, less commonly, legs due to narrowing of the proximal arteries. They may suffer a transient ischaemic attack or stroke due to cerebral ischaemia. Arterial pulses may be decreased, blood pressure measurements may be low or impossible to record in affected limbs and bruits may be audible over the stenoses. Involvement of a carotid artery may be associated with carotidynia (tenderness of the carotid artery), which is a rare but characteristic sign. Involvement of a renal artery results in reduced renal perfusion, stimulating renin production and hence hypertension. TA is a systemic disease and patients often experience fevers, sweats, weight loss and general malaise (Table 4.19).

Table 4.19. American College of Rheumatology classification criteria for TA.

Takayasu's Arteritis
1. Age <40 years
2. Claudication of extremities
3. Decreased pulsation of one or both brachial arteries
4. Difference in systolic blood pressure of >10 mmHg between arms
5. Bruit over subaclavian artery or aorta
6. Arteriographic abnormality involving narrowing or occlusion of aorta, its proximal branches or larger arteries in the proximal upper or lower extremities, not due to atherosclerosis, fibromusclar dysplasia or other causes

For purposes of classification a patient shall be said to have Takayasu's arteritis if at least 3 of these 6 criteria are present. The presence of any 3 or more criteria yields a sensitivity of 90.5% and specificity of 97.8%.

Investigations

Initial investigation is aimed at confirming an inflammatory process involving major arteries.

Blood tests

The CRP and ESR will usually be elevated and there may be a normocytic anaemia. The renal function should be checked, particularly if there is hypertension. An ANCA test will be negative.

Imaging

Assessment of arterial involvement is classically done using percutaneous intravascular contrast angiography but other less invasive techniques are being evaluated (Table 4.20 and Fig. 4.16).

Table 4.20. Investigations to assess arterial involvement in TA.

Test	Reason
Angiography	Percutaneous intravascular contrast angiography has been the gold standard investigation for the diagnosis of TA. Localised narrowing or irregularity of the lumen is the earliest lesion detectable and may develop into stenosis and occlusion. The characteristic finding is the presence of skip lesions where stenoses or aneurysms alternate with normal vessels. Angiography is invasive and provides information on luminal anatomy. It cannot differentiate between active and inactive lesions.
Magnetic resonance angiography	Can provide high resolution imaging of anatomical features including mural thickening, luminal changes and aneurysm formation.
^{18}F-Fluorodeoxyglucose positron emission tomography (^{18}F-FDG-PET)	^{18}F-FDG is taken up by metabolically active cells including those at sites of inflammation. Uptake can be visualized in the walls of inflamed large vessels (>4mm). The role of PET remains to be determined but it may provide information on whether disease is active.
High resolution doppler ultrasound	Provides a non-invasive method of assessing disease especially in the carotid and subclavian arteries. The role remains to be evaluated.

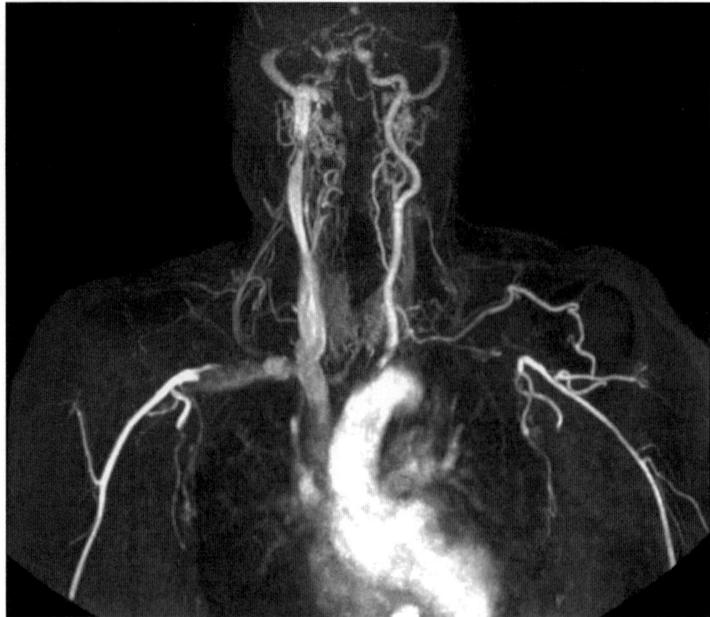

Fig. 4.16. MR angiogram in a patient with Takayasu's aortitis showing lack of blood flow through the left subclavian artery.

Management

Patients need to be educated about the nature of the disease, the requirement for treatment, the side-effects of drugs used and the need for careful monitoring and follow-up.

Immunosuppressive treatment

There are no randomised controlled trials of treatment in TA. Guidelines for the management of large vessel vasculitis have recently been produced by the European League against Rheumatism (EULAR). Treatment in the acute phase is with high dose oral corticosteroids 1 mg/kg (maximum dose 60–80 mg), tapering to 10 mg/day at six months. Methotrexate or azathioprine should be started at the same time as oral corticosteroids; whilst many patients achieve remission on steroids alone, only a minority will remain in remission without use of these second agents. Hypertension should be aggressively managed using conventional anti-hypertensive agents. A relapse should be treated with an increase in prednisolone dose and optimisation of immunosuppression. Patients who are refractory to conventional therapy should be considered for other immunosuppressive agents such as mycophenolate mofetil and biologic agents such as infliximab. There are limited data for the latter but open studies are encouraging.

Surgical treatment

Stenotic lesions may be treated with angioplasty, stenting or bypass procedures. These procedures should only be considered if the stenotic lesions are leading to haemodynamic compromise or if there are aneurysmal lesions which may rupture. Stenting should be considered for renovascular hypertension. Restenosis of lesions is common after initially successful angioplasty.

4.2.2. *Giant Cell Arteritis and Polymyalgia Rheumatica*

Giant cell arteritis (GCA) or temporal arteritis is a common form of vasculitis characterised by involvement of large arteries, particularly extracranial branches arising from the aortic arch. Polymyalgia rheumatica (PMR) is an inflammatory condition characterized by shoulder and pelvic girdle muscle pain and stiffness. Both conditions are rare in individuals less than 50 years of age and have a peak incidence in those over 75 years old. They are more common in females and populations of Scandinavian descent.

Aetiopathogenesis

Inflammation appears to arise in the adventitia of large, extracranial arteries and it is hypothesised that dendritic cells located circumferentially outside the external elastic lamina in these vessels become activated, possibly by a microbial trigger. The activated dendritic cells recruit T cells and activate them locally. This leads to the secretion of T cell cytokines, including IFN-γ which, in turn, activates macrophage differentiation and migration and the formation of giant cells. The multinucleated giant cells secrete metalloproteinases and platelet-derived growth factor that leads to tissue destruction and remodelling resulting in degradation of the internal elastic lamina and occlusive luminal hyperplasia. The inflammation and thickening of the walls of large arteries leads to symptoms reflecting ischaemia or infarction of the tissues served by these vessels. GCA and PMR probably reflect the severe and mild ends, respectively, of a spectrum of clinical phenotypes.

Clinical Features

GCA is characterised by new onset of headaches, frequently temporal in distribution. The temporal artery is often thickened, tender and may be non-pulsatile. The scalp may be tender to touch; patients notice this when they comb their hair. Jaw claudication or tongue claudication may occur when eating. Visual symptoms are important; the classical pattern is of amaurosis fugax in which the patient describes a 'curtain' descending transiently to obscure vision in one eye. Transient visual disturbance may be a prelude to permanent loss. Examination of the eyes to include assessment of visual acuity, visual fields and fundoscopy is important. Notably the combination of headaches and visual symptoms may also be a feature of alternative diagnoses including migraine or meningitis. Occasionally, in patients with GCA, bruits may be heard in the affected arteries, particularly the carotids. Patients very often have polymyalgic features with limb girdle pain and stiffness as described below.

PMR is characterised by pain and weakness affecting the shoulder and hip girdles with prominent morning stiffness. The onset is often quite acute. Patients describe severe aching affecting the muscles and difficulty raising their arms and standing from sitting. In severe cases patients may be unable to get out of bed in the mornings. Despite the symptoms, and in contrast to findings in inflammatory myositis, examination usually shows absence of actual muscle tenderness and normal strength. Patients often experience arthralgias as part of PMR and may even have synovitis; in these cases it can be difficult to distinguish between PMR and polymyalgic onset RA. A proportion of individuals with PMR will progress to develop features of GCA.

In both conditions, non-specific symptoms including fever, malaise and weight loss may be prominent. In all cases the differential diagnoses of malignancy, infection or another immune-mediated inflammatory disease must be considered.

The ACR criteria are often used to help make the diagnosis of GCA (Table 4.21).

Several diagnostic criteria have been proposed for PMR; the Jones and Hazleman (1981) criteria shown in Table 4.22 are often used.

Investigations

The typical finding is one of raised ESR and CRP; these markers are not only useful diagnostically but are very helpful in monitoring response to treatment. The FBC may show a leukocytosis and thrombocytosis, consistent with an inflammatory state.

Patients with suspected GCA should normally have a temporal artery biopsy; the histolopathology may be normal in some individuals with true disease as the lesions are focal ('skip lesions'). The likelihood of a positive biopsy falls

Table 4.21. ACR criteria for classification of GCA.

Criteria	Details
Age	Onset >50 years
New headaches	New onset or new types of headaches
Temporal artery abnormality	Temporal artery tender to palpation or non-pulsatile
Increase in ESR	ESR >50 mm/h by Westergren method
Abnormal artery biopsy	Vasculitis characterised by a predominance of mononuclear infiltrates or granulomas, usually with multi-nucleated giant cells

Three of five criteria required.

Table 4.22. Jones and Hazleman criteria for diagnosis of PMR.

Criteria for diagnosis of polymyalgia rheumatica
Shoulder and pelvic girdle muscle pain without weakness
Morning stiffness
Symptom duration >two months unless treated
ESR >30 mm/h and/or CRP level greater than 6 mg/l
No RA, inflammatory arthritis or malignant neoplasm
No objective signs of muscle disease
Prompt and dramatic response to systemic corticosteroid therapy

All criteria required.

CRP C-reactive protein, ESR erythrocyte sedimentation rate, RA rheumatoid arthritis.

significantly in individuals who have had corticosteroids for more than two weeks. Some centres are using imaging techniques, particularly ultrasound scanning of the temporal arteries, as a further tool to aid diagnosis. The characteristic finding is of a halo sign around involved arteries.

Testing for anti-CCP and RF and for CK levels is important to exclude the differential diagnoses of RA and inflammatory myositis. Negative tests for ANA, ANCA and APLA will help exclude other connective tissue diseases and vasculitides. Immunoglobulins with an electrophoretic strip and urinary Bence Jones protein should be requested to exclude multiple myeloma in all patients and further investigations to exclude a malignancy should be undertaken if there are any suspicious or localising features.

Management

All patients should be educated about the potentially serious nature of the condition and the risk of blindness if arteritis is inadequately treated.

Patients with GCA should initially be treated with high dose oral steroids at a dose of 1 mg/kg/day. If visual symptoms are present then patients should receive iv methylprednisolone, usually at a dose of 1 g/day, for three days prior to treatment with oral prednisolone. The steroid dose should be tapered gradually, titrating against symptoms and ESR or CRP, generally aiming for approximately 20mgs od at two to three months and 10 mg od at six months with a view to completing the course of treatment within approximately 18–24 months. Many rheumatologists also advise low dose aspirin to reduce the risk of thrombosis.

Patients with PMR should be treated with oral steroids at the lower dose of 15 mg/day. Symptoms should improve within one to three days and the diagnosis should be reconsidered if that does not occur. Steroid dose should be tapered, titrating against symptoms and ESR or CRP, generally to reach 10 mg/day by two to three months and then by an average of 1 mg/day every one to two months, with a view to completing the course of treatment within approximately 18–24 months.

Steroid sparing agents, particularly methotrexate or azathioprine are often used in both PMR and GCA if patients relapse whilst the steroid dose is being reduced although the evidence base for their efficacy in these conditions is limited. The need for gastroprotection with a proton pump inhibitor and bone protection with calcium and vitamin D supplementation and a bisphosphonate should be considered in all patients.

Whilst prednisolone treatment can be withdrawn in the majority of patients by two years, a minority experience relapsing or persistent disease that requires treatment for much longer. When managing individuals with apparently relapsing or persistent disease it is very important to exclude other causes for limb girdle pain, such as development of cervical spondylosis or mechanical shoulder problems, or for the elevated ESR or CRP, such as multiple myeloma or infection.

4.2.3. *Polyarteritis Nodosa*

Polyarteritis nodosa (PAN) is a rare vasculitis with necrotising (associated with tissue death) inflammation of medium-sized or small arteries, without glomerulonephritis or vasculitis in arterioles, capillaries or venules.

Aetiopathogenesis

PAN is often the consequence of Hepatitis B Virus (HBV) infection and in these cases there is good evidence for immune complex disease with hepatitis B surface antigen being the triggering factor. HBV-PAN is associated with wild type

HBV, HBe antigenaemia and high HBV replication rates, suggesting that vasculitis could result from deposition of soluble antigen-antibody complexes in antigen excess (HBe). These immune complexes then activate the complement cascade, in turn attracting and activating neutrophils.

The pathological appearances are of a focal necrotizing vasculitis affecting medium and small arteries. The inflammation is characterised by fibrinoid necrosis (necrotic areas with staining pattern of fibrin) and a pleomorphic cellular infiltrate, with predominant macrophages and lymphocytes.

Clinical Features

The condition is multisystem and most organs may be involved. Fatigue, weight loss and myalgias often occur. Skin involvement is one of the most common features, the typical rash being livedo reticularis. Testicular pain and tenderness is typical. Neuropathy is a common feature with a mononeuritis multiplex or sensorimotor neuropathy presenting with changes in sensation and/or motor function. The blood pressure should be checked to detect hypertension and urinalysis performed to detect renal disease. Gastrointestinal tract involvement is uncommon but associated with a poor prognosis. Cardiac involvement may also occur. All patients should be asked about the possibility of HBV infection (Table 4.23).

Investigations

Investigations are performed to aid the diagnosis of PAN, assess organ involvement and monitor patients with known disease. There are no specific serological markers for PAN and definite diagnosis usually rests on demonstration of typical arteriographic abnormalities or histopathological changes, particularly where there is evidence of HBV infection.

Blood tests

FBC may show anaemia of chronic disease and an eosinophilia, although the latter is more suggestive of Churg–Strauss syndrome (CSS). The ESR and CRP will be raised, consistent with an acute phase response. Abnormal renal function suggests renal involvement, abnormal liver function may point towards HBV infection. Serological studies for ANCA and other autoantibodies including ANA, RF and anti-CCP antibodies will generally be negative. Tests for HBV infection will usually be positive. Blood cultures should be performed to exclude a diagnosis of bacterial endocarditis, which can mimic vasculitis.

Table 4.23. ACR classification criteria for PAN.

Criteria	Details
1. Weight loss	>4 kg weight loss not due to dieting or other factors
2. Livedo reticularis	Mottled reticular rash
3. Testicular pain or tenderness	Not due to infection, trauma or other causes
4. Myalgias, weakness or leg tenderness	Diffuse myalgias or muscle weakness or leg muscle tenderness
5. Mononeuropathy or polyneuropathy	Mononeuropathy, mononeuritis multiplex or polyneuropathy
6. Hypertension	Diastolic blood pressure >90 mmHg
7. Elevated urea or creatinine	BUN >40 mg/dl or creatinine >1.5 mg/dl in absence of dehydration or obstruction
8. HBV infection	Presence of Hepatitis B surface antigen or antibody in serum
9. Arteriographic abnormality	Arteriogram showing aneurysms or occlusions of visceral arteries not due to arteriosclerosis, fibromuscular dysplasia or other non-inflammatory causes
10. Histological evidence	Biopsy of small or medium artery showing granulocytes +/– mononuclear cells in artery wall

For purposes of classification a patient shall be said to have PAN if at least three of these 10 criteria are present.
The presence of any three or more criteria yields a sensitivity of 82.2% and a specificity of 86.6%.
BUN blood urea nitrogen, HBV hepatitis B virus.

Imaging studies

CXR will usually be normal in patients with PAN; however, it should be performed to help exclude the differential diagnoses of ANCA associated vasculitis (AAV), malignancy and infection. Angiography is often key to diagnosis; it will show the typical microaneurysms and/or stenoses in the coeliac axis and renal vasculature.

Other investigations

Histopathology of involved tissue is very helpful in confirming the diagnosis if it can be obtained. Initiation of therapy should not be delayed for purposes of obtaining a tissue biopsy. Neurophysiological studies will confirm involvement of peripheral nerves and echocardiography may be helpful in detecting cardiac involvement. Urinalysis should be performed at every visit and a protein:creatinine ratio may also be useful in detecting early renal involvement.

Management

The nature, relationship to HBV infection and prognosis of PAN should be discussed with patients. Drug toxicity may be considerable and patients should be well informed prior to initiation of therapy. Advice about regular follow up is needed.

Treatment of non-HBV PAN

The principles are as for the ANCA associated vasculitides (see below) and are based on immunosuppression with glucocorticoids and cyclophosphamide.

HBV associated PAN

Where PAN is associated with HBV infection then treatment should be with antiviral therapy. There are no controlled trials as the condition is rare. The current preferred protocol is Lamivudine (100 mg/day) combined with plasma exchange to remove immune complexes. This is accompanied by a short course of corticosteroids. Seroconversion from HBe antigenaemia to seropositivity for HBe antibodies is usually achieved and is associated with a decreased risk of relapse.

Monitoring

Patients should be reviewed at least every three months in the longer term to assess disease activity and damage. Objective scoring using the Birmingham Vasculitis Activity Score and Vasculitis Disease Index will help provide an accurate assessment. Regular monitoring for drug toxicity is mandatory where agents such as cyclophosphamide, azathioprine or mycophenolate are being used. As with all chronic inflammatory disease, careful management of cardiovascular risk factors is important.

Prognosis

Properly treated, PAN has a low relapse rate and, overall, a good prognosis. However, the outcome for individuals who have evidence of renal, gastrointestinal, cardiac or neurological involvement at presentation is less good.

4.2.4. *ANCA-Associated Vasculitis*

The ANCA-associated vasculitides are a group of rare medium/small vessel systemic vasculitides characterised by necrotising vasculitis (inflammation of vessel walls associated with tissue death) and the serological presence of ANCA. Three main conditions are considered within the term AAV: Wegener's granulomatosis (WG), Churg–Strauss syndrome (CSS) and microscopic polyangiitis (MPA). Definitions for these conditions were proposed by the Chapel Hill Consensus Conference in 1994 and are generally accepted.

Wegener's granulomatosis

Granulomatous inflammation involving the respiratory tract, and necrotizing vasculitis affecting small to medium sized vessels (e.g. capillaries, venules, arterioles and arteries). Necrotising glomerulonephritis is common.

Microscopic polyangiitis

Necrotising vasculitis, with few or no immune deposits, affecting small vessels (i.e. capillaries, venules, or arterioles). Necrotising arteritis involving small and medium-sized arteries may be present. Necrotising glomerulonephritis is very common. Pulmonary capillaritis often occurs.

Churg–Strauss syndrome

Eosinophil-rich and granulomatous inflammation involving the respiratory tract, necrotising vasculitis affecting small to medium-sized vessels and associated with asthma and eosinophilia.

Pathogenesis

ANCA play a key role in the pathogenesis of systemic vasculitis. ANCA are specific for target antigens located in the primary granules of neutrophils and lysosomes of monocytes, and the plasma membrane secretory vesicles. ANCA are conventionally detected by indirect immunofluorescence and two main patterns are detected: cytoplasmic with a coarse granular pattern throughout the cytoplasm (cANCA) and perinuclear with staining around the nucleus (pANCA). The target antigen for cANCA is proteinase 3 (PR3) and for pANCA is myeloperoxidase (MPO). There is now good clinical and experimental evidence that MPO-ANCA are pathogenic and laboratory evidence that anti-PR3 antibodies can amplify local inflammation. A hypothetical model has been proposed to explain the generation of ANCA-mediated vascular inflammation. It is suggested that cytokines and other priming factors induce neutrophils to express ANCA antigens on the cell surface. ANCA engage with these antigens leading to neutrophil activation. The activated neutrophils interact with endothelial cells and release toxic factors leading to apoptosis and necrosis.

Cytokines are important in pathogenesis of AAV. A Th1 cytokine profile has been reported in WG, with monocytes from clinically active WG patients showing increased secretion of IFN-γ and TNF-α but not IL-4, IL-5 or IL-10. In contrast, in CSS there appears to be a prominent role for Th2 as well as Th1 cytokines with monocytes secreting large amounts of IL-5, which is thought to contribute to the eosinophilia of CSS.

Clinical Features

The conditions are multisystem and most organs may be involved. Typically patients will have constitutional features with a purpuric rash and involvement of the respiratory and renal tract.

Constitutional features

Fevers, sweats, malaise and weight loss are common in all three types of AAV.

Skin

Typically a palpable purpuric rash occurs, often seen over the lower legs or elbows (Fig. 4.17).

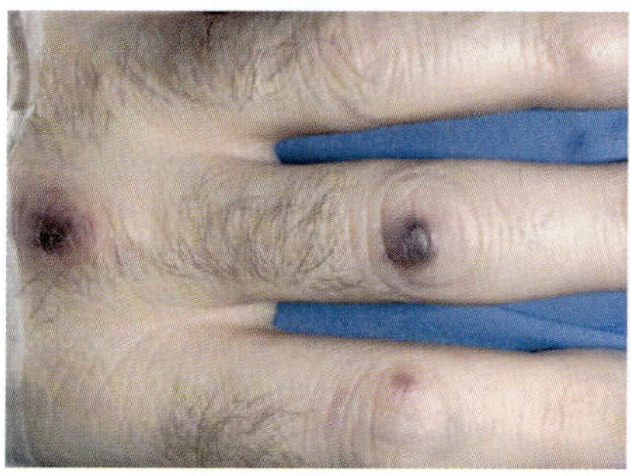
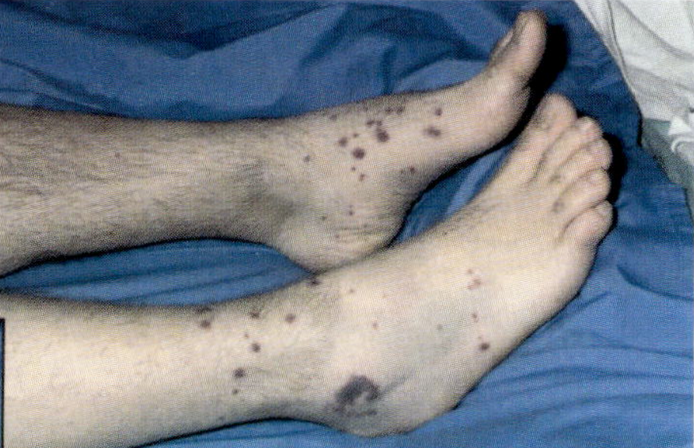

Fig. 4.17. Skin lesions on hands and feet in a patient with Wegener's granulomatosis.

Kidneys

Necrotising glomerulitis occurs in all three types of AAV. Patients may note frothiness of urine (reflecting high protein content), 'smokiness' of urine (reflecting presence of red blood cells) and, in severe renal disease, may become oligouric or anuric. Urinalysis to detect proteinuria and microscopic haematuria is mandatory at presentation and at every clinic visit.

Lungs

Nodules, often large and with cavities, occur within the lungs in WG (Fig. 4.18). Pulmonary haemorrhage is a feature of MPA. Patients with WG or MPA may present with chest pain, breathlessness and haemoptysis. Asthma is a feature of CSS.

Upper respiratory tract

Sinusitis, epistaxis and nasal crusting are features of WG. Chronic nasal disease may result in a 'saddle nose' deformity.

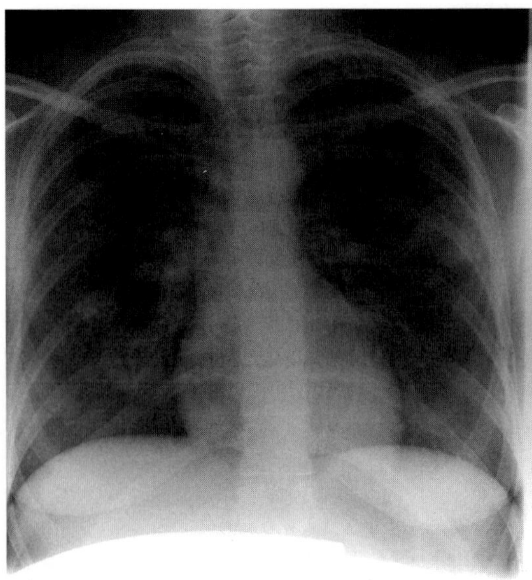

Fig. 4.18. Pulmonary lesions in a patient with Wegener's granulomatosis. Note the large nodules with cavities within the right lung.

Nervous system

Mononeuritis multiplex or a sensori-motor neuropathy is more frequent in CSS and MPA than WG. Patients may develop 'pins and needles' or localised weakness.

Eyes

Scleritis occurs in WG.

Gastrointestinal tract involvement

Oral ulceration is often reported. More extensive involvement of the gastrointestinal tract is uncommon but associated with a poor prognosis.

Classification criteria

The ACR have produced classification criteria for WG and CSS but not MPA (Tables 4.24 and 4.25).

Investigations

Investigations are performed to aid the diagnosis of AAV, assess organ involvement and to monitor patients with known disease. Whilst diagnosis is based on

Table 4.24. ACR classification criteria for WG.

Criteria	Details
1. Nasal or oral inflammation	Oral ulcers or purulent/blood-stained nasal discharge
2. Abnormal chest radiograph	Nodules, fixed infiltrates or cavities seen on chest X-ray
3. Urinary sediment	Microhaematuria or red cell casts in urinary sediment
4. Granulomatous inflammation	Histological changes showing granulomatous inflammation within the wall of artery or arteriole in the perivascular or extravascular area

For purposes of classification, a person shall be said to have WG if at least two of these four criteria are present. The presence of any two or more criteria yields a sensitivity of 88.2% and a specificity of 92.0%.

Table 4.25. ACR classification criteria for CSS.

Criteria	Details
1. Asthma	History of wheezing or diffuse high pitched rales on expiration
2. Eosinophilia	10% on white cell differential count
3. Neuropathy	Mononeuropathy, mononeuritis multiplex or polyneuropathy due to systemic vasculitis
4. Pulmonary infiltrates	Migratory or transient pulmonary infiltrates due to a systemic vasculitis
5. Paranasal sinus abnormality	History of acute or chronic paranasal sinus abnormality or tenderness or radiographic opacification of the paranasal sinuses
6. Extravascular eosinophils	Biopsy including artery, arteriole, or venule showing accumulations of eosinophils in extravascular areas

For purposes of classification, a person shall be said to have CSS if at least four of these six criteria are present.

the overall clinical picture, the presence of ANCA and typical histological changes on tissue biopsy are both very helpful.

Blood tests

FBC will often show anaemia of chronic disease. Eosinophilia is suggestive of CSS. Both the ESR and CRP will be elevated, reflecting the inflammatory response. Renal and LFTs may be abnormal if these organs are involved. An ANCA test may be positive, with a cANCA or pANCA staining pattern and specificity for PR3 or MPO. Whilst the specificity of the antibodies does not absolutely correlate with the clinical diagnosis, antibodies specific for PR3 are strongly associated with WG and those specific for MPO are associated with MPA and are also found in approximately 50% of cases of CSS. Serological tests for ANA, RF and anti-CCP will help to exclude other autoimmune rheumatic diseases and blood cultures and serological tests for HBV, HCV and CMV should also be performed to exclude vasculitis secondary to infection.

Imaging studies

CXR should be requested to look for evidence of cavities, granulomata, pulmonary haemorrhage and to exclude infection or neoplasm. It may be necessary to proceed to high resolution CT scanning of the chest to further define the extent and nature of pulmonary involvement. A CT or MRI scan of the sinuses may demonstrate upper respiratory tract involvement. Angiography is not usually helpful in the diagnosis or assessment of the AAV but may be required to exclude a larger vessel vasculitis or PAN.

Other investigations

Histopathology of involved tissue (often obtained from a renal biopsy) will help to confirm the diagnosis. Treatment should, however, not be delayed until results are available. Neurophysiological tests will be required if patients have features of peripheral nerve involvement. An ECG and echocardiogram should be requested if there are signs of cardiac disease.

Management

The AAV are relapsing remitting conditions and life-long care is required. The nature and prognosis of the AAV should be discussed with patients. Drug toxicity, particularly that of cyclophosphamide, is considerable and patients should be well informed prior to initiation of therapy. The treatment of AAV can be divided into three phases: remission induction, consolidation and remission maintenance.

Immunosuppressive treatment

The use of immunosuppressive drugs is based on a series of randomised controlled trials conducted in Europe over the past decade. Patients can be divided into three groups and the intensity of therapy is based on the severity of organ involvement, particularly renal function (Table 4.26).

Induction/consolidation

Early limited disease: Many patients with early disease or organ-limited disease especially involving the upper respiratory tract may be successfully managed with glucocorticoids and methotrexate. A randomised controlled trial demonstrated that methotrexate and cyclophosphamide were of equal efficacy in remission induction but that methotrexate was less toxic.

Organ-threatening disease: Cyclophosphamide is the gold standard treatment and when combined with glucocorticoids is highly effective in inducing remission. Use of pulses of intravenous cyclophosphamide is preferred to oral dosing as it allows a lower cumulative dose and hence reduced toxicity. Recent trials

Table 4.26. Categories of disease severity and treatment.

Clinical subgroup	Constitutional symptoms	Typical ANCA status	Threatened vital organ function	Serum creatinine (μmol/l)	Treatment Induction
Localised or early systemic	Yes	Positive or negative	No	<150	Methotrexate or Cyclophosphamide Glucocorticoids
Generalised	Yes	Positive	Yes	<500	Cyclophosphamide Glucocorticoids
Severe	Yes	Positive	Yes	>500	Cyclophosphamide Glucocorticoids Plasma exchange

suggest that rituximab, a B cell-depleting monoclonal antibody, may offer an alternative to cyclophosphamide in inducing remission in AAV.

Life-threatening disease: Cyclophosphamide and glucocorticoids are mandatory. A recent trial has shown that adjunctive plasma exchange is beneficial in patients with creatinine >500 mmol/l. Plasma exchange should also be considered in patients with pulmonary haemorrhage.

Remission maintenance: Induction therapy should be continued until remission is achieved and consolidated; typically this takes two to six months. Cyclophosphamide should then be stopped and maintenance therapy continued with either azathioprine or methotrexate. Glucocorticoids should be tapered.

Drug toxicity

Treatment regimens, particularly those including cyclophosphamide, are associated with significant toxicity and care must be taken to minimise this where possible (Table 4.27).

Monitoring

Patients should be reviewed regularly to assess disease activity and damage. Objective scoring using the Birmingham Vasculitis Activity Score and Vasculitis Disease Index will help provide an accurate assessment. Urinalysis must be performed at each visit in order to detect glomerulonephritis in the early stages. Testing for ANCA should also be performed; in many patients the antibody levels fall

Table 4.27. Minimising toxicity of treatment.

Toxicity/morbidity	Management
Dyspepsia/reflux	Proton pump inhibitors
Osteoporosis secondary to glucocorticoids	Calcium, vitamin D, bisphosphonates
Haemorrhagic cystitis secondary to cyclophosphamide	Mesna before and after intravenous cyclophosphamide
Bladder cancer secondary to cyclophosphamide	Mesna before and after intravenous cyclophosphamide
Infertility secondary to cyclophosphamide	Minimise dose. Consider sperm/egg storage
Pneumocystis jirovecii infection	Septrin
Influenza, pneumonia	Influenza and pneumococcal vaccination

following initial treatment and a subsequent rise can presage a relapse in disease. Monitoring for drug toxicity is mandatory where agents such as cyclophosphamide, azathioprine or mycophenolate are being used. As with all chronic inflammatory disease, careful management of cardiovascular risk factors is important.

Prognosis

Untreated, AAV is associated with a very poor prognosis, with 90% mortality at one year for WG. Modern treatment regimens as described above are associated with much less mortality and the five year survival is now 75% for WG, 45–75% for MPA and up to 90% for CSS.

4.2.5. *Henoch–Schönlein Purpura*

Henoch–Schönlein purpura (HSP) is an acute small vessel vasculitis occurring predominantly in childhood with IgA-dominant immune deposits.

Pathogenesis

The aetiology of HSP is obscure. There is a seasonal pattern in some series suggesting an infectious trigger. However, although it is commonly observed that an infection precedes the onset of HSP by several weeks, no specific infectious agent has been identified.

The characteristic pathological lesion is a leukocytoclastic vasculitis (vessel inflammation with exudation of neutrophils, erythrocytes and sometimes fibrin, with nuclear dust) involving small capillaries and post capillary venules in the skin and focal or diffuse proliferative glomerulonephritis. Deposition of IgA in affected vessels is highly characteristic.

Clinical Features

HSP occurs most commonly in children aged between five and seven years and is rare in adults. The condition typically involves the skin, joints, kidneys and gastrointestinal tract (Table 4.28). Patients often also experience prominent fatigue.

Skin involvement

A purpuric rash, which may be palpable, is characteristic and classically occurs on the buttocks and legs (Fig. 4.19).

Joints

Arthralgias or arthritis with swollen joints frequently occur.

Gastrointestinal tract involvement

This is common and due to involvement of mesenteric vessels resulting in bowel ischaemia. Patients experience abdominal pain that is exacerbated by eating, or bloody diarrhoea.

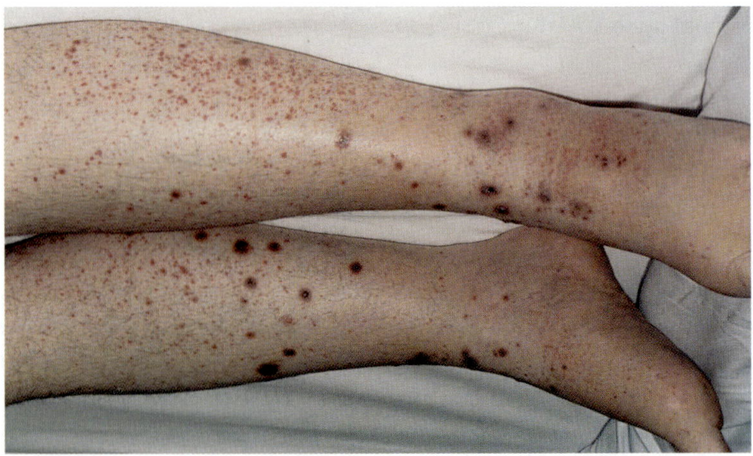

Fig. 4.19. Purpuric rash in a patient with Henoch–Schönlein purpura.

Table 4.28. ACR classification criteria for HSP.

Criteria	Details
1. Palpable purpura	Slightly elevated purpuric rash not related to thrombocytopenia
2. Bowel angina	Diffuse abdominal pain worse after meals, or bowel ischaemia usually with bloody diarrhoea
3. Age at onset <20 years	First symptoms occurring at or before age of 20 years
4. Biopsy findings	Histological changes showing granulocytes in walls of arteries or venules

For purposes of classification a patient shall be said to have HS purpura if at least two of these four criteria are present. The presence of any two or more criteria yields a sensitivity of 87.1% and a specificity of 87.7%.

Kidneys

Glomerulonephritis occurs and may be asymptomatic. Assessment of blood pressure and urinalysis to test for proteinuria and microscopic haematuria are mandatory; abnormalities of either are suggestive of renal involvement. Patients may develop hypertension, nephritic syndrome or nephrotic syndrome; all three are poor prognostic signs.

Investigations

Investigations are performed to aid the diagnosis of HSP, assess organ involvement and monitor patients with known disease. Blood tests are rarely required in children if the presentation is typical. In adults the condition is much rarer and needs to be differentiated from other causes of vasculitis, both primary and secondary.

Blood tests

The ESR and CRP may be elevated. Biochemical tests may indicate renal involvement with a high creatinine value and, if a nephrotic syndrome develops, low albumin value. The FBC may show anaemia of chronic disease but should otherwise be normal; low platelets or other abnormalities may suggest immune thrombocytopenic purpura or leukaemia as the cause for the purpura. Tests for ANA, RF, anti-CCP and ANCA will be negative and will help to exclude autoimmune rheumatic disease and other forms of vasculitis. C3 and C4 complement proteins may be normal or low reflecting consumption. Blood cultures will help to exclude meningococcal septicaemia as a cause of the purpuric rash.

Other investigations

A renal biopsy should be considered in both children and adults if there is significant and persistent proteinuria or haematuria.

Management

Most patients do not need specific therapy as the condition is self-limiting. NSAIDs help the arthralgia but should be avoided in those with significant renal involvement. The role of corticosteroids is controversial. Several trials have shown that, in children, the routine use of corticosteroids early in the disease process does not alter the progression to severe nephritis or gastrointestinal complications. Prednisolone is, however, effective in reducing the severity of abdominal pain and arthralgias. Patients with severe abdominal pain should therefore probably receive corticosteroids. There are no trials to guide therapy in patients with rapidly progressive or established glomerulonephritis and these patients should receive immunosuppressive therapy, following similar protocols to those used for AAV (see above).

Prognosis

Most patients have a good prognosis and the illness is self-limiting, resolving within two to three weeks. However, recurrent attacks of purpura and abdominal pain are common. Chronic renal failure develops in a small proportion of patients and is associated with hypertension, nephritis or nephrotic syndrome at presentation.

Chapter 5

Metabolic Bone Disease and Inherited Disorders of Bone and Connective Tissue

Editor: Paul Wordsworth

Pille Harrison, Paul Wordsworth

5.1. Osteoporosis

Osteoporosis (OP) is a common and potentially disabling skeletal disease. It is caused by compromised bone strength due to low bone mass and progressive microarchitectural deterioration of skeletal tissue, leading to increased bone fragility and fractures. The prevalence of OP is typically measured indirectly through the incidence of fractures resulting from the condition. It is frequently referred to as a 'silent disease' since the deterioration of the skeletal tissue usually progresses without any clear clinical signs until fracture occurs. The most common sites for fracture are the wrist, hip and spine following low-energy trauma but, since the whole skeleton is involved, fractures may occur at any site.

OP is the most common skeletal disorder. It is highly prevalent in postmenopausal women and is strongly associated with old age in both sexes. Its incidence is rising in parallel with the increasing age of the general population. Worldwide, the prevalence of OP as defined by the World Health Organisation (WHO) is approximately 5% in women and 2.4% in men aged 50 years, rising to 50% in women and 20% in men aged 85 years. However, the prevalence and incidence vary greatly in different countries with the highest rates seen in the USA and Europe and lower rates in Africa and Asia. In the UK, around 23% of all women aged ≥ 50 years are osteoporotic.

Aetiopathogenesis

Bone consists of two main types: a compact outer layer of cortical bone, which is 90% calcified bone, and a honeycomb-like inner mesh of spongy trabecular bone, only 25% of which consists of calcified bone (the remainder is bone marrow, connective tissue, fat and blood vessels). As a living tissue, bone is metabolically active throughout life. Initial modelling assures normal bone growth and shape. Constant remodelling, a key adaptive response to stress, occurs throughout life. Both modelling and remodelling depend on the co-ordinated activity of osteoblasts, responsible for bone synthesis, and osteoclasts, necessary for bone resorption. Skeletal growth in childhood is dominated by bone formation leading to gradual increase in bone size and density until peak bone mass is achieved by about 25 years of age. OP is the consequence of an imbalance of bone remodelling over time, in which bone resorption predominates over bone formation. Gradual loss of cortical and trabecular bone can be seen from early adult years, accompanied by deterioration in the structural integrity and increased fragility of trabecular bone in particular. Many factors are involved in the pathogenesis of OP, some of which are genetic and some environmental (Fig. 5.1). Perhaps the most important of these is peak bone mass, which is under strong genetic control. It is largely because men have higher peak bone mass that they are relatively protected from OP. In women, bone loss accelerates after the menopause due to a significant fall in circulating

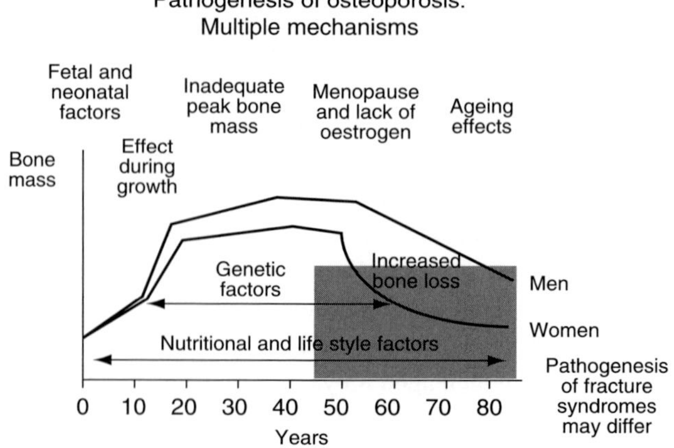

Fig. 5.1. Multiple pathogenetic mechanisms are involved in OP development. Adapted from Russell *et al.*, 2006.

oestrogen levels. This loss is particularly rapid during the first five years and can reach up to 3% per year in the spine. In older men low oestrogen levels also have been correlated with low bone mineral density (BMD) indicating that oestrogens are important regulators of bone formation in both genders. Bone loss in older people is influenced by a number of other factors including increased parathyroid hormone (PTH) levels, vitamin D deficiency and low calcium intake. Discrete monogenic causes of OP are well described. These include osteogenesis imperfecta (OI) and hypophosphatasia, which are covered elsewhere.

Risk factors for OP and fracture

- Genetic: These include female gender and maternal family history of hip fracture. It is estimated that up to 60–85% of the variance in BMD is genetically determined. Genes encoding type 1 collagen, vitamin D receptor, aromatase, low density lipoprotein (LDL)-receptor related protein 5 (LRP5) and the oestrogen receptor have been most widely studied. However, the percentage of OP risk explained by any of these genetic factors individually is relatively small, indicating that many components of the genetic risk remain to be discovered.
- Racial: African-Caribbeans and Asians are much less likely to develop OP than Caucasians.
- Sex hormones: Oestrogen deficiency due to premature menopause and hypogonadism in men are also risk factors.
- Age: Ageing bone is more susceptible to fractures due to decreasing quality of bone. The elderly are also more susceptible to fall-induced fractures as a result of impaired vision, balance and lower muscle mass.
- Environmental: Inadequate physical activity and calcium consumption, cigarette smoking, excess caffeine and alcohol intake have all been linked to OP.
- Drugs: Glucocorticoids are a clear risk factor. Anticoagulants (heparin and warfarin), anticonvulsants, lithium and serotonin re-uptake inhibitors are also associated with development of OP.
- Secondary causes: A large number of other medical conditions predispose to development of OP (Table 5.1).

Clinical Features

OP often progresses without any clinical features and becomes apparent only after a patient has sustained a minimal trauma fracture.

Table 5.1. Secondary causes of osteoporosis.

Class of disease	Examples
Endocrine disease	Cushing's syndrome, type I and type II diabetes, hyperthyroidism, hypogonadism, hyperparathyroidism, hypopituitarism
Gastrointestinal disease	Inflammatory bowel disease, coeliac disease, primary biliary cirrhosis, gastrectomy
Inflammatory arthritis	Rheumatoid arthritis, ankylosing spondylitis, systemic lupus erythemathosus
Malignancy	Multiple myeloma, lymphoproliferative and myeloproliferative diseases, metastatic malignancy
Psychiatric disease	Anorexia nervosa, exercise-induced amenorrhoea
Others	Gaucher's disease, mastocytosis, chronic renal failure

Hip fracture

Among the osteoporotic fractures, hip fracture has the most devastating consequences resulting in pain, loss of mobility and excess mortality. Around 90% of hip fractures result from a simple fall from standing height or less. The average age of an individual experiencing a hip fracture in developed countries is ~80 years and, in line with the increase in life expectancy, the number of hip fractures is predicted to increase dramatically over the next few decades. In the UK and USA the incidence of hip fracture amongst women is twice that amongst men. However, this female preponderance is not common to all populations. The incidence of hip fractures in men is equal to or greater than that in women in Maoris (New Zealand) and Bantus (South Africa).

Vertebral fracture

Vertebral fractures are the most common osteoporotic fractures (Fig. 5.2). The incidence and prevalence of radiologically identified vertebral deformity increases with age. In Europe, one in eight men and women over the age of 50 have vertebral deformity. The prevalence of vertebral fractures is similar in Asian and Caucasian women, appearing less common in black and Hispanic populations. Vertebral fractures occur most commonly in the lower thoracic segment and at the thoracolumbar junction and are the result of compressive loading associated with daily activities like lifting. Only ~30% of new vertebral fractures relate to falls and only 10–30% of vertebral fractures present symptomatically. Those

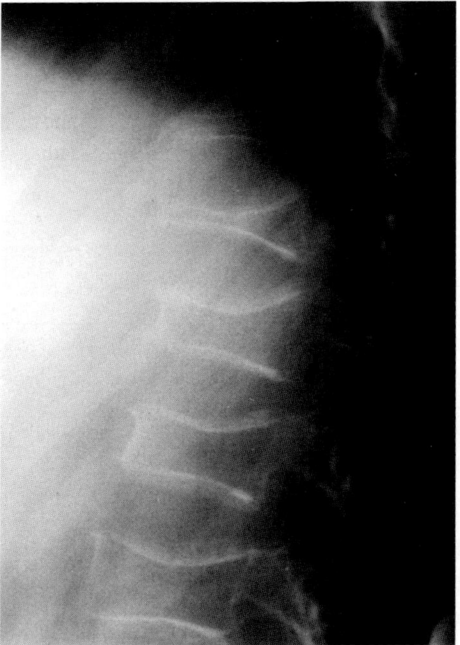

Fig. 5.2. Severe OP of the spine with typical biconcave vertebrae and crush fractures.

that do may affect quality of life by limiting activities and restricting participation. In general, pain and disability worsen with each new vertebral fracture and with increasing spinal deformity.

OP in pregnancy

OP associated with pregnancy and lactation is a rare condition that usually presents with fragility fracture most commonly in the third trimester or just after delivery in primagravid women. Most frequently one or more vertebral fractures are observed that can cause severe and prolonged pain and height loss in the affected women.

Mortality

The effect of fractures on mortality depends very much on the type of fracture. Hip fracture has the most serious consequences since 10–20% more women die than expected for age within the first year and the excess of mortality is even greater for

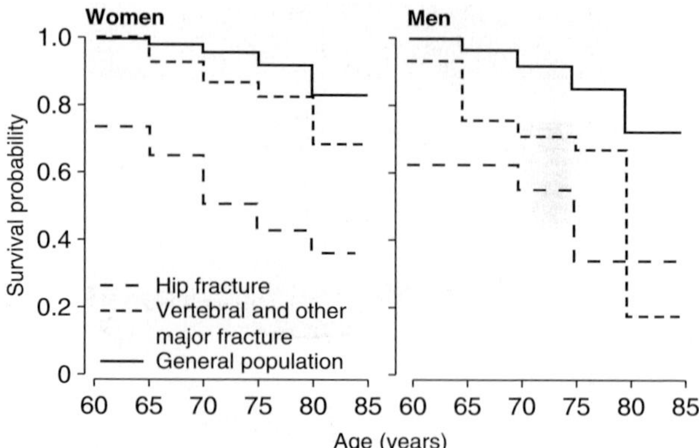

Fig. 5.3. Cumulative survival probability by sex and type of fracture. Adapted from Cummings *et al.*, 2002.

men. The risk of death is greatest immediately after the fracture and decreases over time (Fig. 5.3). The majority of these deaths can be attributed to co-morbidities from other chronic diseases and are not caused by the fracture *per se*.

Investigation

Imaging

In 1994, the WHO released recommendations for defining OP and osteopenia based on BMD, currently assessed by axial dual energy X-ray absorptiometry (DEXA) scan (Fig. 5.4). The absolute bone density, T-score and Z-score are recorded. The T-score compares the patient's BMD with that of a healthy population of young women and represents the number of standard deviations from the mean BMD in the young female population. The Z-score compares the patient's BMD with that of an age and ethnicity matched population, again representing the numbers of standard deviations from the mean BMD in the comparator population. The diagnoses of osteopenia and OP are based on the T-scores as a way of identifying those individuals with an increased risk of fracture (Table 5.2).

FRAX assessment

Fracture risk is not exclusively determined by bone mass but also depends on the bone quality, geometry and turnover. In early 2008, WHO provided a new web-based fracture risk assessment tool, FRAX: (http://www.shef.ac.uk/FRAX/)

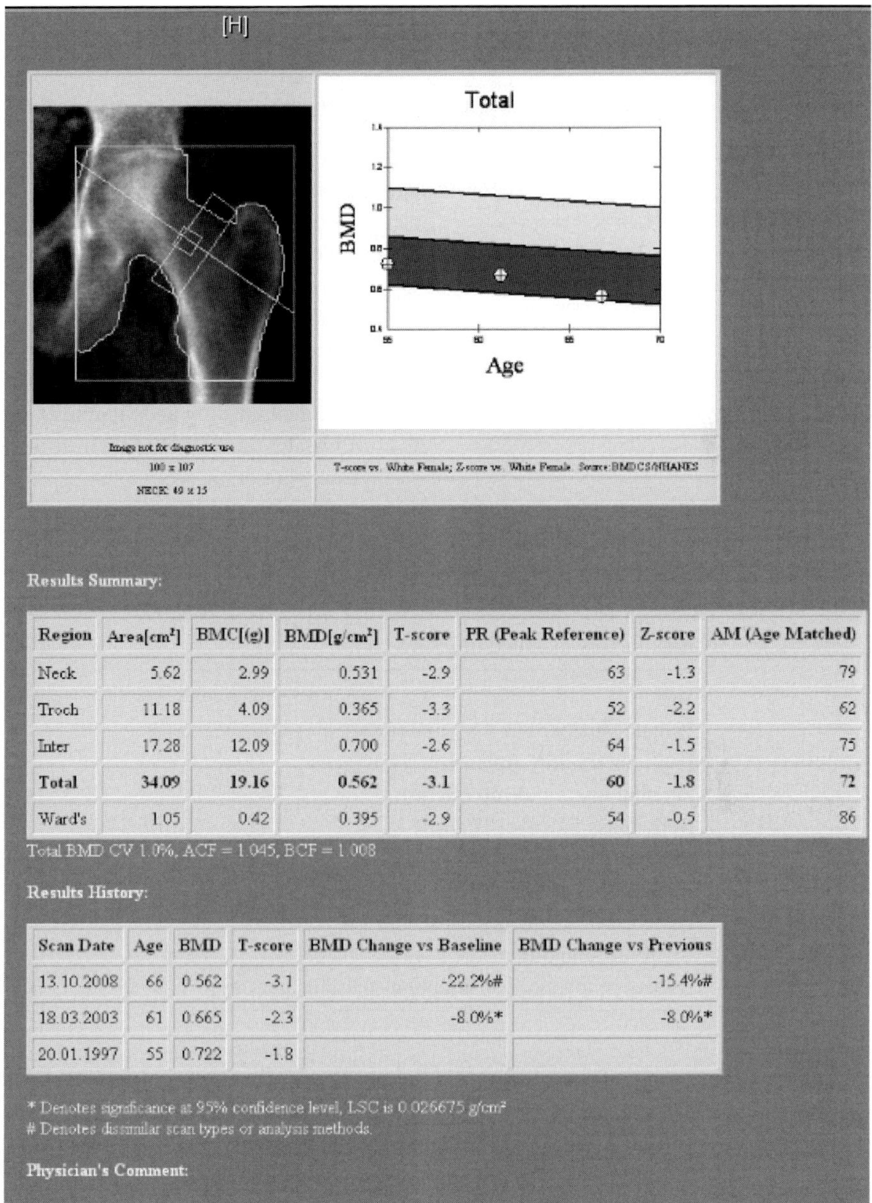

Results Summary:

Region	Area[cm²]	BMC[(g)]	BMD[g/cm²]	T-score	PR (Peak Reference)	Z-score	AM (Age Matched)
Neck	5.62	2.99	0.531	-2.9	63	-1.3	79
Troch	11.18	4.09	0.365	-3.3	52	-2.2	62
Inter	17.28	12.09	0.700	-2.6	64	-1.5	75
Total	**34.09**	**19.16**	**0.562**	**-3.1**	**60**	**-1.8**	**72**
Ward's	1.05	0.42	0.395	-2.9	54	-0.5	86

Total BMD CV 1.0%, ACF = 1.045, BCF = 1.008

Results History:

Scan Date	Age	BMD	T-score	BMD Change vs Baseline	BMD Change vs Previous
13.10.2008	66	0.562	-3.1	-22.2%#	-15.4%#
18.03.2003	61	0.665	-2.3	-8.0%*	-8.0%*
20.01.1997	55	0.722	-1.8		

* Denotes significance at 95% confidence level, LSC is 0.026675 g/cm²
# Denotes dissimilar scan types or analysis methods.

Physician's Comment:

Fig. 5.4. DEXA scan of a hip in a female patient with longstanding rheumatoid arthritis. The T-score reflects bone density in relation to peak bone mass in healthy young adults of the same gender. The Z-score is related to individuals of the same gender and age.

Table 5.2. BMD values, fracture risk and recommended action measures according to T-score defined by WHO.

Grade	T-score	Fracture risk	Action
Normal	>–1	Low	Lifestyle advice
Osteopenia	–1 to –2.5	Above average	Lifestyle advice, Optimise calcium and vitamin D Calculate risk using FRAX
OP	<–2.5	High	Lifestyle advice Optimise calcium and vitamin D Consider pharmacological measures
Severe OP	<–2.5 + one or more fractures	High	Lifestyle advice Optimise calcium and vitamin D Consider pharmacological measures Pain control

Table 5.3. Risk factors for osteoporotic fractures included in the FRAX tool.

Risk factors included in FRAX tool
Age
Female gender
Previous fragility fracture
Parental history of hip fracture
Body mass index <19 kg/m^2
Long term steroids
Rheumatoid arthritis
Presence of secondary causes for OP
Cigarette smoking
Excessive alcohol consumption (>3 units per day)

(WHO Collaborating Centre for Metabolic Bone Diseases, University of Sheffield, Sheffield, UK), that combines easily ascertained, validated risk factors with femoral neck BMD T-score to calculate 10-year absolute fracture risk for hip fractures and major osteoporotic fractures (Table 5.3). FRAX can be used with women and men of several different ethnicities. It is most helpful in treatment decisions for patients with osteopenia, where risk stratification is necessary. Previous bone damage and frequency of falls are also important contributors to fracture risk and are not considered by the FRAX calculator.

The FRAX assessment does not specify who should be treated; this remains a matter of clinical judgement. In the USA, for example, the new National Osteoporosis Foundation's Clinician's Guide recommends pharmacological treatment for postmenopausal women and men aged >50 years with osteopenia (based on a BMD T-score at spine or hip between −1.0 and –2.5) who have a 10 year absolute fracture risk, as determined by FRAX, of ≥3% for hip or ≥20% for major osteoporotic fractures.

Laboratory tests

A number of laboratory tests are recommended in order to exclude secondary OP (Table 5.4).

Bone turnover markers (BTM) measure the rate of bone remodelling, allowing a dynamic assessment of skeletal status. They are not generally used in routine clinical practice but have potential for monitoring treatment in the future. The most commonly used markers are listed in Table 5.5. BTM during childhood and adolescence can be up to ten times higher than concentrations found in a healthy young adult. Following a fracture, BTM may remain elevated for up to one year. Immobility leads to rapid losses in bone mass and increase in bone resorption markers (as high as 40% after a week of bed rest).

Management

Management of OP encompasses both its prevention and treatment. This is achieved through the implementation of preventive lifestyle measures and appropriate effective pharmacological intervention.

Table 5.4. Initial laboratory assessment for OP.

Laboratory test	Secondary causes of OP
Full blood count	Inflammatory disease
Erythrocyte sedimentation rate	Inflammatory disease, multiple myeloma
C-reactive protein	Inflammatory disease
Urea, electrolytes and creatinine	Chronic renal impairment
Liver function tests	Liver disease
Calcium, phosphate and alkaline phosphatase	Vitamin D deficiency, hyperparathyroidism
Thyroid stimulating hormone	Thyroid dysfunction
Serum and urine protein electrophoresis	Multiple myeloma

Table 5.5. Biochemical markers of bone turnover.

	Markers of bone formation	Markers of bone resorption
Serum	Bone alkaline phosphatase Osteocalcin Type I collagen extension propeptides (P1CP, P1NP)	N-terminal (S-NT_X) and C-terminal (S-CT_X) cross-linking telopeptide of type I collagen
Urine		Pyridinoline Deoxypyridinoline U-NT_X, U-CT_X Hydroxyproline

P1CP procollagen 1 carboxyterminal peptide, P1NP procollagen 1 aminoterminal peptide, S-NTx serum aminoterminal cross-linking telopeptide of type I collagen, S-CTx serum carboxyterminal cross-linking telopeptide of type I collagen, U urinary.

Lifestyle changes

The risk of sustaining a fragility fracture increases with advancing age. This risk can be reduced by correcting eye problems such as cataracts and reducing the risk of falls by making adjustments in the home environment (ensuring adequate lighting, avoiding slippery surfaces).

Regular, weight-bearing and resistance exercise is important throughout life for maximizing peak bone mass, preventing bone loss and maintaining muscle strength and balance. Individually tailored exercise programmes, including Tai Chi and yoga, have been shown to be particularly useful in preventing falls in the elderly. A minimum twenty minutes of load bearing exercise at least three times a week is recommended. Calcium and vitamin D are essential for optimum bone health throughout life and adequate supplementation has been demonstrated to improve BMD and reduce fracture risk. Current evidence indicates that the risk for fragility fracture is greatest in those who consume under 400 mg of calcium daily. Calcium and vitamin D supplementation should be considered in all patients before and during treatment with bone sparing compounds, including the bisphosphonates, selective oestrogen receptor modulators (SERMs) and recombinant PTH (teriparatide). Patients should be advised to stop smoking and to minimise their alcohol intake (Table 5.6).

Pharmacological treatment

The currently available treatments for OP are very effective in preventing bone loss and reducing fracture risk (Table 5.7). Although most therapeutic measures retard the rate of bone loss, they are unable to convert abnormal osteoporotic

Table 5.6. Measures for the prevention of OP and the grade of evidence of these recommendations based on literature review. A–C denote level of recommendations, A being highest. (Adapted from Royal College of Physicians UK recommendations).

Intervention	BMD	Vertebral fracture	Hip fracture
Exercise	A	B	B
Calcium ± vitamin D	A	B	B
Dietary calcium	B	B	B
Smoking cessation	B	B	B
Reduced alcohol consumption	C	C	B

bone back to normal bone. Anabolic agents such as PTH (teriparatide) stimulate new bone formation by continually activating osteoblasts. In contrast, inhibitors of bone resorption reduce osteoclastic activity. These include bisphosphonates, SERMs and calcitonin. Strontium ranelate has a unique mechanism of action that targets both bone resorption and formation, resulting in increased bone mass.

Bisphosphonates

Bisphosphonates are the most commonly used compounds for the treatment of OP. Alendronate, risedronate, ibandronate and etidronate are oral agents licensed in the UK for the prevention and treatment of OP. Ibandronate, zoledronate and pamidronate may be given intravenously.

The bio-availability of bisphosphonates following oral administration is poor and therefore they should be taken on an empty stomach with plenty of water and in an upright position that should be sustained for ≥30 minutes in order to prevent oesophageal erosion. The following points should be considered prior to prescribing a bisphosphonate:

- Oral preparations should be avoided in patients who have had recent peptic ulcers (within ~ one year) or are known to have abnormalities of oesophagus and other conditions that delay gastric empting (achalasia, stricture).
- Calcium levels should be checked in patients at higher risk for hypocalcaemia including those with vitamin D deficiency, impaired parathyroid and renal function. Adequate calcium and vitamin D intake should be provided.
- Transient flu-like symptoms lasting up to 48 hours can occur after administration of IV bisphosponates that contain nitrogen (ibandornate, zoledronic acid, pamidronate). Symptoms are usually mild and are less likely to occur with subsequent dosing. Paracetamol and non-steroidal anti-inflammatory drugs (NSAIDs) have been used for symptom relief.

Table 5.7. Treatment measures and evidence of efficacy in treating postmenopausal women. A–C denote level of recommendation, A being highest. Adapted from Royal College of Physicians guidelines.*

Intervention	Vertebral	Non-vertebral	Hip	Administration	Dose
Alendronate	A	A	A	Oral	70 mg weekly
Calcitonin	A	B	B	Intranasal	200 IU daily
Calcitriol	A	A	C	Oral	250 ng twice daily
Calcium + vitamin D	A	A	B	Oral	1.2 g calcium and 800 IU vitamin D daily
Etidronate	A	B	B	Oral	400 mg daily for 14 days every 3 months
HRT	A	A	B	Various	Multiple preparations available
Raloxifene	A	–	–	Oral	60 mg daily
Risedronate	A	A	A	Oral	35 mg weekly or 5 mg daily
Denosumab*	+	+	+	Subcutaneous	60 mg every six months
Ibandronate*	+	+	–	Oral	150 mg monthly
				Intravenous	3 mg every three months
Strontium ranelate*	+	+	+	Oral	2 g daily
Teriparatide*	+	+	+	Subcutaneous	20 µg daily for 18–24 months

* No advice was included in original guidelines but + denotes evidence and – denotes lack of evidence for efficacy.
HRT hormone replacement therapy.

- Bisphosphonates should not be used in patients with significant renal impairment, i.e. creatinine clearances <30 mL/min (ibandronate, risedronate) or <35 mL/min (zoledronic acid, alendronate). No dosage adjustment is needed for patients with mild renal impairment. Serum creatinine should be checked before each zoledronic acid dose.
- Aetiology and pathogenesis of the bisphosphonate related osteonecrosis of the jaw is poorly understood. It generally occurs more commonly in patients with advanced malignancies (incidence ranging from 2–11% patients with skeletal metastases who receive higher doses and IV treatment). The incidence of bisphosphonate related osteonecrosis of the jaw among patients treated for OP is probably between 1/10,000 to 1/100,000. These agents are best avoided where there is clear evidence of poor dental hygiene and recurrent oral sepsis.
- Recent links between oesophageal cancer and bisphosphonate use have been well documented. However, the risk:benefit ratio for the vast majority of OP patients will favour the use of bisphosphonates, as fractures are far more common than oesophageal cancer.

Strontium ranelate

Strontium ranelate has a novel dual mechanism of action by decreasing bone resorption and promoting bone formation and has been demonstrated to reduce risk for vertebral and non-vertebral fractures (including hip) especially in women over 75 years of age. Strontium ranelate is well tolerated and, as it is not metabolised, the compound has limited potential for interactions with other commonly used drugs.

Raloxifene

Raloxifene is a SERM that acts as an oestrogen agonist in bone and lipid metabolism. Raloxifene is recommended for the prevention of osteoporotic fractures in postmenopausal women. It has been shown to reduce the incidence of vertebral fractures but has no demonstrable benefit in non-vertebral fractures. It significantly reduces the risk of breast cancer. However, raloxifene has been associated with increased risk of venous thromboembolism and may worsen vasomotor symptoms.

Hormone replacement therapy

Hormone replacement therapy (HRT) was previously considered the main treatment for postmenopausal OP but has lost favour because of the increased risk of breast cancer and heart disease. It has an important role in young women with premature menopause and following hysterectomy/oopherectomy in order to prevent early post-menopausal bone loss in situations where other therapies are contraindicated or not tolerated.

Calcitonin

Calcitonin is an endogenous peptide, produced by thyroid C cells. Parenteral calcitonin has been shown to increase BMD and reduce new vertebral fractures. Tolerance can be poor with side effects like nausea, diarrhoea and flushing that are less prominent with intranasal use.

Parathyroid hormone

In the UK, recombinant forms of human PTH, Teriparatide or Preotact, are recommended for women over the age of 65 years who have severe OP who cannot tolerate bisphosphonates or in whom bisphosphonates have failed to prevent fracture. They are administered by subcutaneous injection for a maximum of 18–24 months.

Denosumab

Denosumab is a monoclonal antibody to receptor activator nuclear factor kappa B ligand (RANKL) and is a promising anti-resorptive agent. In women with post-menopausal OP denosumab 60 mg subcutaneously every six months reduces the risk of vertebral, hip and non-vertebral fracture compared to placebo.

Future agents for the treatment of osteoporosis

Several novel anti-resorptive agents are being developed. Glucagon, like peptide 2, is an intestinal hormone which, given at bed time, substantially decreases bone resorption and does not seem to have an effect on bone formation. Clinical trials with Odanacatib, an inhibitor of cathepsin K, are currently ongoing. Cathepsin K is a proteolytic enzyme produced by osteoclasts required for bone matrix resorption. Cathepsin K deficiency caused by homozygous mutations is a cause of increased bone density known as pyknodysostosis in humans. Novel anabolic agents include antibodies that target molecules (sclerostin and Dkk1) participating in Wnt signalling, a pathway that regulates gene transcription of proteins that are important for osteoblast function.

5.2. Osteomalacia and Parathyroid Disorders

5.2.1. *Osteomalacia*

Osteomalacia is a generalised bone disease most commonly caused by disorders of vitamin D metabolism. It is characterised by impairment of mineralisation of the bone matrix leading to a qualitative defect rather than the quantitative deficiency found in OP. When this pathophysiological process occurs in the growing skeleton, it is referred to as rickets. The prevalence of osteomalacia is variable. It is estimated to be around 1% in unselected autopsy cases in Detroit, USA, but as high as 18% in nursing home residents and hip fracture patients.

Aetiopathogenesis

Vitamin D and bone

Bone formation occurs in distinct stages. Unmineralised matrix (osteoid, composed largely of type 1 collagen) is laid down by osteoblasts in response to numerous growth factors, including bone morphogenetic factors, transforming growth factor (TGF)-β and the Wnt/LRP5 signalling system. Subsequently, this matrix becomes mineralised by the precipitation of calcium hydroxyapatite, initiated in matrix vesicles derived from chondrocytes and osteoblasts.

In vitamin D deficiency there is no difficulty in laying down the bone matrix collagen but it is not properly mineralised. In osteomalacia, most surfaces of trabecular and cortical bone are covered with thick unmineralised osteoid seams. This is very different from OP where only relatively small amounts of unmineralised osteoid are present.

Vitamin D mediates its effects on bone in a number of different ways. It directly regulates osteoblast gene expression, controlling expression of factors such as osteocalcin and osteopontin. Vitamin D also has a more indirect effect by regulating calcium absorption in the gut. Hypocalcaemia due to vitamin D deficiency is detected by the calcium-sensing receptor in the parathyroid glands, stimulating the release of PTH, a condition termed 'secondary hyperparathyroidism'. In longstanding vitamin D deficiency the increased PTH secretion may become autonomous; this is referred to as 'tertiary hyperparathyroidism'. PTH has numerous actions that will increase calcium levels:

- increased 1 α hydroxylation of $25(OH)D_3$ to the active metabolite $1,25(OH)_2D_3$
- increased calcium absorption from the gut mediated by $1,25(OH)_2D_3$
- increased renal calcium re-absorption

- increased renal phosphate excretion
- increased osteoclast activity

Both hypomineralisation and high bone turnover due to the increased osteoclast activity contribute to the increased fracture risk in patients with vitamin D deficiency.

Causes of vitamin D deficiency

Osteomalacia usually results from poor vitamin D intake, synthesis or metabolism (Fig. 5.5).

Reduced vitamin D intake and/or synthesis in the skin

- Dietary
- Malabsorption (e.g. coeliac disease, pancreatic insufficiency)

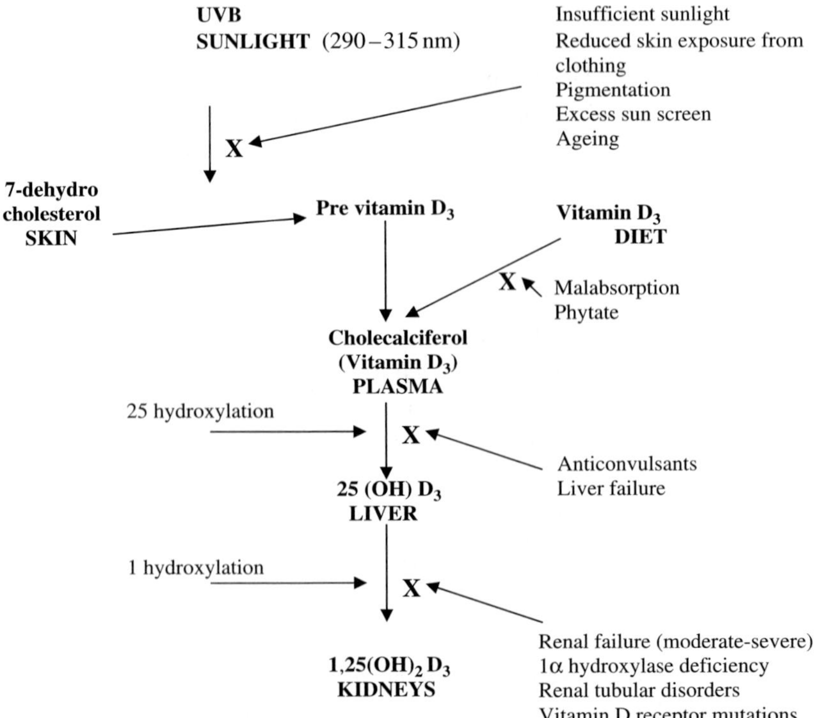

Fig. 5.5. Vitamin D metabolism and some potential causes of deficiency.

- Insufficient sunlight (housebound elderly people, immigrants to northern latitudes)
- Ageing

Impaired vitamin D metabolism

- Liver disease
- Renal disease
- Anticonvulsant therapy (induce hepatic enzymes that metabolise vitamin D)

Rare causes of osteomalacia

- Renal tubular defects (e.g. X-linked hypophosphataemia, Fanconi syndrome)
- Impaired bioactivity of alkaline phosphatase (hypophosphatasia)
- Inhibitors of calcification (e.g. aluminium)
- An abnormal pH at the site of calcification (e.g. renal tubular acidosis)
- Vitamin D dependent rickets (VDDR). Two forms exist: one is caused by loss of function mutations in 1 α hydroxylase (type 1 VDDR) and the other by defects in the vitamin D receptor (type 2 VDDR).
- Oncogenic rickets associated with abnormal levels of fibroblast growth factor (FGF) 23 produced by certain tumours, particularly of blood vessel origin. FGF23 mediates phosphate excretion through the kidney.
- Autosomal dominant hypophosphataemia may also result from mutations in FGF23 that reduce its physiological clearance, thereby increasing serum concentrations.

Clinical Features

Although there are many different forms of osteomalacia, the clinical features are generally similar. Unlike OP, which commonly progresses silently for a long time and becomes evident only when fractures occur, osteomalacia is typically symptomatic in almost all affected patients. The symptoms include:

- Proximal muscle weakness
- Symmetrical diffuse bone pain and tenderness, worse with weight bearing
- Insufficiency fractures more commonly in axial skeleton and lower extremities.

Deformities are most marked in childhood 'rickets' where there is enlargement of the epiphyses, a rickety rosary (due to rib enlargement at the costochondral junctions) and angular deformities of the limbs (e.g. bow legs) (Fig. 5.6). In severe hypocalcaemia there may be paraesthesiae or tetany in the hands and feet.

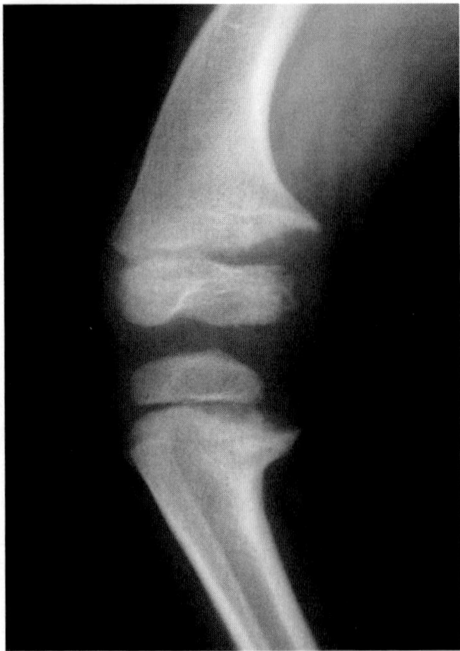

Fig. 5.6. Hypophosphataemic rickets in a child demonstrating the typical widening of the growth plate and splaying of the metaphysis and bowing of the legs.

Investigations

The diagnosis of osteomalacia presents few problems once it has actually been considered but is too often neglected. The availability of assays for vitamin D has rendered the need for bone biopsy largely redundant. The diagnosis can usually be established definitively on the basis of a combination of clinical features and biochemistry. Radiographs are unlikely to be contributory unless there is long-standing disease. The following may be helpful in diagnosis:

- Low levels of circulating $25(OH)D_3$
- Low or normal serum levels of calcium and phosphate (except in renal failure)
- Increased alkaline phosphatase (occurs relatively late)
- Low BMD measured by DEXA scan (due to reduced mineralisation of the bone matrix)

- Radiographic evidence of secondary hyperparathyroidism presenting as subperiosteal resorption, endocortical scalloping and increased cortical thinning and porosity. Presence of Looser's zones or pseudofractures (Fig. 5.7).
- Bone biopsy is only occasionally needed for diagnosis (usually in rare forms of bone disease).

Investigations in renal glomerular osteodystrophy

In chronic renal failure there is defective renal 1 α hydroxylation of $25(OH)D_3$ causing reduced calcium absorption from the gut and reduced mineralisation of bone. Secondary hyperparathyroidism leads to increased osteoclastic bone resorption and, in severe cases, osteitis fibrosa. Radiographs show subperiosteal erosion of the phalanges and evidence of bone resorption in the femoral neck and pelvis. There is biochemical evidence of renal failure, hypocalcaemia, elevated plasma phosphate and raised alkaline phosphatase.

Heritable forms of osteomalacia

Heritable forms of osteomalacia require more complex further assessment, which is best undertaken in a specialist unit.

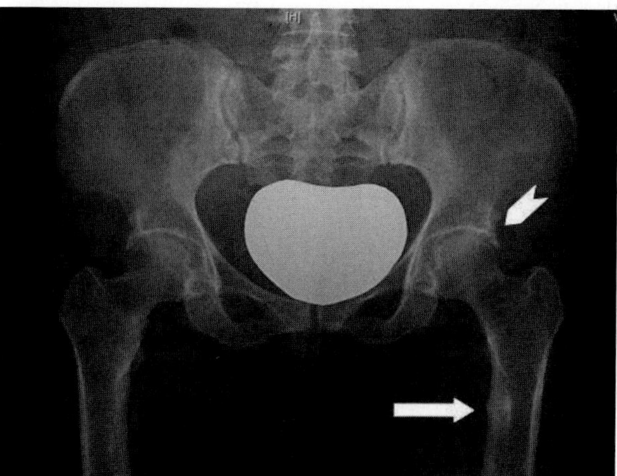

Fig. 5.7. Pelvic radiograph from an individual with X-linked hypophosphataemia. There is ossification of the capsule of the hip joint (chevron) and pseudofractures (Looser zones) are apparent in the proximal femora (arrows).

Management

The management of osteomalacia will depend on the underlying cause. It is important to treat any underlying condition such as coeliac disease.

Nutritional osteomalacia typically responds promptly to treatment with vitamin D (ergocalciferol or cholecalciferol). Daily doses of 1000 IU of vitamin D3 or up to 3000 IU of vitamin D2 are usually effective. Alternatively, higher dose preparations may be given on a weekly, monthly or even three-monthly basis. Vitamin D2 for injection is available for 'boosting' very low vitamin D levels or is sometimes given three-monthly to maintain levels.

Other types of osteomalacia, such as VDDR type 2, may require much larger doses of vitamin D. Use of the active metabolites of vitamin D (e.g. $1\alpha(OH)D_3$ or $1,25(OH)_2D_3$) may be required to treat bone disease in individuals with renal disease.

5.2.2. *Primary Hyperparathyroidism*

In addition to secondary hyperparathyroidism described above, overactivity of the parathyroids may occur as a primary event. This usually affects the parathyroid glands alone but rarely may be part of one of the multiple endocrine neoplasia (MEN) syndromes. In the latter, hyperparathyroidism is associated with pancreatic and pituitary tumours in MEN type 1 and with medullary carcinoma of the thyroid and phaeochromocytoma in MEN type 2. Isolated primary hyperparathyroidism is most commonly identified as a result of multiple channel biochemical screening. It is often asymptomatic with a benign course but sometimes may present with severe features of hypercalcaemia.

Aetiopathogenesis

The parathyroid glands play a central role in maintaining optimal calcium levels through the G protein coupled calcium-sensing receptor. In response to hypocalcaemia this receptor stimulates the production of PTH by parathyroid cells. In contrast, elevated calcium suppresses PTH. This regulatory mechanism is dysregulated in primary hyperparathyroidism where excessive PTH production is autonomous, often from an adenoma. The effects of increased PTH secretion have been described in Section 5.2.1 and include increased 1α hydroxylation of vitamin D, increased calcium absorption from gut and re-absorption via kidneys as well as increased osteoclast activity.

Clinical Features

Primary hyperparathyroidism is most commonly detected during routine biochemical screening when it is typically asymptomatic. Prolonged mild hyperparathyroidism is an important cause of OP. The most frequent clinical presentations are with bone disease (osteitis fibrosa) or renal stones due to hypercalcuria. There may be bone pain, deformity and fractures, particularly in the long bones and ribs. Renal stones, caused by oversaturation of the urine with calcium phosphate, are more common than nephrocalcinosis but progressive renal failure may occur in the latter. Hypercalcaemia may cause an osmotic diuresis with nocturia, thirst and dehydration headache as consequences. Other features include anorexia, constipation and depression. Corneal calcification, proximal myopathy, pancreatitis and pyrophosphate arthropathy may also occur.

Investigation

The finding of raised plasma calcium and lowered phosphate is typical but raised alkaline phosphate is only seen in the presence of bone disease. PTH levels can be measured reliably. A high value or even one in the normal range in the presence of hypercalcaemia is suggestive of hyperparathyroidism since PTH should be suppressed by hypercalcaemia. Distinction must be made from hypercalcaemia of malignancy where PTH-related protein levels will be raised and PTH suppressed. Radiographic features include the following:

- OP on DEXA scan
- Widespread subperiosteal bone erosion (especially phalanges)
- 'Pepper pot' appearance of the skull
- Bone cysts, particularly in long bones and ribs.

Hypercalcuria and hyperphosphaturia are evident. Renal stones and nephrocalcinosis may be identified on plain abdominal radiographs but are more sensitively identified by ultrasonography.

Management

Many individuals in whom mild hyperparathyroidism is detected incidentally require no specific treatment although they should be monitored. Parathyroidectomy is technically demanding but greatly facilitated by the techniques of selective venous sampling and isotope scanning to localise tumours accurately pre-operatively. There is still substantial debate about the overall role of surgery for the less severe forms of the condition.

5.2.3. *Hypoparathyroidism and Conditions Associated with PTH Signalling Abnormalities*

Parathyroid Hormone Deficiency

The commonest cause of parathyroid deficiency is following inadvertent removal during thyroidectomy. Autoimmune hypoparathyroidism is less common and may be associated with adrenal insufficiency and susceptibility to systemic candidiasis. Hypocalcaemia and hyperphosphataemia occur. Confusion, dementia, cataracts and cranial calcification are recognised. Treatment with calcium and $1{,}25(OH)_2D_3$ can be strikingly effective.

Other Conditions Associated with PTH Signalling Abnormalities

Several related conditions with varying degrees of PTH deficiency and resistance are recognised. Detailed discussion is beyond the scope of this chapter but they provide useful insights into the pathophysiology of many other bone disorders:

- Mutations in calcium-sensing receptor (causing familial hypocalcaemia)
- Mutations in G protein signalling system downstream of G protein coupled receptors may cause PTH resistance (pseudohypoparathyroidism). This may be associated with musculoskeletal features such as short stature and short fourth and fifth metacarpals.
- The skeletal abnormalities noted above in pseudohypoparathyroidism may also occur in the absence of biochemical abnormalities when the condition is known as pseudo-pseudohypoparathyroidism.
- Activating mutations in G protein system can cause monostotic fibrous dysplasia or polyostotic fibrous dysplasia (McCune–Albright syndrome), in which multiple endocrine defects and skin pigmentation also occur.

5.3. Paget's Disease of the Bone

Paget's disease of the bone is a chronic focal disorder caused by excessive and abnormal remodelling of ageing bone that can lead to deformity and enlargement of single or multiple bones. The pelvis (70%), femur (55%), lumbar spine (53%), skull (42%) and tibia (32%) are most commonly affected. It can be monostotic or polyostotic and the bone lesions often continue to increase in size if untreated.

Paget's disease of the bone is common, affecting 2–3% of the population over the age of 60. The disease is particularly prevalent in the UK, Australia, New Zealand, South Africa, Central Europe and North America. In contrast, it is rare in Scandinavia, China, Japan and other countries in Southeast Asia. Over the past 25 years, substantial reduction in the prevalence and clinical severity of the disease has been observed in the UK and New Zealand. However, this is not the case in the USA and Italy, where the incidence of Paget's disease of the bone has remained comparatively stable.

Aetiopathogenesis

The initial bone lesions in Paget's disease demonstrate evidence of increased bone resorption with increased number and size of multinucleated osteoclasts. These osteoclasts also contain characteristic nuclear inclusion bodies that resemble virus particles. Despite this, extensive research has failed to identify a viral cause for the disease. The coupling of bone formation and resorption, which is a feature of normal bone turnover, is maintained in Paget's disease where the primary lytic phase, mediated by activated osteoclasts, is followed by bone formation. This reparative response of the bone leads to increased bone and blood vessel formation and marrow fibrosis. Histologically, the disorganised new bone has a mosaic appearance with a mixture of woven and lamellar bone. Radiographically, the resorptive and reparative phases are quite distinct. In the resorptive phase a lytic lesion (resorption front) may be seen. Subsequently, the bone becomes enlarged, deformed and distorted with grossly irregular trabecular architecture. The exact cause of the disease is currently unclear, both genetic and environmental factors contribute to the pathogenesis. Familial aggregation has been observed and the risk of the disease developing in first-degree relatives is about seven to ten times higher than in the general population. Some cases of familial Paget's disease are caused by activating mutation in RANK. This cell surface receptor on osteoclast precursors is responsible for their differentiation and activation after stimulation by RANKL (typically produced by active osteoblasts). The related condition, juvenile Paget's disease, is caused by mutations in the natural inhibitor of RANKL known as osteoprotegerin. Finally, germline mutations in the sequestosome 1 gene (*SQSTM1*) are quite commonly found in Paget's disease. *SQSTM1* encodes the p62 protein involved in downstream signalling from RANK but the precise mechanisms involved are unclear, particularly why it often leads to patchy bone involvement rather than affecting the whole skeleton (Fig. 5.8).

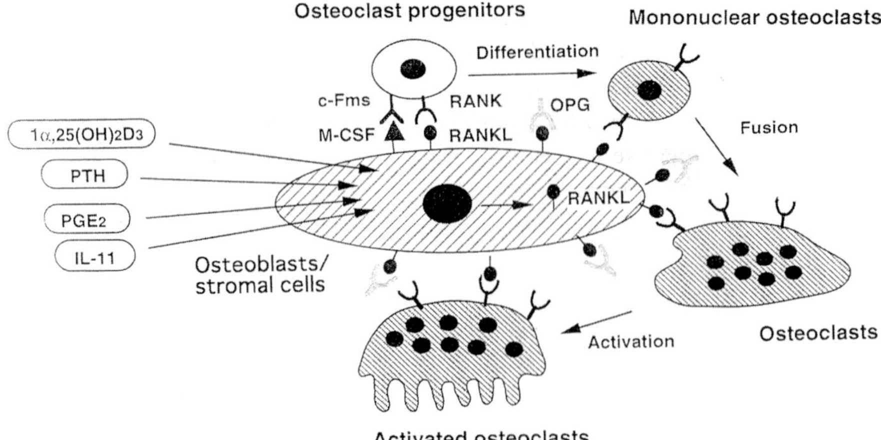

Fig. 5.8. Factors involved in the differentiation and activation of osteoclast precursors. RANKL produced by active osteoblasts plays a central role through activation of RANK on the cell surface. This is inhibited by the decoy receptor osteoprotegerin (OPG). Activating mutations in RANK or loss of function mutations in OPG can lead to Paget's disease-like syndromes in man.

Table 5.8. Complications of Paget's disease of the bone.

Frequency	Complication
Common	Bone deformity
	Spontaneous and fissure fractures
	Secondary osteoarthritis
	Spinal stenosis
	Hearing loss and cranial nerve palsies
Rare	Hydrocephalus
	Paraplegia
	Malignant transformation

Clinical features

Most patients with Paget's disease are asymptomatic; diagnosis is often based on incidental findings of raised alkaline phosphatase or an abnormal radiograph. However, 10–15% of patients have bone pain which is deep and aching in nature, persists at rest and is worse at night. Other patients present with complications of the disease (Table 5.8).

Around 10% of patients develop fractures. Estimates of incidence of malignant transformation vary widely from 0.9–20% with the most common histological type of tumour being an osteogenic sarcoma. This possibility should be considered in patients with longstanding disease with worsening bone pain that is poorly responsive to medical treatment, new soft tissue swelling around bone or occurrence of sudden fracture.

Investigations

Serum total alkaline phosphatase is raised in 95% of untreated patients but normal concentrations do not exclude the diagnosis. Both serum alkaline phosphatase and urinary hydroxyproline excretion are highly correlated with extent and activity of Paget's disease. Other BTMs offer little extra information except in patients with liver disease, where measurement of procollagen 1 aminoterminal peptide (P1NP) concentration provides a more accurate reflection of metabolic activity.

Radiographs reveal characteristic features of local resorption, bone enlargement, deformity, distorted trabecular architecture and fissure fractures (typically on the convex bone surface) (Figs. 5.9a and 5.9b). Radionuclide bone scan is more sensitive in the detection and assessment of the extent of bone lesions (Fig. 5.9c).

In rare cases bone biopsy is needed to confirm the diagnosis.

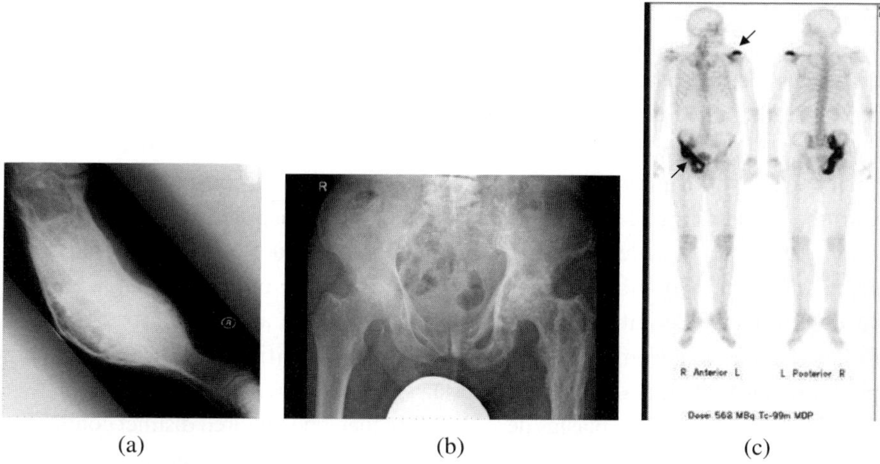

(a) (b) (c)

Fig. 5.9. (a) Extensive Paget's disease with marked expansion and bowing of the tibia. (b) Paget's disease involving the left pubis, ischium and left proximal femur. (c) Radionuclide bone scan showing Paget's disease of the right hemipelvis. There is also Paget's disease at the left scapula, most active at the acromion.

Management

Many cases of Paget's disease do not require treatment. However, if the lesions are symptomatic or are considered likely to cause complications, then a bisphosphonate should be prescribed. Risedronate given at a dose of 30 mg orally for two months or a single dose of 5 mg IV zoledronic acid are commonly used. Non-steroidal anti-inflammatory and analgesic agents will provide symptomatic relief from associated pain. Calcitonin intranasally and subcutaneously has been used successfully for the medical management of spinal stenosis complicating Paget's disease. Non-pharmacological measures may be helpful including physiotherapy, hydrotherapy and orthotics. Surgery is required mainly for the management of complications of Paget's disease. This may include joint replacement for osteoarthritis, fracture fixation, osteotomy and prophylactic surgery in patients with symptomatic pseudofractures. Pre-operative bisphosphonates or calcitonin reduces vascularity and blood loss associated with these procedures.

5.4. Heritable Disorders of the Musculoskeletal System

Heritable defects of the skeleton and associated soft tissues may be due to qualitative or quantitative defects in a wide range of genes. These include structural genes for matrix components, genes involved in post-translational modification of these proteins and other genes controlling growth and development. Many mesenchymal tissues may be affected, including the skeleton, ligaments, tendons, blood vessels and other internal viscera. Some disorders also affect the skin and other ectodermal tissues. It is not always possible to distinguish disease phenotypes easily and similar phenotypes may arise from mutations in different genes ('phenocopies'). Milder variants of many of these conditions may also merge with the broad range of normality seen in the general population.

Monogenic disorders of the soft connective tissues vary greatly in their severity but are particularly important in some because of their potential cardiovascular effects. Conditions such as Marfan syndrome and the various types of Ehlers–Danlos syndrome (EDS) can usually be identified clearly by applying predominantly clinical diagnostic criteria.

The osteochondrodysplasias describe more than one hundred distinct conditions affecting either bone itself or the cartilage precursor from which it develops. Osteogenesis imperfecta results from abnormalities of type I collagen. In the chondrodysplasias the abnormalities of the skeleton are generally secondary to abnormal cartilage development, resulting in a wide range of phenotypes. Broadly speaking, these conditions can be categorised according to the part of the bone that is affected (epiphysis, metaphysis, diaphysis) and whether the spine is also involved (Fig. 5.10).

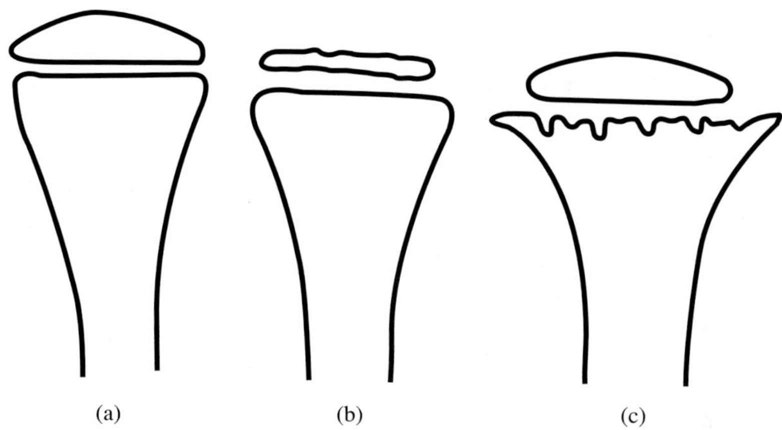

Fig. 5.10. Simple radiographic distinction of chondrodysplasias from (a) normal, according to whether there is involvement of, (b) the epiphysis, or (c) the metaphysis and/or spinal involvement (if all three were involved the description would be spondylo-epi-metaphyseal dysplasia).

Table 5.9. Classification of skeletal dysplasias based on stature and skeletal disproportion.

Stature	Skeletal dysplasias
Short proportionate	Pyknodysostosis Mucopolysaccharidoses
Short trunk	Spondyloepiphyseal dysplasia tarda (X-linked)
Short-limbed, lethal	Achondrogenesis Thanatophoric dwarfism Osteogenesis imperfecta (type II)
Short-limbed, nonlethal	Achondroplasia Hypochondroplasia Diastrophic dysplasia
Short limbs and trunk	Spondyloepiphyseal dysplasia (congenita) Kniest dysplasia Pseudoachondroplasia
Mild short stature/normal	Multiple epiphyseal dysplasia Stickler syndrome Hereditary multiple exostoses Metaphyseal chondrodysplasia (Schmid) Osteogenesis imperfecta (type I)

Table 5.10. Classification of heritable disorders of the skeleton and associated tissues into families according to the underlying metabolic and genetic defects.

Protein/enzyme	Gene	Disease
Collagen 1	*COL1A1* or *COL1A2*	Osteogenesis imperfecta (I–IV) and Ehlers–Danlos syndrome (arthrochalasia)
Collagen 2	*COL2A1*	Achondrogenesis (II) Kniest dysplasia Spondyloepiphyseal dysplasia (congenita) Stickler syndrome
Collagen 3	*COL3A1*	Ehlers–Danlos syndrome (vascular)
Collagen 5	*COL5A1* *COL5A2*	Ehlers–Danlos syndrome (classic)
Collagen 7	*COL7A1*	Epidermolysis bullosa congenita
Collagen 9	*COL9A1* *COL9A2* *COL9A3*	Multiple epiphyseal dysplasia (EDM II)
Collagen 10	*COL10A1*	Metaphyseal chondrodysplasia (Schmid type)
Collagen 11	*COL11A1* *COL11A2*	Stickler syndrome
Cartilage oligomeric matrix protein (COMP)	*COMP*	Pseudoachondroplasia Multiple epiphyseal dysplasia (Fairbank type)
Fibroblast growth factor receptors	*FGFR3*	Achondroplasia Hypochondroplasia Thanatophoric dwarfism
	FGFR2	Apert syndrome Crouzon syndrome
Diastrophic dysplasia sulphur transferase	*DTDST*	Diastrophic dysplasia
Parathyroid hormone receptor-1	*PTHR-1*	Metaphyseal dysplasia (Jansen)
Fibrillin 1	*FBN1*	Marfan syndrome
Fibrillin 2	*FBN2*	Congenital contractural arachnodactyly

Briefly, epiphyseal and metaphyseal dysplasias tend to exhibit short-limbed dwarfism while in spondyloepiphyseal dysplasias the trunk is disproportionately short (Table 5.9).

These conditions can also be categorised according to their underlying biochemical/genetic causes into disorders of matrix components and their metabolism or growth factors and their receptors (Table 5.10).

For completeness some conditions associated with abnormal bone density are also included in this section. Inherited disorders of bone mineralisation have been considered in the section on osteomalacia.

5.4.1. *Marfan Syndrome*

This classic disorder of connective tissue is best known because of its association with potentially catastrophic structural failure of the proximal cardiovascular tree. It is an autosomal dominant trait caused by mutations in the fibrillin gene (*FBN1*), affecting about one in 15,000 births (30% of all cases result from new mutations). It ranges in severity from the most aggressive cases, in which there is congenital cardiomyopathy, through to individuals exhibiting little more than moderate dilatation of the proximal aorta in later life. Life expectancy is greatly reduced (average age of death in the late 40s) with 80% of deaths due to cardiac involvement. The outlook has been improved with prophylactic use of β-blockers and earlier consideration of elective cardiac surgery in those with significant aortic dilatation.

Pathogenesis

Mutations in *FBN1* are the primary cause of Marfan syndrome. *FBN1* has 65 exons encoding the 347 kDa profibrillin 1 molecule which is subsequently processed to FBN1. Mutations associated with Marfan syndrome are fairly evenly distributed throughout *FBN1* but those in exons 24–32 are particularly associated with more severe cardiac disease and neonatal cardiomyopathy. Many different mutations are described, including those that reduce the quantity of FBN1 and others which affect protein folding.

Fibrillins are cysteine-rich glycoproteins with multiple repeats homologous to the calcium-binding epidermal growth factor domain (cbEGF). FBN1 is widely distributed in the extracellular matrix and is the major constituent of the 10–12 nm microfibrils associated with elastin in many connective tissues. It is the main component of the suspensory ligament of the ocular lens and in elastic tissues it forms a scaffold for the deposition of tropoelastin. Abnormalities in

FBN1 may cause disruption of the elastin network of elastic tissues secondary to abnormalities of the microfibrillar architecture. Conceptually it is therefore easy to explain such features as dislocation of the ocular lens in Marfan syndrome as the logical consequences of structural failure of these elastic tissues.

It is difficult, however, to explain all the abnormalities of Marfan syndrome simply by invoking deficiency of the elastin architecture. Some clues have come from the study of related disorders, such as Loeys–Dietz syndrome. Loeys–Dietz syndrome was distinguished only recently from Marfan syndrome in a small number of families with a phenotype that included excessively tortuous and fragile large arteries. Genetic mapping excluded *FBN1* as the mutant locus but implicated one of the receptors for TGF-β suggesting that abnormal TGF-β signalling might play a role in the development of the arterial abnormalities. Latent TGF-β binding protein is among those proteins that are normally associated with FBN1 microfibrils. In fibrillin-deficient mice TGF-β activation and signalling is abnormal and the effects of the deficient fibrillin on the proximal aorta can be reversed with TGF-β neutralising antibodies. It is now abundantly clear that disordered regulation of TGF-β signalling plays a highly important role in the pathogenesis of Marfan syndrome in man. The angiotensin II type 1 receptor blocker, losartan, inhibits signalling through the TGF-β receptor and has beneficial effects in animal models of Marfan syndrome. Large-scale trials looking at efficacy of angiotensin receptor blockers in suppressing aortic dilatation in human disease are now being conducted.

Clinical Features

The most immediately obvious clinical features of Marfan syndrome are a tall lean body habitus with disproportionately long limbs, scoliosis, slender fingers and high-arched palate. Many other features, such as striae, hypermobility, scoliosis (Fig. 5.11), flat feet and pneumothorax occur in patients with Marfan syndrome but are also common in the general population. Careful evaluation both of skeletal and non-skeletal manifestations is crucial to accurate diagnosis.

Cardiovascular

Weakness of the elastic tissues of the aortic root leads to progressive aortic dilatation and eventually to aortic regurgitation. Aortic dissection occurs most frequently in the ascending aorta and is particularly common when the aortic diameter exceeds 5 cm (compared with an upper limit of normal of approximately

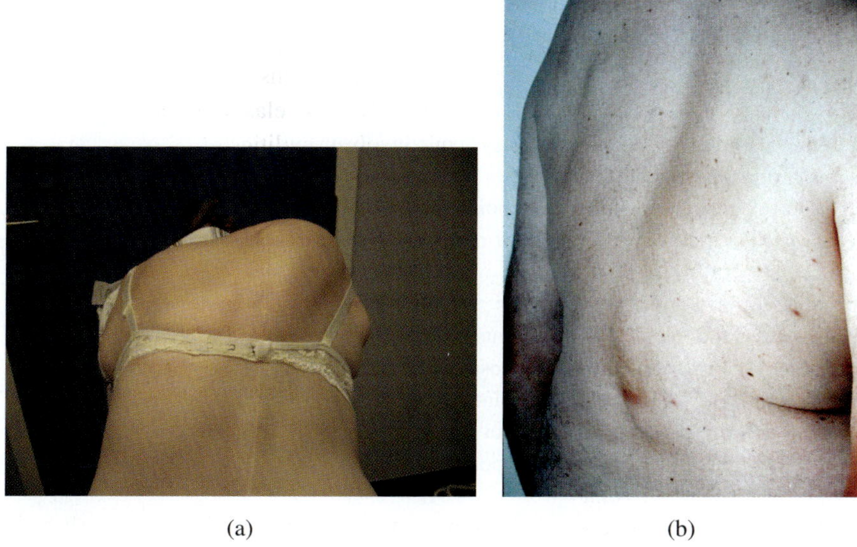

(a) (b)

Fig. 5.11. Scoliosis in Marfan syndrome. (a) Typical thoracic scoliosis with posterior rib hump exacerbated by forward flexion. (b) Localised thoracolumbar junction scoliosis.

3.5 cm for a young adult male). Mitral valve prolapse affects two thirds of patients, commonly producing modest mitral valve regurgitation.

Eye

Dislocation of the ocular lens due to weakness of the suspensory ligament is found in 55% of patients with classic Marfan syndrome but may require slit lamp examination to identify. It may be congenital and will nearly always be apparent by the age of 12 years. It can be precipitated by head trauma which is a reason for limiting participation in contact sports. Dislocation may be in any direction (i.e. not necessarily upward and outward as has classically been taught). Myopia due to excessive length of the globe requires optometry for detection.

Systemic features

Most of these are musculoskeletal in nature and it may require some expertise to determine whether they are truly present or within the normal range. For diagnostic purposes systemic features carry different weighting as shown in Table 5.11.

Table 5.11. Major diagnostic criteria used in Brussels revision of Ghent criteria for the diagnosis of Marfan syndrome (2010).

Major diagnostic criteria for diagnosis of Marfan syndrome
Systemic features (≥7/20 constitutes systemic involvement)
Pectus carinatum = 2 points
Pectus excavatum or asymmetry = 1 point
Reduced upper to lower body segment ratio (< 0.86) + disproportionate arm span to height (<1.05:1) = 1*
Spontaneous pneumothorax = 2 points
Positive wrist and thumb sign = 3 points (wrist OR thumb alone = 1 point)
Scoliosis >20° or thoracolumbar kyphosis = 1 point
Elbow contracture 15° or more = 1 point
Hindfoot deformity = 2 points (flat foot = 1 point)
Skin striae (lumbar or shoulders) = 1 point
Myopia >3 diopters = 1 point
Protrusio acetabuli = 2 points
Mitral valve prolapse = 1 point
Dural ectasia on MRI = 2 points
Facial features (3/5 dolichocephaly, enophthalmos, downward slanting palpebral fissure, retrognathism, malar hypoplasia) = 1 point
Ocular system
Dislocated lens (ectopia lentis)
Cardiovascular system
Dilatation of ascending aorta (> two standard deviations above the mean for body surface area) involving at least the sinus of Valsalva
Dissection of ascending aorta
Family/genetic history
First-degree relative independently satisfying diagnostic criteria
Presence of mutation in FBN1 likely to cause Marfan syndrome
Linkage to a haplotype around FBN1

MRI magnetic resonance imaging.
* In absence of scoliosis.

Pronounced thoracolumbar lordoscoliosis is common and may be very localised. Pectus abnormalities may be severe. Spondylolisthesis affects up to 10% of patients. The arm span to height ratio is typically greater than 1.05 to 1 and the upper body segment (crown to symphysis pubis) to lower body segment (symphysis pubis to floor) ratio is reduced below 0.86 in adults. The feet are long, slender and flat often with pronounced medial displacement of the medial malleolus. Radiographs may be necessary to evaluate spinal curvature and are essential to identify protrusio acetabuli.

Diagnosis

Classic Marfan syndrome is relatively straightforward to diagnose but all too often the diagnosis is made inappropriately purely on the basis of tall stature and minor features, such as high arched palate or long slender fingers (arachnodactyly). Referral to a specialist genetic and/or cardiovascular service should be made when the condition is suspected so that cardiac ultrasound (US), optometry, slit lamp examination and magnetic resonance imaging (MRI) scan can be carried out as needed.

The 'Brussels' revision of the diagnostic classification criteria for Marfan syndrome give increased weighting to cardiovascular and ocular signs, relative to musculoskeletal features (see Tables 5.11 and 5.12). They also take account of the utility of genetic testing; *FBN1* mutations can be identified in up to 90% of patients with classic Marfan syndrome although in many cases the diagnosis can be established without recourse to gene analysis.

Other conditions that may present with a similar phenotype include familial aortic dissection, isolated Marfan-like body habitus (in which musculoskeletal features dominate and there is no enlargement of the aorta or lens dislocation), familial mitral valve prolapse, familial isolated ocular lens dislocation, the MASS phenotype, Loeys–Dietz syndrome and Shprinzen–Goldberg syndrome. *FBN1* mutations may be found in some of these other conditions.

Management

Expert assessment and management of the cardiovascular system is essential because progressive aortic root dilatation and mitral valve prolapse occur frequently. In childhood cardiac surgery is most commonly required for progressive mitral regurgitation. Regular monitoring of the aortic root dimensions by ultrasonography is essential. Diameters >5 cm are associated with markedly increased risk of dissection; prophylactic surgery on the ascending aorta and aortic valve should then be considered, particularly if there is an adverse family history of dissection. It is customary to use β-blockers in patients with proven Marfan syndrome since these can slow the rate of aortic distension. The potential role of angiotensin converting enzyme (ACE) inhibitors and angiotensin receptor blockers is under investigation but not routine currently. The increased use of elective cardiac surgery has undoubtedly improved prognosis substantially.

Table 5.12 Brussels revision of the Ghent diagnostic criteria for Marfan syndrome (2010).

Brussels revision of Ghent diagnostic criteria for Marfan syndrome
If no family history
Marfan syndrome is present if:
1) Aorta >2SD or dissection PLUS ectopia lentis
2) Aorta >2SD or dissection PLUS *FBN1* mutation or linkage in pedigree
3) Aorta >2SD or dissection PLUS systemic features (≥ seven points – see Table 5.11)
4) Ectopia lentis without aortic dilatation but PLUS *FBN1* mutation known to be associated with aortic dilatation in other individuals
If there is a definite family history in first-degree relative
Marfan syndrome is present if:
5) Ectopia lentis PLUS family history of Marfan syndrome
6) Systemic features (≥ seven points) PLUS family history of Marfan syndrome
7) Aorta >2SD for adults (>3SD for children) PLUS family history of Marfan syndrome
Alternative diagnoses include
1) Isolated ectopia lentis syndrome (ectopia lentis, aorta <2SD, without systemic (≥ seven points) and no *FBN1* mutation of the sort associated with aortic involvement
2) MASS phenotype if aorta <2SD, systemic features (≥ five points, including at least one skeletal) and no ectopia lentis
3) Mitral valve prolapse syndrome if mitral valve prolapse but aorta <2SD

FBN1 = fibrillin 1 gene, SD = standard deviation above the mean for age and surface area.

Specific orthopaedic care may be required for those with more severe forms of scoliosis, particularly if this is evident before the adolescent growth spurt. Foot problems are common; these can usually be managed with corrective footwear but sometimes need surgery.

Refractive errors need careful correction and retinal detachments are common. Dislocated lenses affect 55% of those with classic Marfan syndrome and will usually be apparent by the end of the first decade of life if they are to occur. They sometimes need removal and are prone to opacification.

Many individuals with Marfan syndrome also experience complex psychological issues, relating to their height, diminished life expectancy and reduced capacity for normal activities. These should be specifically sought and addressed because they are frequently not recognised.

5.4.2. *Ehlers–Danlos Syndrome*

This heterogeneous group of conditions is characterised by varying degrees of joint laxity, hyperelasticity of the skin, abnormal scarring and fragility of internal viscera (Fig. 5.12). Seven distinct variants are recognised by the 1997 'Villefranche' classification but more than half of those with features of EDS do not fit well into specific types (Table 5.13). Some of the rarer forms of EDS are well characterised clinically and at the biochemical level. However, the less well defined but very common 'joint hypermobility syndrome' is heterogeneous clinically and biochemically and merges with the normal population.

Pathogenesis

Most forms of EDS, with the exception of benign joint hypermobility syndrome, are caused by abnormalities in the structural collagen genes (type 1, type 3 or type 5) or in their modifying enzymes.

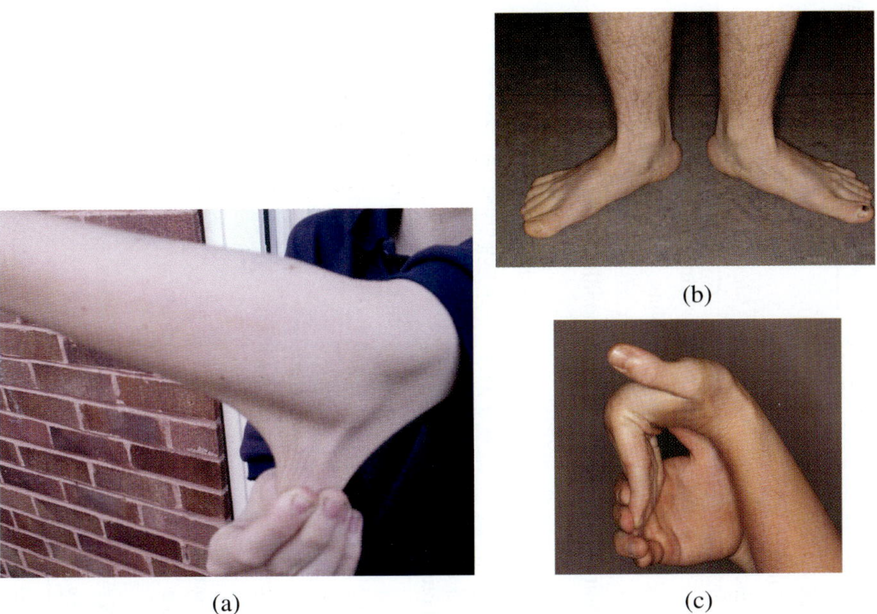

(a) (b) (c)

Fig. 5.12. Ehlers–Danlos syndrome showing (a) hyperelasticity of the skin, (b) flat feet and (c) pronounced hypermobilty of the fingers.

Table 5.13. Main types of EDS based mainly on the 1997 Villefranche nosology.

Villefranche Classification (where applicable)	Main features	Inheritance	Collagen or other gene affected	Biochemistry
Classic	Hyperextensible skin Hypermobile joints Wide atrophic scars	AD	V	Haploinsufficiency of Type V collagen usually
Hypermobility	Marked hypermobility of joints	AD	Usually unknown	Not known
Vascular	Rupture of middle-sized arteries, bowel and uterus Premature ageing in some	AD	III	Abnormal type III collagen synthesis
Oculoscoliotic	Scoliosis Fragile eyes with keratoconus	AR	*PLOD*	Lysyl hydroxylase deficiency
Arthrochalasia	Congenital dislocation of the hips Short stature	AD	I	Exon 6 deletion Absent cleavage site for N terminal peptide
Dermatosparaxis	Severe fragility Osteoporosis	AR	*ADAMTS2*	Procollagen (I) N-protease deficiency
Occipital horn syndrome	Soft skin Bladder diverticula Occipital horns	XLR	*ATP7A*	Secondary defect of Cu-dependent lysyl oxidase
Tenascin X deficiency	Similar to EDS II but without atrophic scars	AR	*TNXB*	Absence of tenascin X

AD autosomal dominant; AR autosomal recessive, XLR X-linked recessive.

Abnormalities of type 5 collagen

Classic EDS is caused by dominant mutations in the type V collagen genes, encoding type 5 collagen which is a minor component of collagen fibrils in the skin. These abnormalities of type 5 collagen influence collagen fibre size which may be evident on electron microscopy.

Abnormalities of type 3 collagen

In the vascular form of EDS there is deficiency of type 3 collagen, the major form in blood vessel walls. Most of the corresponding mutations in *COL3A1* result in the production of faulty over-modified type 3 collagen which is retained intracellularly rather than secreted. In at least two-thirds of cases this is the result of a cysteine for glycine mutation disrupting the collagen triple helical domain.

Abnormalities of type 1 collagen

Specific type I collagen mutations are described in arthrochalasia where deletion of the protease cleavage site for the N-propeptide of the procollagen I chain causes abnormal collagen processing. In contrast, in the extremely rare dermatosparaxis there is homozygous deficiency for the enzyme procollagen I N-proteinase (ADAMTS-2) that cleaves this N-terminal peptide. A small proportion of patients with classic EDS or joint hypermobility syndrome also have demonstrable mutations in the type I collagen genes.

Lysyl hydroxylase deficiency

Deficiency of the enzyme lysyl hydroxylase causes the oculoscoliotic variant of EDS in which there is defective post-translational modification of collagen interfering with the collagen cross-links that are essential for the tertiary structure of collagen.

Tenascin X deficiency

Homozygous deficiency of tenascin X, an essential regulator of collagen deposition by dermal fibroblasts, causes a form of hypermobility. Tenascin X deficiency commonly complicates 21-hydroxylase deficiency caused by small chromosomal deletions in the major histocompatibility complex because the gene lies in close proximity to the 21-hydroxylase gene.

Clinical Features

Joints

Musculoskeletal features are highly varied in EDS but joint laxity may be prominent and is assessed using the Beighton scoring system as described in Chapter II. In some variants the joints may be unstable and children may be late to walk. In others, particularly arthrochalasia, joint dislocation occurs. There is a common perception that joint hypermobility causes joint pain although this is not yet proven. It has been suggested that pain may arise from peri-articular soft-tissues that are susceptible to low-grade trauma on account of the hypermobile joints or from an increased incidence of degenerative changes within the joint.

Skin

In classic disease the skin feels velvety and is excessively extensible although it returns to normal after stretching. There may be redundant skin folds and the skin may be fragile.

In the vascular form of EDS the skin is thin and translucent with the blood vessels showing through. Atrophic ('cigarette paper') scars are prominent features of the classic and oculoscoliotic forms. Easy bruising is prominent in most cases but is more diagnostic in the upper than lower limbs. In dermatosparaxis skin fragility is severe with hernias and marked redundant skin folds.

Blood vessels

The most severe outcomes are in patients with the vascular form of EDS where there is greatly increased risk of premature death from rupture of major blood vessels or other hollow internal viscera. Pregnancy related deaths occur in 10–25% of pregnancies. Although complications of vascular EDS are uncommon in childhood, 80% of individuals suffer complications by the age of 40 years and the median life expectancy is 48 years.

Heart

Mitral valve prolapse may occur but is probably little increased in frequency over the general population rate. Proximal aortic dilatation has been described but this is rarely progressive.

Eye

Ocular fragility is a feature of the oculoscoliotic form and rupture of the eyeball can follow minor trauma. In some cases of EDS the sclerae may appear blue and there is sometimes overlap with OI.

Diagnosis

Deficiency of type III collagen and lysyl hydroxylase are usually detected from fibroblast cultures but can be detected by DNA analysis. Abnormalities of type V collagen and type I collagen are typically detected by DNA sequencing although in general clinical practice this is not routinely required since the diagnosis can usually be made on clinical grounds.

Management

Practical steps to encourage general muscular fitness, core stability and enhanced joint proprioception should be supervised by physiotherapists. Appropriate analgesia should be used and, where necessary, cognitive and other approaches to the management of chronic pain may be helpful. Monitoring of the heart valves and proximal aorta is not routinely needed. Women with the vascular form of EDS must be counselled about risks of pregnancy and referred to specialist maternity services.

5.4.3. *Osteogenesis Imperfecta*

Osteogenesis imperfecta (brittle bone syndrome) affects tissues containing type I collagen, including skin, bone, ligaments and tendons. It is an important cause of heritable OP and may also cause significant short stature and deformity. Its birth incidence is about one in 20,000. There is a wide range of severity from lethal short-limbed dwarfism through to a barely perceptible increased fracture risk.

Pathogenesis

Type 1 collagen is a heterotrimer of two $\alpha 1(I)$ and one $\alpha 2(I)$ chain which form a triple helical structure. In the collagen triple helical domain the amino acid sequence is glycine-X-$Y_{(n)}$ where X is often proline and Y hydroxyproline. The requirement for glycine at every third residue is determined by the limited space at the centre of the triple helix. Glycine is the smallest amino acid, lacking a side-chain which therefore allows it to pack into the core of the molecule. The triple helical trimers are packaged in parallel in fibrils cross-linked by interchain bonds. Post-translational modifications of collagen include hydroxylation and glycosylation of amino acids. These modifications are arrested by triple helix formation, which proceeds from the carboxy-terminus of the molecule. Larger amino acids such as cysteine substituting for glycine in the third position of the triple helical part of the molecule disrupt helix formation leading to over-modification of the mutant collagen and rendering it biologically unsound. Since the presence of only one abnormal procollagen chain is sufficient to damage the function of the collagen trimer, mutations of this type may effectively reduce the amount of normal type I collagen by 90%. In contrast, null mutations, resulting in complete failure of translation of one allele, will typically result in a 50% reduction of type 1 collagen and a correspondingly less severe phenotype. In general, such null mutations in *COL1A2* cause a somewhat more severe phenotype (type IV OI) than those in *COL1A1*.

Clinical Features

There are at least eight distinct forms of OI, of which type I disease is the most common and also the mildest.

Type I OI

In type I OI fractures are rarely present at birth. Subsequently they may be numerous, particularly in childhood and the post-menopausal period, but fractures usually heal normally without deformity. Many adults with type I OI experience an extended period of remission from fractures during adult life when bone mass is greatest. Life expectancy for this variant is near normal. Extra-articular features include blue sclerae and a premature complete arcus, premature hearing loss (conductive or sensory), varying degrees of joint laxity, skin hyperelasticity and abnormal scarring, similar to EDS. Involvement of the teeth (dentinogenesis imperfecta) affects some patients, causing discolouration of the teeth, which may be opalescent and break easily.

Type II OI

Type II OI is lethal *in utero* or in the perinatal period. It is one of the commonest causes of short-limbed dwarfism and is characterised by multiple fractures *in utero* and grossly defective mineralisation of the skull. Typically this form is associated with glycine to cysteine mutations in type I collagen.

Type III OI

Type III OI is a severe form of the disease and probably causes the most clinical problems. It is associated with severe stunting of growth, major deformity of the spine and long bones. Multiple fractures occur (frequently evident from birth) and these are typically associated with significant deformity (Fig. 5.13). Mobility is impaired sometimes by the severe fracture tendency but often by severe deformity of the limbs and most of these patients are wheelchair bound. Life expectancy is greatly reduced and respiratory complications are common.

Type IV OI

Type IV OI is intermediate in severity between type I and type III. Stature is short and there may be deformity. In contrast to type I disease, the sclerae in this variant are white.

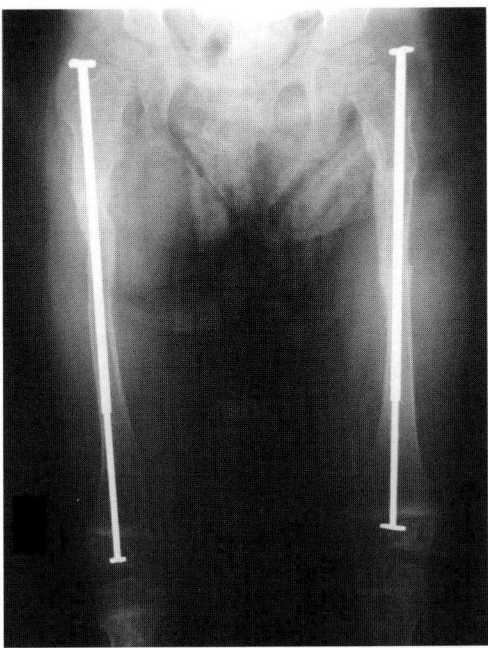

Fig. 5.13. Severe osteoporosis in a child with type III osteogenesis imperfecta. Intramedullary rods have been introduced in an attempt to prevent further fractures and to allow walking.

Diagnosis

The more severe variants of OI can be identified *in utero* or in the perinatal period using ultrasonography and/or perinatal radiographs. In contrast, other variants may present in childhood with fractures and may initially escape diagnosis. The combination of low impact fractures with characteristic extra-skeletal features (particularly blue sclerae, abnormal teeth, joint laxity and/or abnormal scarring) usually assists the diagnosis. However, distinction may be difficult from non-accidental injury particularly since unusual fractures and fractures of different ages can occur in both. Wormian bones (multiple bony islands in the skull) may be evident on skull radiographs. DNA sequencing of the type I collagen genes can successfully identify mutations in up to 90% of cases. Although this may be useful in some cases it is not routinely necessary.

Management

Survival is normal in type I disease and near normal in type IV disease and the major management issues relate to multiple fractures. These should be managed using normal orthopaedic techniques since fracture healing is essentially normal. In the more severe type III disease deformity and fracture risk typically dictate a wheelchair-bound lifestyle. The patient should be encouraged to self-propel if possible because of the benefits of activity on the skeleton. In those using a self-propelling wheelchair the disparity between the strong and fairly normal-looking upper limbs and the weak, wasted lower limbs is often dramatic.

Regular intravenous pamidronate infusions are beneficial for children with severe forms of OI. Oral bisphosphonates also increase bone density in those with milder forms of the disease although beneficial effects on fracture rates are less clear.

Nearly all cases of lethal OI are caused by new dominant mutations in type I collagen but a risk of recurrence due to parental germinal mosaicism cannot be discounted entirely. Early detection by chorionic villus sampling or ultrasonography may be desirable in subsequent pregnancies.

5.4.4. *Achondroplasia*

This is the commonest form of short-limbed dwarfism with a birth incidence of about 1 in 10,000. However, in the past many other types of chondrodysplasia have been erroneously classified as achondroplasia, which may have led to erroneous estimates of its frequency. It is dominantly inherited and can be relatively easily distinguished by clinical and radiographic features.

Pathogenesis

Achondroplasia is caused by a highly specific mutation in the transmembrane domain of fibroblast growth factor receptor (FGFR)-3 which normally exerts a negative regulatory action on chondrocytes in the growth plate. This mutation facilitates dimerisation and activation of the receptor, thereby suppressing chondrocyte growth and reducing longitudinal growth. The mutation is exclusively paternally derived and there is a strong paternal age effect. The rare but related condition, thanatophoric dysplasia, is a lethal form of short-limbed dwarfism in which mutations in the kinase domain of FGFR3 cause constitutive activation of the receptor without the need to engage its cognate ligand. The phenotype is correspondingly more severe.

Clinical Features

Achondroplasia can be diagnosed within the first year of life when there is a clear disparity between the large skull and short limbs (particularly in the proximal segment of the limb- 'rhizomelic shortening'). The condition particularly affects the metaphyses but radiographic changes are apparent in both the epiphysis and the metaphysis. There is bulging of the vault of the skull with a flat nasal bridge. Excess mortality in infants is largely due to cervical cord compression but hydrocephalus may also occur. In infancy there is pronounced lumbar lordosis, sometimes with wedging of the first lumbar vertebra (Fig. 5.14). This corrects by the age of six years. The vertebral canal is tight due to short pedicles (see Fig. 5.14) and in later life this may lead to complications of spinal stenosis requiring surgical decompression. Flexion deformities of the elbows are common. The fingers are broad and short with divergence between the third and fourth fingers ('trident hand'). Adult height is typically about 130 cm in males.

Diagnosis

The clinical and radiographic features are so characteristic that the diagnosis is rarely in doubt. It can easily be distinguished from hypochondroplasia and pseudochondroplasia, both of which have a normal facial appearance. Diagnostic US will identify the condition *in utero*. The FGFR3 mutation that is responsible for 98% of cases can be identified by DNA analysis but this is rarely necessary.

Management

Most individuals with achondroplasia are highly independent. There is a small chance of hydrocephalus developing in infants and serial MRI scans may be

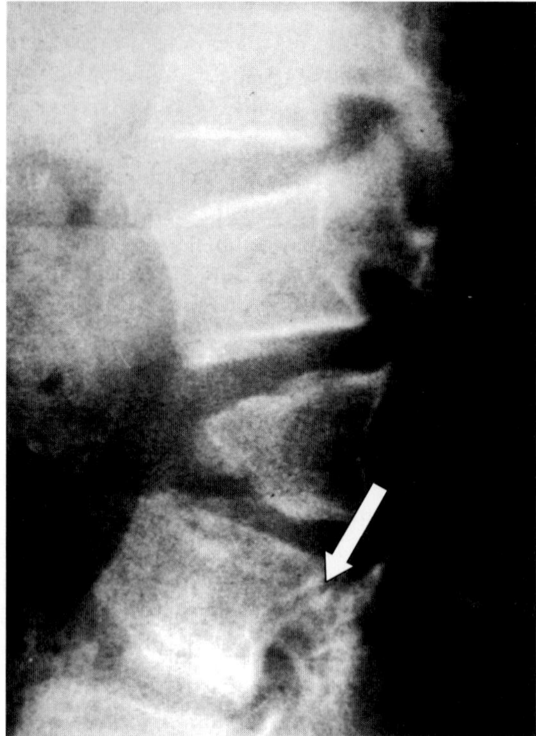

Fig. 5.14. Radiograph of the thoracolumbar junction in a child with achondroplasia. The wedge-shaped L1 vertebra is typical but corrects by the age of six years. The pedicles (arrow) are short and may lead to spinal stenosis in later life.

necessary. Leg lengthening and corrections of varus deformities in the legs using Ilizarov technology may be considered in childhood. Spinal surgery to relieve spinal stenosis may have to be repeated at several levels. Since people with achondroplasia often marry each other, offspring with the severe/lethal homozygous phenotype may occur. These can be detected by chorionic villus sampling in early pregnancy.

5.4.5. *Epiphyseal/Spondyloepiphyseal Dysplasias*

These are characterised by abnormalities in the growing ends of the bones in which the abnormalities are primarily in the cartilage with secondary abnormalities of ossification. Spinal involvement varies between the types.

Pathogenesis

Many of these conditions result from defects in the structural genes for protein components of the cartilage matrix. Type 2 collagen is quantitatively the most important protein in cartilage and, by analogy with type 1 collagen and OI, there is a family of type 2 collagenopathies that underpin some forms of epiphyseal/spondyloepiphyseal dysplasias. Very specific mutations in calcium-binding domains of cartilage oligomeric matrix protein (COMP) (affecting its secondary structure and secretion from chondrocytes into the extra-cellular matrix) underlie one potentially severe form of epiphyseal dysplasia known as pseudoachondroplasia (Fig. 5.15). In contrast, milder forms of epiphyseal dysplasia arise from mutations in type IX collagen, a minor species found in cartilage that facilitates interactions with cartilage proteoglycans. Some rare forms result from abnormal sulphation of proteoglycans in the cartilage ground substance or from abnormalities in matrilin.

Clinical Features

There is variable shortness of stature mainly due to shortness of the long limb bones. Where the spine is less obviously affected the overall effect is towards disproportionate short-limbed short stature. Where the spine is also affected the condition is referred to as a spondyloepiphyseal dysplasia (Fig. 5.16). Distinguishing radiographic features are often best seen in the developing

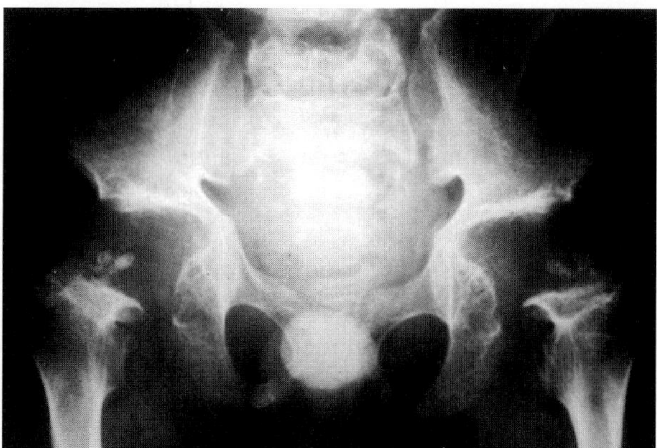

Fig. 5.15. Radiographic appearances of the hips in a child with pseudoachondroplasia. The epiphysis is small and late to appear while the acetabulum is clearly dysplastic.

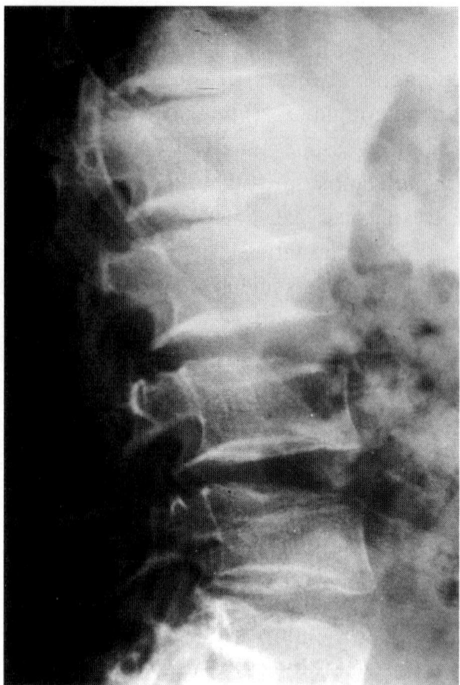

Fig. 5.16. Flattening of the vertebral bodies in a form of X-linked dominant spondylo-epiphyseal dysplasia. There is also a characteristic heaping up of bone in the posterior part of the vertebral body.

skeleton in children rather than in adults. There may also be deformity of the joints which can appear knobbly (particularly the hands) and premature degenerative arthritis is common.

The type 2 collagenopathies have a broad range of phenotypes and include the following:

- achondrogenesis (type 2) which is lethal *in utero*
- spondyloepiphyseal dysplasia congenita, which causes severe short stature, coxa vara with severe arthritis and marked spine and limb involvement
- Kniest dysplasia in which there is pronounced short stature, arthropathy, myopia and cleft palate
- Stickler syndrome in which stature is variable but often normal. Typically, there is little spine involvement but peripheral joint arthropathy. Ocular involvement is prominent with myopia, retinal detachment and degeneration of the vitreous.

Diagnosis

The key to accurate diagnosis is careful clinical assessment for the extent and severity of the phenotype coupled with limited skeletal survey. Comparison with radiographic atlases is often essential. DNA analysis can be very valuable but is relatively expensive. Referral to specialist genetic services is recommended. Difficulties may occur in knowing which individuals to investigate. Generally those below the 0.5th percentile, whose height is serially crossing centiles or in whom there is also evidence of skeletal disproportion should be investigated further.

Management

Subjects with these disorders often require no specific treatment other than an accurate diagnosis and reassurance. Limb deformities and shortening may be suitable for correction by Ilizarov techniques. Premature osteoarthritis as a result of mechanical factors increases the need for joint replacement in these disorders.

5.4.6. *Metaphyseal/Spondylometaphyseal Dysplasias*

In these conditions the growth plate itself is primarily affected, with a variety of different phenotypes that may also include extra-skeletal features. Structural proteins, such as type X collagen in the Schmid type of metaphyseal chondrodysplasia, may be involved. This syndrome is characterised by moderate short stature (~ 145 cm) with pronounced coxa vara and considerable bowing of the legs. In some exceptionally rare recessive forms of metaphyseal dysplasias (Jansen type metaphyseal) abnormalities in the growth plate are mediated through abnormal signalling through the PTH receptor which also causes biochemical abnormalities. Since the growth plate rather than the epiphysis is involved there is rather less predisposition to accelerated arthritis in patients with these types of skeletal dysplasias.

The diagnosis can usually be made from a combination of the family history, clinical signs and appropriate radiographs. Radiographic features are more diagnostic in the growing skeleton where there is widening and splaying of the metaphysis (similar to rickets). Such radiographic changes will not be evident in the adult although angular bone deformities will persist. Biochemical screening to exclude rickets is mandatory. DNA analysis may be helpful in some cases.

As with other forms of skeletal dysplasias subjects often require no specific treatment. Leg lengthening or surgical correction of limb deformities may sometimes be appropriate.

5.4.7. *Diaphyseal Dysplasias*

Perhaps the most important of these conditions is multiple hereditary exostoses (diaphysial aclasis). In this condition cartilage outgrowth originating from the growth plate may occur at single or multiple sites in the skeleton, causing bony outgrowths of variable sizes that can potentially interfere with joint functions (Fig. 5.17). It is an autosomal dominant trait caused by mutations in exostosin, which plays a role in cartilage growth and may function as a tumour suppressor. The potential of these lesions occasionally to undergo malignant change over time is well documented. Any lesion which becomes inflamed or enlarges rapidly should be assessed by US to gauge the thickness of the cartilage cap. Surgical removal may be necessary.

Another rare recessive disorder of the diaphysis is Camurati–Engelmann syndrome, a form of hyperostosis in which pronounced thickening of the cortex

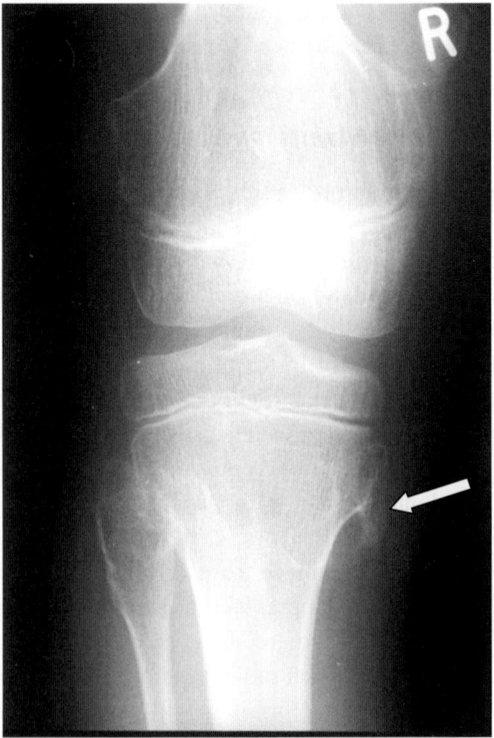

Fig. 5.17. An exostosis on the proximal tibia in a child with hereditary multiple exostoses. Note that the bone grows away from the growth plate.

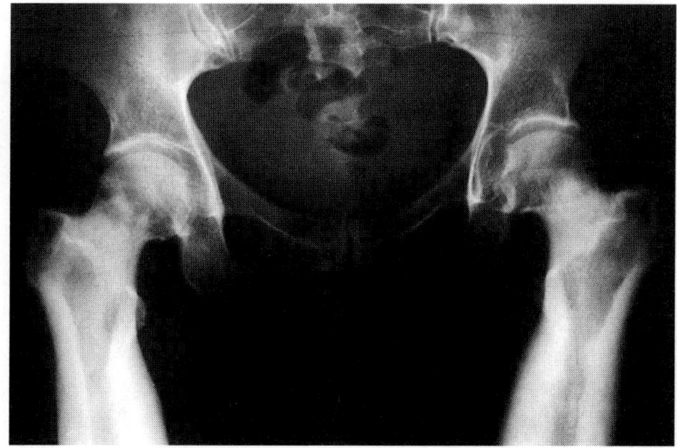

Fig. 5.18. Thickened femoral cortices in Camurati–Englemann syndrome.

of the bone (Fig. 5.18) is caused by activating mutations in TGF-β, which has bone anabolic affects. It is associated with a myopathy.

5.4.8. *Disorders of Bone Density*

Monogenic disorders of bone metabolism have given crucial insights into how the tightly regulated system of bone turnover may be disrupted. Activating and inactivating mutations in genes involved in both osteoblastic and osteoclastic activity are described, along with others that disrupt the linkage of osteoblast and osteoclast activity. The following limited list gives a flavour of the rich pathophysiology of these conditions.

Abnormalities of bone formation

Endosteal hyperostosis causes homogeneous increase in bone density as a result of activating mutations in LRP5, a receptor involved in Wnt signalling that is crucially involved in osteoblast activation (Fig. 5.19). Familial high bone mass is also related to mutations in LRP5. In contrast, inactivating mutations in LRP5 cause OP in the osteoporosis pseudoglioma syndrome, in which there is also failure of normal development of the retina. Natural variation of the LRP5 gene is also associated with variation in bone density in the general population. A natural inhibitor of LRP5, known as Dickkopf, is produced by myeloma cells which partly accounts for the OP of myelomatosis. Abnormalities in natural inhibitors of bone morphogenetic proteins also cause increased amounts of bone formation.

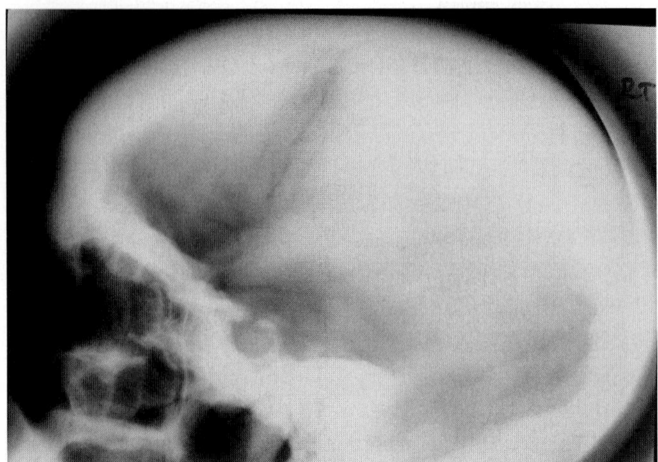

Fig. 5.19. Homogeneous increase in density and thickness of the skull bones in the Worth -type of endosteal hyperostosis. The thickening of the bones in the skull base may cause cranial nerve palsies.

Thus, inactivating mutations in sclerostin underlie conditions such as sclerostosis and van Buchem hyperostosis. In contrast, activating mutations in the bone morphogenetic protein (BMP) receptor, activin A receptor type 1, cause fibrodysplasia ossificans progressiva in which there is disordered formation of new bone eventually leading to extensive ossification of the muscles and related soft tissues (Fig. 5.20).

Abnormalities of bone resorption

Osteopetrosis (often known as 'marble bone disease') is caused by defective osteoclast function generally due to abnormalities of the mechanisms by which the acidic resorption lacuna is generated by the osteoclast. In the severe infantile form of the disease there is loss of function of the osteoclast-specific proton pump; in the less severe adult forms there are abnormalities of the chloride channel (CLCN7) necessary for the maintenance of electrical neutrality (Fig. 5.21) and in another type there is deficiency in the carbonic anhydrase gene required for the generation of hydrogen ions intracellularly. A related disorder, pycnodydostosis, also reduces osteoclast activity but in this case as a result of deficiency in the proteolytic enzyme cathepsin K, which is required for bone resorption. Despite causing increased bone density these disorders are associated with

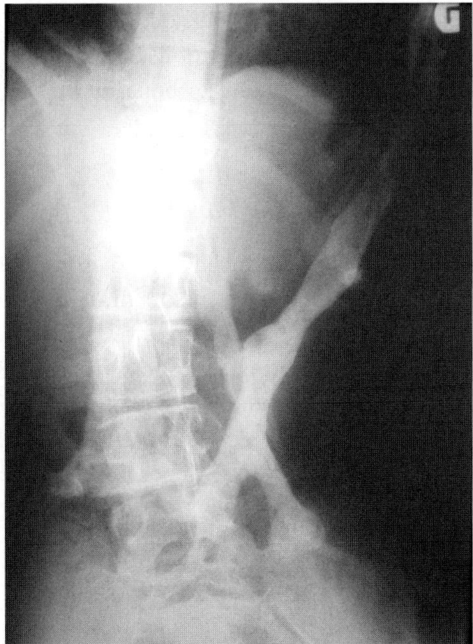

Fig. 5.20. Elaborate new bone formation in the trunk of an individual with fibrodysplasia ossificans progressiva.

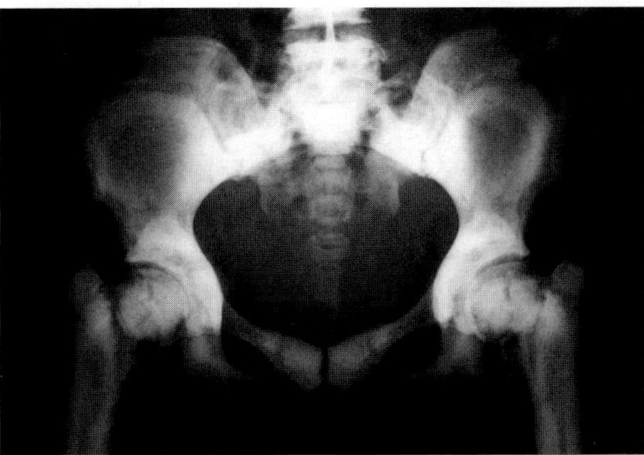

Fig. 5.21. Classic radiographic appearance of the pelvis in a form of osteopetrosis caused by mutations in the CLCN7 chloride channel. Note the dense bones and bone within a bone ('endobone') appearance.

qualitative deficiency of bone and a variable increased fracture tendency. Infantile osteopetrosis causes severe compromise of the bone marrow cavity by thickening of the bone trabeculae leading to bone marrow failure. This may be amenable to bone marrow transplantation.

Disorders of the RANK/RANK ligand axis

Under normal conditions RANKL produced by active osteoblasts stimulates the maturation and activation of osteoclast precursors through their RANK receptors. This interaction is modulated by the production of a decoy receptor (osteoprotegerin) that blocks RANKL. Activating mutations in RANK and inactivating mutations in osteoprotegerin can both lead to disproportionate activation of osteoclasts. These defects underlie two conditions, familial expansile osteolysis and idiopathic hyperphosphatasia (juvenile Paget's disease) respectively.

Chapter 6

Regional Pain Problems

Editor: Margaret Callan

Margaret Callan, Jeremiah Healy, Justin Lee

6.1. Shoulder Pain

Anatomy and Aetiopathogenesis

The shoulder girdle includes the articulation between the humerus and the glenoid cavity of the scapula and the acromioclavicular joints. The articulation between the humeral head and the glenoid is stabilised by the glenoid labrum, the glenohumeral ligaments, the rotator cuff tendons and the glenohumeral joint capsule. Above this the coracoacromial arch is formed by the coracoid process anteriorly, the acromion posteriorly and the coracoacromial ligament bridging the two structures. The rotator cuff tendons surround the shoulder joint with supraspinatus (abductor) passing superiorly, subscapularis (internal rotator) anteriorly and infraspinatus and teres minor (external rotators) posteriorly. The tendons are separated and protected from the structures of the coracoacromial arch by the subacromial bursa, which communicates with the more peripheral subdeltoid bursa. Deltoid itself passes over the bursae to its origin on the lateral clavicle, acromion and scapular spine. The long head of biceps runs along the bicipital groove on the humerus to the supraglenoid tubercle of the scapula whereas the short head passes anteriorly to insert directly to the coracoid process.

Pain affecting the shoulder area may arise from the bone, the glenohumeral or acromioclavicular joints, the tendons or subacromial bursa. Pain felt in the shoulder region may also be referred from the neck (particularly in the case of lesions involving the C4-C6 roots) or from subdiaphragmatic lesions. Finally, isolated shoulder pain, particularly in a child, has frequently been reported as the presenting feature of a haematological malignancy (Table 6.1).

Table 6.1. Common causes of shoulder pain.

Diagnosis	Underlying process
Glenohumeral arthritis	Osteoarthritis, rheumatoid arthritis
Acromioclavicular arthritis	Osteoarthritis
Subacromial bursitis	Impingement, rheumatoid arthritis, polymyalgia rheumatica
Tendinopathy or tendon tear	Impingement, degeneration, trauma
Calcific tendonitis	Calcium phosphate (hydroxyapatite) crystal deposition within tendons
Adhesive capsulitis	Unknown
Fracture	Trauma, osteoporosis, tumour
Tumour	Primary or secondary malignancy, benign bone tumour
Referred pain	Cervical spine pathology, subdiaphragmatic pathology

The glenohumeral joint may be involved in osteoarthritis or in inflammatory forms of arthritis such as rheumatoid arthritis. The acromioclavicular joint often develops osteoarthritic changes and this is particularly associated with repetitive heavy lifting or trauma. The tendons and subacromial bursa may become compressed between the head of the humerus and the coracoacromial arch, a process termed 'impingement'. The constant pressure on the subacromial bursa and tendons can lead to subacromial bursitis and tendinopathy. Thus the three conditions termed impingement, tendinopathy and subacromial bursitis often exist together. The rotator cuff tendons may also be damaged by trauma, leading to tears, or may be affected by degenerative change resulting in tendinopathy and progressing to degenerative tears. Calcification within rotator cuff tendons may precipitate an inflammatory response leading to episodes of acute shoulder pain. The subacromial bursa may become inflamed in association with tendon damage or in a variety of primarily inflammatory conditions including polymyalgia rheumatica and rheumatoid arthritis. The joint capsule itself may be involved in a process known as 'adhesive capsulitis' resulting in restriction of shoulder movement in all directions. Bone pathology, including local fracture and tumours may also present with shoulder pain.

Clinical Assessment

Patients will generally give a history of pain localised to the shoulder, upper back or upper arm. Pain from rotator cuff tendon pathology or subacromial bursitis is commonly felt only in the upper arm in the region of the deltoid. Examination should focus on determining the aetiology of the pain and should follow the 'look, feel, move' approach as described in Chapter 2. The examiner should assess the glenohumeral joint, the acromioclavicular joint and the rotator cuff. Examination should also include an assessment of the cervical spine and neurological examination of the upper limbs to exclude a cervical origin of the pain.

Many patients can be managed, in the first instance, on the basis of the clinical assessment without the need for further investigation. An X-ray of the shoulder may show a fracture or bone tumour and can be helpful in diagnosis of glenohumeral or acromioclavicular arthritis. Reduction in space between the acromion and humeral head suggests the possibility of rotator cuff degeneration. An X-ray will also demonstrate tendon calcification and so is an appropriate test for individuals with acute shoulder pain (Fig. 6.1). For the majority of patients the clinical signs will suggest tendon pathology or bursitis rather than arthritis and ultrasound (US) imaging is more appropriate than X-ray provided the US operators have appropriate expertise. A magnetic resonance imaging (MRI) scan will provide detail about the joints, rotator cuff and capsule; it is less dependent on operator expertise but is more expensive.

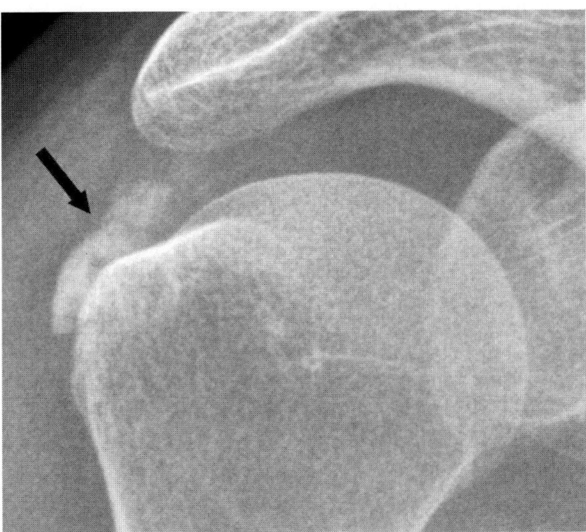

Fig. 6.1. Calcification of the supraspinatus tendon (arrow) as it passes over the humeral head and below the acromium. The subacromial bursa lies between the rotator cuff tendons and the arch formed by the acromium and the coracoacromial ligament.

Management

Management of osteoarthritis is considered elsewhere and the same principles apply with respect to the shoulder. Where the diagnosis relates to rotator cuff tendonitis/tendinosis or to subacromial bursitis then the first line of management is with non-steroidal anti-inflammatory drugs (NSAIDs) and with physiotherapy. If this is not helpful then subacromial injection of corticosteroid and lignocaine may relieve the symptoms and facilitate physiotherapy. It may be necessary to perform more than one injection and these are usually spaced at intervals of two to three months. Hydrodilatation, involving injection of ~25 ml fluid (including local anaesthetic and corticosteroid) into the shoulder joint, performed under imaging guidance, may be helpful in the case of adhesive capsulitis. Referral to an orthopaedic surgeon is indicated where there is a significant tear of the rotator cuff musculature, particularly in a relatively young patient. It may also be appropriate to refer for subacromial decompression where there are ongoing symptoms relating to impingement, or for manipulation under anaesthetic to facilitate restoration of movement in cases of adhesive capsulitis.

6.2. Neck Pain

Anatomy and Aetiopathogenesis

The cervical spine extends from the atlas (C1) and axis (C2) down to the vertebra prominens (C7), which has a long and easily palpable spinous process. The dens (odontoid peg) of the axis passes upwards through the atlas and is held in position adjacent to the anterior arch of the atlas by the transverse ligament. The individual vertebral bodies are separated from each other by intervertebral discs and articulate with each other via facet joints. The spinal cord passes from the brain down the vertebral foramen and gives rise to the eight cervical nerve roots. C1 exits above the first cervical vertebra and so on with C8 exiting from below C7. The C1 (suboccipital nerve) is purely motor. The remaining nerve roots provide sensory innervation to the occiput, neck and upper limbs and motor innervation to the muscles of the neck and arms.

The neck may be affected by degenerative disease of the spine with loss of intervertebral disc height, disc prolapse and development of facet joint arthritis. This condition is often referred to as cervical spondylosis and may result in compression of exiting nerve roots or, in severe cases, in compression of the cord itself resulting in cervical myelopathy. The upper part of the cervical spine may be involved in rheumatoid arthritis where loss of integrity of the transverse ligament of the atlas results in atlantoaxial subluxation, again with the possibility of

Table 6.2. Common causes of neck and back pain.

Diagnosis	Underlying process
Prolapsed intervertebral disc	Degenerative disease, trauma
Facet joint arthritis	Osteoarthritis
Vertebral body compression	Osteoporosis, local malignancy
Atlantoaxial subluxation	Rheumatoid arthritis
Sacroiliitis	Ankylosing spondylitis, psoriasis, inflammatory bowel disease
Osteomyelitis	Infection
Discitis	Infection

cervical cord compression. Much less commonly the cervical vertebrae may be the site of secondary neoplastic deposits or the vertebral bodies and discs may become infected (osteomyelitis and discitis). The neck is a common site for pain felt within the musculature, sometimes termed 'myofascial pain', and there are often associated tender 'trigger points'; the aetiology of this condition is not well understood (Table 6.2).

Clinical Assessment

A history of fevers, malaise, weight loss or previous malignancy signals the possibility of an infectious or malignant process. These features or a history of progressive neurological involvement should all prompt urgent assessment.

The neck should be inspected for deformity or spasm of musculature and the cervical spine itself palpated for tenderness. Patients should be assessed for their capacity to forward flex and extend, to laterally rotate both to the left and the right and to laterally flex their neck. Impairment of this last movement is usually associated with disease of the lower cervical spine. A neurological examination of the upper limbs should be performed to provide information about possible nerve root involvement. If cervical cord compression is a possibility then neurological examination of the lower limbs should also be performed to look for upper motor neurone signs including an extensor plantar response. The musculature of the neck and in particular the fibres of the trapezius passing laterally should be palpated to identify painful trigger points.

A plain X-ray of the cervical spine will provide some information about the presence of degenerative disease (Fig. 6.2). Views in flexion and extension allow for an assessment of the degree of atlantoaxial subluxation; the anterior aspect of the dens should lie within 4 mm of the anterior arch of the atlas

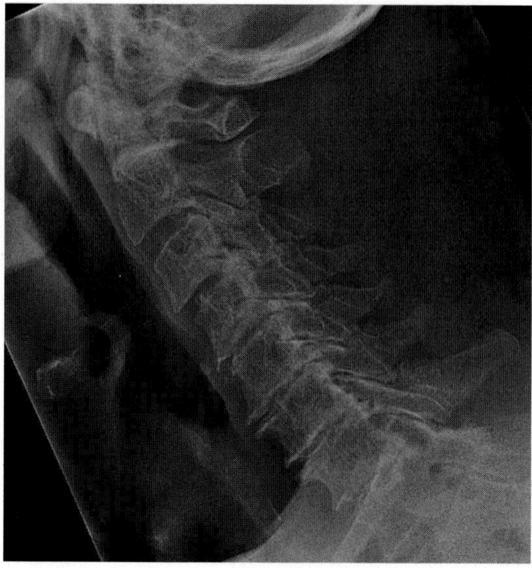

Fig. 6.2. Lateral X-ray of cervical spine demonstrating cervical spondylosis. Note loss of intervertebral disc height and anterior osteophyte formation particularly within the lower cervical spine.

(Fig. 6.3). An MRI scan will give much more detailed anatomical information than a plain X-ray and should always be requested if there is concern about local infection or malignancy or about significant neurological impairment. A computed tomography (CT) scan is generally less informative but may be of some value where an MRI scan is contraindicated and is very helpful in assessing for erosive disease (usually involving the odontoid peg) and atlantoaxial subluxation in patients with rheumatoid arthritis. Electromyography is also a useful tool for identifying nerve root lesions.

Management

The majority of patients who present with neck pain are found to have some degree of cervical spondylosis and may have associated myofascial pain. In general they may be treated with physiotherapy, analgesics and NSAIDs. Where muscle spasm is very severe then a benzodiazepine may be prescribed for a few days. Local injection of myofascial trigger points with lignocaine can be of benefit in some patients. Cervical epidurals or nerve root blocks are not commonly

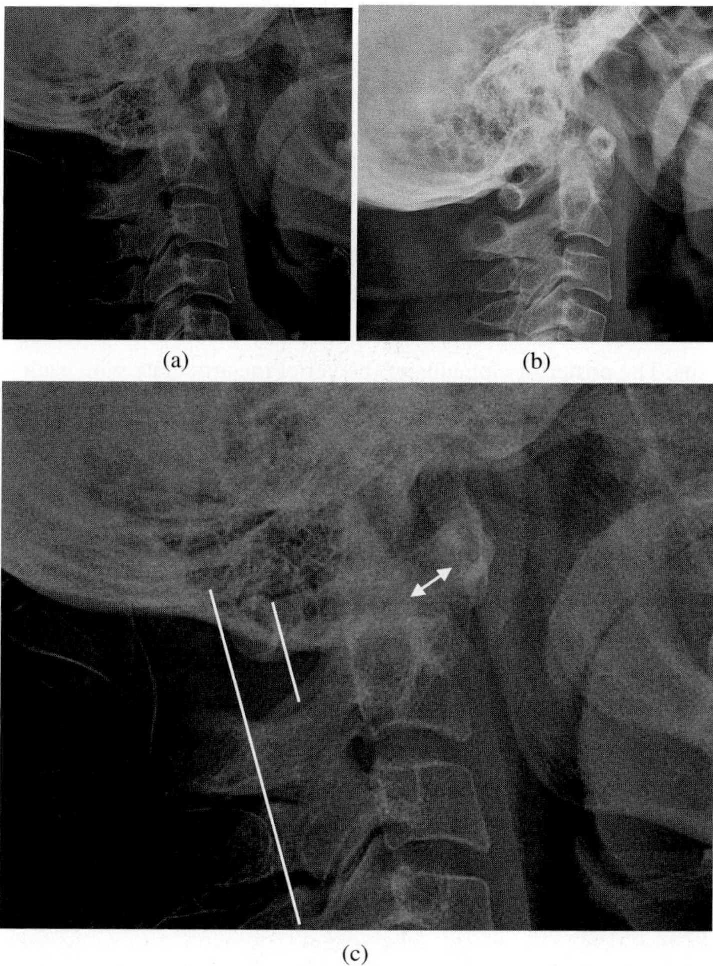

(a) (b)

(c)

Fig. 6.3. Lateral X-rays of cervical spine obtained in (a) flexion and (b) extension views. Note the different positions of the odontoid peg in the two views, consistent with atlanto-axial instability. This is considered significant where the distance between the odontoid peg and the anterior arch of the atlas is 4 mm or greater as demonstrated by the arrow in (c).

performed but have their place in management of persistent severe symptoms; patients should be referred to an appropriate pain service for these procedures. Referral for surgery may be considered if there is evidence of significant nerve root compression or cord compression. Likewise, patients with rheumatoid arthritis with atlantoaxial subluxation should be referred for a surgical opinion.

6.3. Mid and Low Back Pain

Anatomy and Aetiopathogenesis

The thoracic spine includes the 12 thoracic vertebrae whilst the lumbar spine comprises five lumbar vertebrae, the lowest of which articulates with the sacrum (Fig. 6.4). The sacrum in turn is formed from five fused sacral vertebrae, the lowest of which articulates with the coccyx. The sacrum articulates with the ilia via the sacroiliac joints. Within the thoracic and lumbar spine the vertebrae are separated from each other by intervertebral discs which are formed from a gelatinous core known as the nucleus pulposus surrounded by a fibrous ring termed the anulus fibrosus. The posterior elements of the vertebrae articulate with each other via the facet joints. The spinal cord passes down the spinal canal within the thoracic

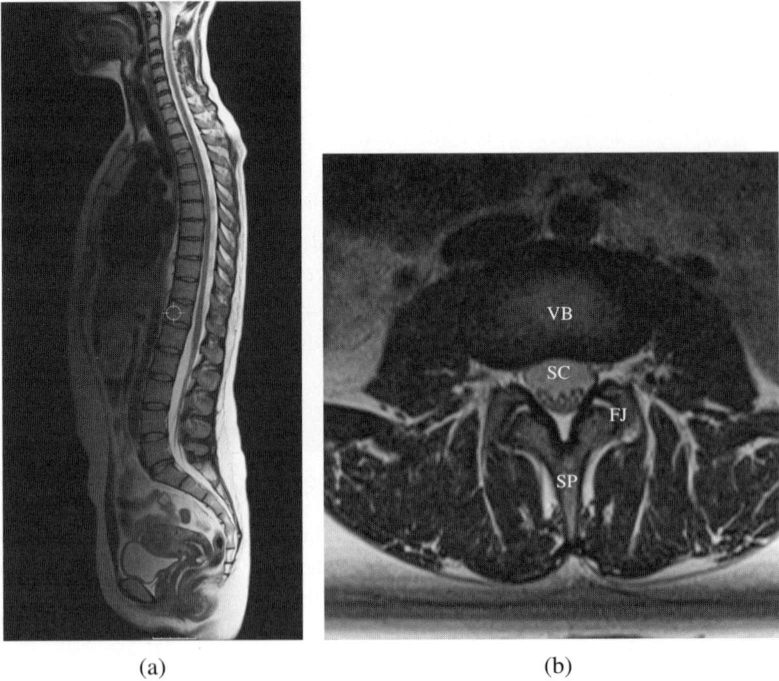

Fig. 6.4. MRI scan of spine. (a) Sagittal view showing cervical, thoracic, lumbar and sacral vertebrae. (b) Cross-sectional view through the lumbar spine showing the position of the vertebral body/disc (VB), spinal canal with nerve roots (SC), facet joints (FJ) and spinous process of the vertebra (SP).

spine and usually terminates at the L1 level; the lower nerve roots pass down through the lumbar vertebral canal as the cauda equina. Individual roots exit at each level and, in contrast to the nomenclature within the cervical spine, the root exiting below the T1 vertebral body is known as the T1 root and so on throughout the thoracic and lumbar spine. The nerve roots provide sensory innervation to the trunk and legs and motor innervation to the muscles in these regions.

Many different conditions may manifest as mid or low back pain. Degenerative disease of the spine refers to the changes within the intervertebral discs and facet joints that may accompany aging. Degenerative changes within the disc may result in circumferential disc bulge (involving >50% disc circumference) or disc herniation (focal herniation involving <25% disc circumference, broad based herniation involving 25–50% disc circumference). Circumferential disc bulges usually occur in older individuals whilst focal disc prolapses are more typical in younger people. They usually occur within the lower lumbar spine and may result in important stenosis of the canal or neural foramina resulting in neural compression. In some cases, loss of integrity of the annulus fibrosis allows the nucleus pulposus to pass posteriorly through the outer annulus fibrosus into the spinal canal. The discharging material results in chemical irritation of the nerve roots, which may present similarly to compression of the roots. Arthritis of the facet joints may be associated with the development of effusions or hypertrophied bone. It can cause pain locally or may contribute to spinal or foraminal stenosis and neural compression and be a source of referred pain.

Osteoporosis involving the thoracic or lumbar vertebral bodies may be symptomatic when compression fractures occur. Within the thoracic spine the tendency of the vertebral bodies to develop anterior wedging following fracture results in forward angulation of the spine known as kyphosis.

Inflammatory disease within the spine initially affects the sacroiliac joints and occurs in ankylosing spondylitis and in some patients with psoriasis or inflammatory bowel disease. The condition may progress to a true spondylitis involving the spine itself; details are given in the section on spondyloarthritis in Chapter 3.

Infections of the vertebral bodies (osteomyelitis) and intervertebral discs (infectious discitis) are rare but important causes of back pain. Although staphylococcus is the most common organism found in such patients, other organisms including *Mycobacterium tuberculosis* may be causative.

Metastatic malignant disease and myeloma may involve the thoracic or lumbar spine and may present with back pain, with or without evidence of vertebral collapse.

Compression of the spinal cord or cauda equina may be caused by any of the above pathologies. Cord compression will result if the compressive lesion is above the level of termination of cord at L1-L2 and will be characterised by upper motor neurone signs in the lower limbs with hyperreflexia and upgoing plantar responses. A cauda equina syndrome will result if the compressive lesion is below the level of termination of the cord at L1-L2. Patients with a cauda equina syndrome usually experience back pain and may also have sciatic type symptoms, variable motor and sensory deficits in the legs, saddle sensory disturbance and bladder and bowel dysfunction with poor anal sphincter tone. Since the condition affects the cauda equina nerve roots rather than the cord itself the neurological signs will be those of lower rather than upper motor neurone lesions. Patients with features of cord compression or cauda equina syndrome need to be investigated and treated urgently.

Clinical Assessment

Back pain is a very common complaint and it is important to identify those cases where there may be serious spinal pathology. Possible indicators of such pathology have become known as the 'red flags' but are simply indicators of possible infectious or malignant disease or important neurological involvement. They include a history of fever, weight loss, general ill health, previous diagnosis of cancer, progressive neurological deficit, disturbed gait, saddle anaesthesia or bowel or bladder dysfunction. These patients need prompt investigation with relevant blood tests and an MRI scan of the lumbar spine.

The term 'yellow flags' is used to describe psychosocial factors that are indicative of long-term chronicity and disability. These include a negative attitude that is harmful or disabling, avoidance behaviour resulting from fear of pain that results in reduced activity, an expectation that passive treatment will be beneficial with a reluctance to engage actively in physical based therapies, a tendency to depression, low morale, social withdrawal and social or financial problems. Whilst these patients do not generally need detailed or urgent investigation with blood tests and MRI scans they do need prompt treatment to minimise the risk of chronicity (Table 6.3).

The spine should be examined using the 'look, feel, move' approach as described in Chapter 2. The modified Schober's test is a useful tool for assessing capacity to forward flex the lumbar spine and the straight leg raise and femoral stretch tests can detect impingment of lower and upper lumbar nerve roots respectively. A neurological examination of the legs should be performed, looking for abnormalities of tone, power and sensation to light touch. The knee, ankle and plantar reflexes should be elicited.

Table 6.3. Red and yellow flags in the assessment of back pain.

Red flags	Yellow flags
Fever	Negative attitude
Weight loss	Fear avoidance behaviour with low activity
Previous diagnosis of cancer	Expectations of benefit from passive treatment
Progressive neurological deficit	History of depression
Disturbed gait	Social isolation or other social problems
Saddle anaesthesia	Financial problems
Bladder or bowel dysfunction	

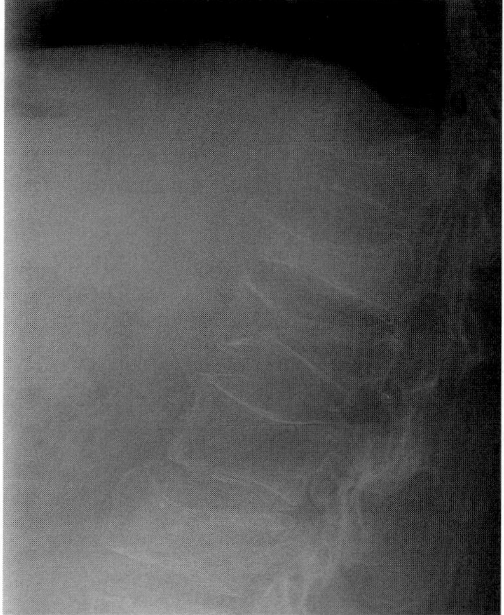

Fig. 6.5. Plain X-ray of the thoracolumbar spine demonstrating osteopenia of bones and multiple vertebral compression ('wedge') fractures.

Thoracic and lumbar spine X-rays are relatively uninformative although they may give general information about the presence of degenerative spinal disease and will be helpful in identifying vertebral compression fractures (Fig. 6.5). Where 'red flags' are present or the symptoms are severe and persistent then an MRI scan is indicated (Fig. 6.6). A CT scan is much less informative although it may be of some value where an MRI scan is contraindicated and can be helpful

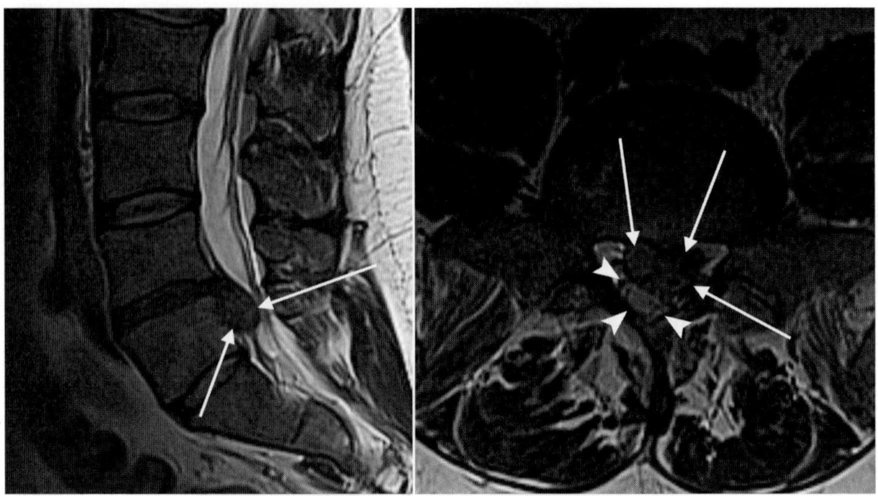

Fig. 6.6. MRI scan showing sagittal and axial cross-sectional views of the lumbar spine demonstrating disc prolapse (long arrows) displacing the thecal sac (arrowheads) posteriorly.

in identifying bony lesions such as an osteoid osteoma. Likewise, a nuclear medicine bone scan is effective in identifying bony lesions including metastases. Specific imaging of the sacroiliac joints should be performed if there is a concern about the possibility of sacroiliitis. Blood tests should be performed if there is any suspicion of infectious or malignant disease to look at the white cell count, inflammatory markers, immunoglobulins and tumour markers. Electrophysiological studies may be helpful in the detection of nerve root lesions.

Management

The majority of patients will have evidence of degenerative disease of the spine without evidence of serious infectious or malignant pathology or important neurological compromise. The symptoms may respond to simple analgesics or NSAIDs. Where significant muscle spasm is present then a short course of diazepam, for two to four days, may be beneficial. The patient should be referred to a physiotherapist and encouraged to engage in a programme of strengthening exercises. Where pain is more severe or persistent then referral to a pain clinic may be indicated for an epidural, selective nerve root injection or facet joint injections. In a small proportion of individuals, referral to a surgeon may be required for consideration of discectomy, laminectomy or spinal fusion.

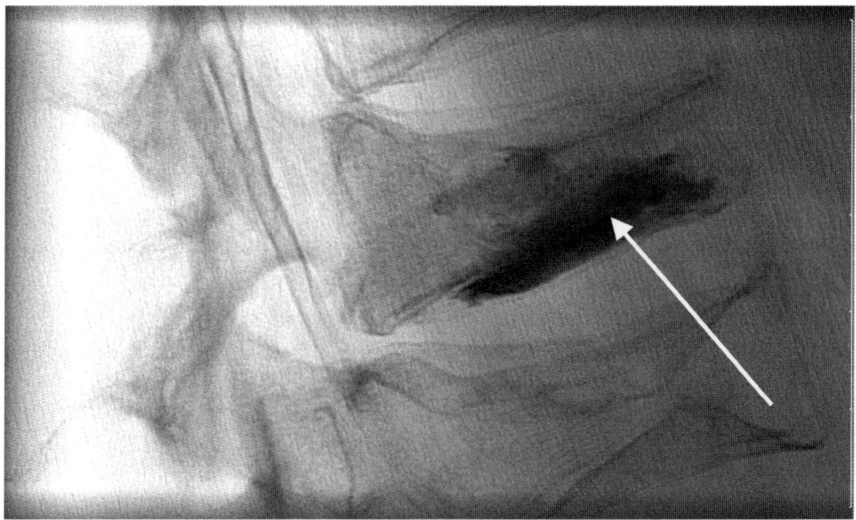

Fig. 6.7. Fractured vertebral body following injection of 'cement' (indicated by arrow) during vertebroplasty. The cement has filled a cleft adjacent to the inferior end plate.

Patients who have vertebral compression fractures should be treated with appropriate analgesics. If pain persists there may be a role for percutaneous vertebroplasty. In this procedure a needle is inserted into the vertebral body via the pedicle and semi-liquid surgical cement is injected (Fig. 6.7). This provides some support for the fractured vertebra and is effective in relieving pain in the majority of individuals. An alternative procedure in which a small balloon is inflated within the vertebral body and the resultant cavity is filled with cement is termed kyphoplasty. This latter procedure may be more effective in restoring vertebral height than a vertebroplasty particularly if undertaken within four weeks of the fracture; however, at this stage some patients and physicians will prefer to wait to see whether pain will improve with conservative management. The possibility of underlying osteoporosis or malignancy must be considered in patients with vertebral compression fractures.

6.4. Nerve Entrapment Syndromes

Compression of the median nerve at the wrist and the ulnar nerve at the elbow are the most common nerve entrapment syndromes (Table 6.4). Compression of the

Table 6.4. Median and ulnar nerve entrapment syndromes.

	Median Nerve	Ulnar Nerve
Usual site of compression	Wrist	Elbow
Testing for sensory abnormalities	Palmar aspect of thumb, index, middle and radial side of ring finger	Palmar aspect of little finger and ulnar side of ring finger
Testing for motor abnormalities	Resisted thumb abduction Resisted thumb opposition	Resisted finger spreading Crossed finger test
Specific tests	Tinel's test over carpal tunnel at wrist Manual compression of carpal tunnel Phalen's test	Tinel's test over ulnar groove at elbow and Guyon's canal at wrist Froment's test

tibial nerve in the tarsal tunnel or of the lateral femoral cutaneous nerve as it passes under the inguinal ligament is less commonly seen. It is thought that compression results in reduction of epineural blood flow, leading to ischaemia and reduced capacity to conduct nerve impulses. Severe or chronic compression can lead to irreversible damage with increased likelihood of motor involvement. Compression occurs at sites where the nerves pass through confined spaces and is made more likely in the context of local inflammation, space occupying lesions, increases in adipose tissue or oedema. Thus inflammatory arthritis, local trauma, ganglion cysts, obesity, pregnancy and hypothyroidism may all be associated with an increased risk of peripheral nerve entrapment syndromes. Whilst peripheral nerve entrapment syndromes are common, care must always be taken to distinguish between a peripheral and a more proximal lesion involving the nerve roots.

6.4.1. *Carpal Tunnel Syndrome*

Anatomy and Aetiopathogenesis

The median nerve passes through the carpal tunnel, which is bordered dorsally by the bones of the carpus and ventrally by the flexor retinaculum and also provides a passageway for the flexor digitorum and pollicis tendons. The median nerve carries sensory fibres for the radial part of the palm and the radial 3 1/2 digits. However, there is anatomical variation between individuals and extensive overlap between territories supplied by the different nerves. The distal part of the index and middle fingers are usually exclusively supplied by the median nerve.

The nerve also carries motor fibres supplying the first and second lumbricals and the muscles of the thenar eminence (opponens pollicis, abductor pollicis brevis, flexor pollicis brevis), memorable by the acronym 'LOAF'.

Clinical Assessment

Patients usually present with 'pins and needles' or numbness affecting the hand and often report an aching sensation over the ventral aspect of the wrist. They are rarely able to be specific about the precise part of the hand that is affected. Examination should seek to determine whether there is a reduction in sensory capacity over the palmar aspect of the radial 3 1/2 digits and whether there is any wasting of the thenar eminence or weakness of the thumb abductor or opponens muscles (test resisted thumb abduction and opposition). Tapping on the volar aspect of the wrist over the carpal tunnel may elicit tingling in the distribution of the nerve (Tinel's sign). Compression of the carpal tunnel for 30 seconds by the examiner's thumbs may also reproduce symptoms as may full flexion of the wrist for 60 seconds (Phalen's test). The likelihood of the diagnosis is higher if the ratio of wrist thickness:wrist width is >70% (square wrist sign). A suspected diagnosis needs to be confirmed by electrophysiological tests; these nerve conduction studies are then used to grade the condition as mild, moderate or severe.

Management

Where the condition is mild or moderate it may be treated conservatively in the first instance. Underlying precipitating factors such as weight gain, thyroid abnormalities or inflammatory arthritis should be diagnosed and treated. Patients should be given a wrist support that will hold the wrist in a neutral position and told to wear the orthosis at night. Local injection of corticosteroid into the carpal tunnel can be effective in alleviating the symptoms although the effects may be temporary. Where the symptoms do not respond to conservative measures or where they are graded as severe on electrophysiological testing then referral to a hand surgery department for carpal tunnel decompression (release of the flexor retinaculum) should be made.

6.4.2. *Ulnar Nerve Entrapment Syndrome*

Anatomy and Aetiopathogenesis

The ulnar nerve is usually compressed at the elbow, either within the olecranon groove or cubital tunnel. The nerve may also be compressed as it bifurcates into the deep motor and superficial sensory branches within Guyon's canal, which lies on the ulnar aspect of the volar surface of the wrist. Within the forearm the ulnar nerve supplies the flexor carpi ulnaris and the fibres of flexor digitorum profundus that serve to flex the ring and little fingers. Following its bifurcation the sensory fibres innervate the skin of the hypothenar eminence, little finger and ulnar aspect of the ring finger and the motor fibres innervate the 3rd and 4th lumbricals, interossei, the muscles of the hypothenar eminence as well as the adductor pollicis and deep head of flexor pollicis brevis.

Clinical Assessment

Patients usually present with paraesthesia affecting the ring and little fingers. In more severe cases motor function is impaired leading to loss of strength of the intrinsic hand muscles and consequent 'clawing' of the hand. There may also be loss of strength of flexor carpi ulnaris if the site of compression is at the elbow rather than the wrist. Nerve entrapment at the wrist may involve only the sensory or motor branch depending on the precise site of pathology.

Examination should be directed at determining whether there is sensory deficit over the little finger and ulnar portion of the ring finger and whether there is loss of power of flexor carpi ulnaris (tested with resisted wrist flexion) and of the intrinsic muscles of the hands. The latter may be tested by asking the patient to cross the middle finger over the index finger (crossed finger test), by resisted abduction of the little and index fingers (spreading fingers against resistance) or by asking the patient to grip paper between their adducted thumb and palm of hand or index finger; this will induce flexion at the thumb interphalangeal (IP) joint as described in Chapter 2 (Froment's sign). Tapping over the ulnar nerve at the elbow or in Guyon's canal at the wrist may reproduce the symptoms (Tinel's test). The course of the ulnar nerve should also be palpated to try and identify pathologies that might be causing compression.

The diagnosis can be confirmed by electrophysiological studies. Further investigation should include X-rays and US scans of the elbow and/or wrist as appropriate to attempt to identify the aetiology of the compression. X-rays will show bony spurs or fragments at the elbow or fracture of the hook of the hamate or dislocation of the small joints of the wrist. An US scan may demonstrate a neurogenic tumour or an extrinsic mass such as a ganglion.

Management

The majority of patients will experience sensory without motor symptoms, have compression at the elbow and can be treated conservatively. The condition will usually respond to simple measures aimed at reducing stress on the ulnar nerve at the elbow. Thus patients should avoid sleeping with their elbows flexed, leaning on bent elbows or holding a telephone to their ear for long periods of time. Elbow extension splints can be used to prevent individuals from flexing the affected arm although many patients find these splints cumbersome and inconvenient. NSAIDs may be helpful in some cases. If there is no response to conservative measures and particularly if the symptoms progress or involve motor function then a referral for surgery, which usually involves decompression with or without anterior transposition of the ulnar nerve at the elbow, should be considered.

6.4.3. *Tarsal Tunnel Syndrome*

Anatomy and Aetiopathogenesis

Tarsal tunnel syndrome results from compression of the tibial nerve posterior and inferior to the medial malleolus, as it passes through the tarsal tunnel. The floor of the tunnel is formed by the tibia, talus and calcaneum with the roof being provided by the flexor retinaculum. Other structures passing through the tunnel include the posterior tibial artery and the flexor hallucis longus, flexor digitorum longus and tibialis posterior muscles/tendons. The tibial nerve divides after passing through the tunnel into medial and lateral plantar nerves. Sensory branches from the tibial, medial and lateral plantar nerves supply the heel and plantar aspect of the foot. Motor branches supply many of the small muscles within the feet including the flexor muscles for the toes, lumbricals and interossei muscles.

Clinical Assessment

Patients report pain, ‘pins and needles’ and numbness that usually affect the heel and plantar aspect of the foot. More rarely there is weakness and atrophy of individual foot muscles. Valgus deformity of the hindfoot may increase tension within the nerve and exacerbate symptoms. Tinel’s test or Phalen’s test over the tarsal tunnel may be positive. The diagnosis can be confirmed by electrophysiological studies.

Management

Similarly to management of the upper limb nerve entrapment disorders, orthoses, corticosteroid injections and surgery all play a role in treatment. Foot orthoses should aim to correct valgus deformities of the hind foot. Night splints that place the foot in plantar flexion with varus may be helpful although they are cumbersome. Local injection of corticosteroid and lignocaine to the tarsal tunnel may be effective. Surgical decompression is rarely required.

6.4.4. *Meralgia Paraesthetica*

Anatomy and Aetiopathogenesis

Meralgia paraesthetica describes a mononeuropathy involving the lateral femoral cutaneous nerve (sometimes know as the lateral cutaneous nerve of the thigh). The nerve passes along the psoas muscle and through a tunnel created by the lateral attachment of inguinal ligament and anterior superior iliac spine and provides sensory innervation for the anterolateral thigh. It does not have any motor fibres. It is usually compressed as it passes under the inguinal ligament and the condition may be precipitated or exacerbated by obesity, pregnancy, use of tight clothing or sleeping in the foetal position. More rarely symptoms result from more proximal compression by a space occupying lesion.

Clinical Assessment

Patients usually present with numbness and sometimes with pain that affects the anterolateral thigh. The condition is usually unilateral. Tinel's test over the lateral inguinal ligament may be positive. Extending the hip to stretch the nerve or deep palpation just below the anterior superior iliac spine may both reproduce pain. Muscle strength should be normal. Electrophysiological studies may be required to confirm the diagnosis. Imaging studies will be needed if there is concern about a proximal space occupying lesion as a cause for neural compression.

Management

Most patients may be managed conservatively with advice to lose weight and to avoid tight clothing. Local injection with corticosteroid and lignocaine placed around the nerve as it passes under the inguinal ligament may be helpful in more resistant cases. Surgical intervention is rarely necessary.

6.5. Disorders of Tendons and their Sheaths

A tendon is a band of fibrous tissue that attaches a muscle to a bone and serves to transmit the force of the muscle contraction to the bone. The matrix of the tendon is composed predominantly of collagen. The 'tenocytes' are the tendon cells; they are arranged longitudinally along the course of the collagen fibre bundles and are fibroblast-like cells, capable of producing the surrounding collagen and proteoglycans. The tendon matrix is continually remodelled although the rate of matrix turnover is very varied, with increased levels of collagen synthesis occurring in the more highly stressed tendons. The enthesis refers to the tendon-bone insertion where there is a gradual conversion from tendon to fibrocartilage to bone. Sections of tendons may be enclosed by sheaths lined with synovial tissue, particularly as they pass through fibro-osseous tunnels (compartments formed from bone and overlying fibrous retinaculum) and this enhances their capacity to glide freely at these sites. The Achilles tendon and infrapatella tendons do not have a true synovial sheath but are enclosed by a thin membrane of connective tissue known as a paratenon.

The term tendinopathy covers both degenerative (tendinosis) and inflammatory conditions of the tendons (tendonitis). In general, histopathological studies suggest that tendinosis rather than tendonitis is the dominant pathological process; changes occur in the morphology and numbers of resident cells with neovascularisation and alterations of the matrix whereas infiltration with inflammatory cells is rarely seen. Despite the lack of inflammatory cells, some pro-inflammatory mediators, including cytokines such as interleukin (IL)-1 and IL-6 may be present, so the picture is often mixed to some extent.

Enthesopathy refers to pathology at the tendon enthesis and these conditions also come under the broad heading of tendinopathies. The term 'enthesitis' is commonly used instead of that of 'enthesopathy' but can be inaccurate as histopathological studies suggest that the condition is frequently degenerative rather than inflammatory in nature.

The term tenosynovitis is used where the synovial sheath around a tendon becomes infiltrated with inflammatory cells and the synovial tissue is stimulated to proliferate in a manner analogous to that which occurs within synovial joints. The term 'paratenonitis' or 'paratendonitis' is used to describe inflammatory change within the paratenon of the Achilles tendon.

Abnormalities may also occur within the fibrous retinacular tissues that form part of the fibro-osseous tunnels leading to stenosis of these tunnels. The term 'tenovaginitis' has been used to describe presumed inflammation within the fibrous tissue although this may also be a misnomer as histopathological studies suggest that fibrocartilaginous metaplasia rather than inflammatory infiltrates are characteristic.

Tendinopathies most commonly involve the supraspinatus tendon at the shoulder, the common extensor or flexor tendons at the elbow, the infrapatella tendon at the knee and the tibialis posterior and the Achilles tendons at the ankle. Tenosynovitis or paratenonitis often occur in association with tendinopathies of the tibialis posterior and Achilles tendons respectively. Abnormalities within the fibrous retinacular tissues are thought to underlie the conditions known as De Quervain's disease and 'trigger digits' (Table 6.5).

Systemic inflammatory conditions may lead to the development of truly inflammatory tenosynovitis or enthesitis. Tenosynovitis is a very common feature of rheumatoid arthritis and psoriatic arthritis and usually responds to systemic treatment for these conditions or to paratendinous corticosteroid injection. Enthesitis and plantar fasciitis are also well recognised in psoriatic arthritis and spondyloarthritis and may likewise respond to systemic treatment or local corticosteroid injection.

6.5.1. *Lateral Elbow Tendinopathy*

Anatomy and Aetiopathogenesis

Lateral elbow tendinopathy is the best term to describe the condition often known as 'tennis elbow', lateral epicondylitis or lateral elbow enthesitis. It usually occurs in middle aged individuals with a history of repetitive wrist use and is much more common in supermarket shelf stackers and sandwich makers than in tennis players. The tendinopathy involves the wrist extensor muscles, or occasionally the supinator muscle, close to their attachment at the lateral epicondyle.

Table 6.5. Common pathologies of tendons and fascia.

Region	Tendon(s) commonly involved	Common name
Shoulder	Supraspinatus tendon	–
Elbow	Common extensor tendons	Tennis elbow
	Common flexor tendons	Golfer's elbow
Wrist	Abductor pollicis longus	De Quervain's disease
	Extensor pollicis brevis	
Hand	Flexor digitorum	Trigger fingers or thumb
	Flexor pollicis	
Knee	Infrapatella tendon	Jumper's knee
Ankle	Tibialis posterior tendon	
	Achilles tendon	

Clinical Assessment

Patients experience pain close to the lateral epicondyle, which is worse with activity and relieved by rest. Tenderness is usually felt over and just distal to the lateral epicondyle. Pain is precipitated by resisted wrist extension and resisted middle finger extension, with the elbow in an extended position and the forearm pronated. Provided the clinical picture is typical then there is usually no need for any specific investigations to be performed.

Management

There is a lack of evidence suggesting that specific treatment alters the long-term outcome from lateral elbow tendinopathy and approximately 80% of individuals recover within one year without treatment. However, there is some evidence that topical or oral diclofenac is beneficial in the short term and that local, peritendinous corticosteroid injection also provides short-term relief. Much smaller studies have suggested a possible role for topical nitrates, which may stimulate collagen synthesis, dry needling of the tendon or autologous blood injections at the site of tendinopathy. There is a role for physiotherapy and application of a counterforce brace applied 10 cm distal to the elbow may also be symptomatically helpful. Surgery is rarely indicated but can be beneficial in refractory cases.

6.5.2. *Medial Elbow Tendinopathy*

Anatomy and Aetiopathogenesis

Medial elbow tendinopathy refers to a similar condition affecting the tendons inserting to the medial epicondyle and is often referred to as 'golfer's elbow'. The involved tendons are those of the wrist flexors and forearm pronator. It occurs much less commonly than lateral elbow tendinopathy but is likewise associated with repetitive stressing of the relevant muscles and tendons, being reported for example in workmen using hammers and screwdrivers as well as in tennis players and golfers.

Clinical Assessment

Patients present with pain affecting the medial elbow that is worse with activity and relieved by rest. Tenderness is usually felt over and just distal to the medial epicondyle and pain is reproduced by resisted wrist flexion and forearm pronation. In typical cases there is no need for investigations to be performed.

Management

Treatment is as described above for lateral elbow tendinopathy.

6.5.3. *Patella Tendinopathy*

Anatomy and Aetiopathogenesis

This condition usually affects the attachment of the patella tendon to the inferior pole of the patella although the attachment of the quadriceps tendon to the superior pole of the patella or of the patella tendon to the anterior tuberosity of the tibia may also occur. The condition is often referred to as 'jumper's knee' and is associated with repetitive stressing or overloading of the patella tendon as may occur in sporting activities such as basketball.

Clinical Assessment

Patients report an aching type of pain affecting the anterior part of the knee. In mild cases the pain classically occurs after activity but in those more severely affected it may also occur during activity. Examination usually shows tenderness over the inferior pole of the patella although in some cases the signs are localised to the superior pole of the patella or the tibial tuberosity. X-rays are not helpful in making the diagnosis. A US scan may show focal or generalised thickening of the tendon with hypoechogenicity and increased flow on colour Doppler. An MRI scan can also be used to identify abnormal areas within the tendon and may, in addition, demonstrate an associated stress response in the patella and adjacent oedema within the infrapatella fat pad.

Management

Patients should be advised to modify their level of activity and to apply ice topically after activity. A counterforce strap may reduce stress on the tendon during activity. Patients should be referred to physiotherapy for a stretching and strengthening programme. NSAIDs may be helpful in alleviating symptoms. A peritendinous injection of local corticosteroid may be considered if the symptoms do not respond to conservative measures, although care must be taken to avoid damaging the tendon and the patient should be advised to avoid activity for 14 days after the injection. Where the condition is severe and tendon rupture occurs then this requires referral to an orthopaedic surgeon for repair.

6.5.4. *Achilles Tendinopathy*

Anatomy and Aetiopathogenesis

Within the lower calf the gastrocnemius and soleus muscles merge to form the Achilles tendon, which runs within a paratenon sheath and inserts to the calcaneal tuberosity. A relative watershed in blood supply exists approximately 3–4 cm proximal to the calcaneal insertion and this portion of the tendon is most susceptible to tendinopathy and rupture.

The Achilles tendon is particularly subject to stress in individuals with heel or forefoot varus, pronated or cavus feet and tibia vara, and pathology is associated with overuse or overloading, particularly in older and recreational athletes.

Two principal types of pathology affect the Achilles tendon and these often coexist. Paratenonitis describes inflammatory change within the paratenon whilst tendinopathy describes the changes, usually degenerative in nature, within the tendon. Severe tendinosis may lead to partial or complete tendon rupture.

Clinical Assessment

Individuals with paratenonitis usually present with pain and swelling over the tendon with the symptoms being exacerbated by activity. Tendinopathy itself is often aymptomatic although individuals may notice a nodular lesion within the tendon at the site of the degenerative change. Examination should be undertaken with the patient lying prone with the feet hanging over the edge of the couch. The entire tendon should be palpated for tenderness and nodules. In the majority of cases there is no need for further investigations. However, if more detailed information is required and particularly if there is concern about tendon tear or rupture then either a US or MRI scan should be requested.

Management

Patients should be advised to avoid sporting activities involving forceful plantar flexion, such as running, and should use local ice to treat symptoms. NSAIDs may help to relieve symptoms. A heel pad may relieve the stress on the Achilles tendon. Patients should be advised about stretching exercises and should be referred to physiotherapy for eccentric strengthening exercise and help in gradually escalating sporting activity if relevant. Peritendinous injections of corticosteroid are generally avoided because of a possible associated risk of tendon damage and rupture. Occasionally surgery is required for excision of adhesions, decompression of the tendon or repair of tendon rupture.

6.5.5. *Posterior Tibial Tendinopathy*

Anatomy and Aetiopathogenesis

The tibialis posterior muscle arises from the interosseous membrane and posterior surface of the tibia in the proximal third of the lower leg. The fibres coalesce to form the tendon in the lower third of the leg and this curves around the posterior aspect of the medial malleolus to pass through the tarsal tunnel and insert to the navicular, giving off fibrous expansions to the calcaneus, cuneiforms, cuboid and metatarsals. The tibialis posterior muscle serves to plantar flex and invert the foot. The pathological processes may involve a tenosynovitis and a tendinopathy and both tend to occur at the level of the medial malleolus where a synovial sheath is present and where the blood supply to the tendon is relatively poor. The condition may progress leading to flattening of the longitudinal arch of the foot.

Clinical Assessment

Patients usually present with medial ankle pain and difficulty walking. They may have swelling and tenderness posterior or inferior to the medial malleolus, or more distally along the course of the tendon. Their foot position may be abnormal with a tendency to valgus at the ankle, flattening of the arch and splaying of the forefoot. They will not be able to stand on their toes easily and this manoeuvre will tend to reproduce pain at the site of the tendon pathology. An US scan is helpful in confirming the diagnosis and assessing the severity of the tendiopathy.

Management

If the condition is acute then NSAIDs and local icing may be beneficial. Supportive insoles, boots or a short leg cast will help to rest or immobilise the tendon. In general corticosteroid injections are avoided because of concerns about increasing the risk of tendon damage and rupture. Referral to a surgeon may be appropriate in severe cases for consideration of debridement or tendon reconstruction.

6.5.6. *De Quervain's Disease*

Anatomy and Aetiopathogenesis

De Quervain's tenosynovitis is more properly called De Quervain's disease and refers to thickening and stenosis of the fibrous sheath of the first dorsal (extensor) compartment which encloses the tendons of extensor pollicis brevis and abductor pollicis longus. The histopathological findings are of proliferation of fibrous tissue and myxoid degeneration within the fibrous sheath. The thickening of the fibrous sheath creates friction as the tendons move through the first dorsal compartment and this is thought to cause inflammation within the synovial sheath. The condition affects women much more commonly than men and often presents in the months following childbirth. It may be exacerbated by repetitive pinching action of the thumb although whether this is actually causative is controversial.

Clinical Assessment

Patients complain of pain affecting the radial aspect of the wrist that is worse on activity. There may be local swelling and tenderness. Finkelstein's test involves asking the patient to enclose their thumb in their fist and subjecting the wrist to ulnar deviation. Whilst this may be mildly uncomfortable in normal individuals, the manoeuvre usually induces significant pain in the context of De Quervain's disease. There is rarely a need for specific investigation but if the diagnosis is in doubt then US scanning of the wrist can demonstrate changes within the relevant fibrous sheath. Care should be taken to distinguish between this condition and osteoarthritis of the first carpometacarpal (CMC) joint.

Management

The condition is usually self-limiting within a period of approximately 12 months. NSAIDs can provide symptomatic relief. A thumb post type orthosis may also be helpful. Corticosteroid injections into the tendon sheath may be beneficial although care should be taken not to damage the tendon or to inject too superficially; the latter can be associated with skin thinning. Referral to a surgeon for release of the first dorsal compartment is very rarely required.

6.5.7. *Trigger Digits*

Anatomy and Aetiopathogenesis

'Trigger digits' result from the compromised movement of the flexor tendons to the thumb and fingers. The flexor tendons to the thumb and fingers are encompassed in a synovial lining as they pass through a fibrous sheath. The latter runs from the level of the metacarpal heads to the distal phalanges and is attached to the underlying bones and volar plates of the joints. Thickenings within the fibrous flexor sheath are termed 'the pulleys'. The A1 pulley is the first annular thickening of the sheath and overlies the metacarpophalangeal (MCP) joint. Other annular and cruciate pulleys lie more distally along the course of the tendon.

'Trigger digits' are thought to arise because of a mismatch between the size of the tendon and the pulleys. The condition usually affects the flexor pollicis longus or flexor digitorum superficialis tendons, usually at the site of the A1 pulley. The prime lesion is thought to be fibrocartilaginous metaplasia of the pulley. The abnormal, thickened pulley then causes friction where the tendon passes under it and this may result in some local inflammation and, ultimately, in the development of a fusiform swelling in the tendon itself. The latter results from 'bunching' of the tendon fibres consequent upon the recurrent compression and friction. Occasionally adhesions may form within the tendon sheath, further compromising movement of the tendon.

Clinical Assessment

Trigger digits commonly affect women in their 50s and 60s and usually involve the thumb or ring finger. They are more common in the context of diabetes or hypothyroidism. Patients may experience pain and tenderness, usually on the palm at the level of the MCP joint, and a local nodule may be palpable. The finger may lock when flexed and, on attempted extension, may release suddenly with a popping sensation.

Management

NSAIDs may provide some symptomatic relief in painful cases. In general, the condition is best treated with a peritendinous injection of corticosteroid and lignocaine; the outcome from this intervention is usually very good although it is more variable in the context of diabetes mellitus. On occasions it may be necessary to proceed to either percutaneous or open tendon release.

6.6. Plantar Fasciitis

Anatomy and Aetiopathogenesis

The plantar fascia originates from the medial tubercle of the calcaneus and spreads out over the plantar aspect of the foot to the metatarsal heads and toes, serving to support the longitudinal arch of the foot and to absorb the 'shock' associated with weight bearing on the foot. Degenerative and secondary proliferative changes within the fascial tissue are particularly common at the site of its insertion to the calcaneum and may lead to the clinical condition known as plantar fasciitis. The condition is more likely to develop in the context of obesity or repetitive low-level trauma (joggers). It is also commonly found in individuals with a spondyloarthritis and may have a more primarily inflammatory aetiology in this context

Clinical Assessment

Patients usually experience heel pain that is particularly severe when they first weight bear in the mornings. There is often some improvement with initial activity but subsequent deterioration with higher levels of activity during the course of the day. They may develop an abnormal gait in an effort to avoid weight bearing on the affected heel. Examination will show tenderness over the heel, particularly over the medial tubercle of the calcaneus. Pain may be exacerbated by forcibly dorsiflexing the toes or asking the patient to stand on their toes. There is rarely a need to request specific investigations although a US or MRI scan will demonstrate thickening of the plantar fascia and MRI scanning may show evidence of inflammation.

Management

The condition is usually self-limiting within 12 months. During this time NSAIDs may provide symptomatic relief. Injection with corticosteroid has also been shown to provide short-term relief from symptoms. There may be some benefit from stretching both the calf musculature and the plantar fascia. Heel pads, particularly those that minimise weight bearing over the medial calcaneum, may be helpful. There is only very rarely a role for surgery in management of this condition.

6.7. Bursitis

Bursa is the latin word for 'purse' and bursae comprise synovial lined sacs containing small amount of synovial fluid. Within the body they are flattened and provide a smooth slippery structure that allows friction-free gliding of skin, muscles or tendons over bone. There are over 150 bursae within the human body, some of which are particularly likely to become inflamed. As part of the inflammatory process the synovial cells proliferate and increase production of matrix and synovial fluid leading to distension of the bursa (Table 6.6).

Inflammation of a bursal sac often occurs in the context of repetitive use or trauma and may also develop as part of a systemic inflammatory disease such as rheumatoid arthritis or gout. Chronic renal failure is likewise associated with an increased tendency to bursitis. Bursitis may also be infectious in aetiology. These cases usually involve superficial bursae and are often associated with a history of local perforating trauma. Individuals with a history of diabetes, corticosteroid use and alcoholism are particularly at risk. Patients with an infected bursa may have a history of fevers and malaise and signs may include prominent local erythema or peribursal cellulitis. The causative organism is usually a staphylococcus, with a streptococcus being the second most commonly found bacterium. Mycobacterial infection of bursae is also frequently described. Where infection is suspected, fluid must be aspirated from the bursa and sent for microscopy and culture. If there is any difficulty in obtaining fluid within the clinic then a US guided aspiration should be requested. Where an infectious aetiology is suspected or confirmed then treatment with appropriate antibiotics should be initiated and, depending on the patient's clinical condition, it may be appropriate for these to be given intravenously.

Table 6.6. Common sites for bursitis.

Region	Bursa commonly involved	Common name
Elbow	Olecranon bursa	–
Pelvis	Iliopsoas bursa	–
	Subgluteus maximus bursa	Trochanteric bursitis
	Ischial bursa	Weaver's bottom
Knee	Prepatella bursa	Housemaid's knee
	Infrapatella bursa	Clergyman's knee
	Pes anserine bursa	–
Ankle	Retrocalcaneal bursa	–
Forefoot	Intermetatarsal bursa	–

6.7.1. *Subacromial Bursitis*

The subacromial bursa is commonly inflamed in association with shoulder impingement syndromes and this is discussed in Section 6.1.

6.7.2. *Olecranon Bursitis*

Anatomy and Aetiopathogenesis

The olecranon bursa lies superficially, just posterior to the olecranon, and serves to protect the skin from the underlying bone. Its superficiality renders it particularly vulnerable to infection although it is also commonly inflamed in rheumatoid arthritis and gout.

Clinical Assessment

Patients present with pain and swelling over the extensor aspect of the elbow. Imaging is not usually required for diagnosis. If infection is suspected then fluid should be aspirated and sent for microscopy and culture. An US scan can be helpful in guiding the aspiration of the fluid.

Management

If present, infection should be treated as outlined in the introductory paragraph of this section. Where olecranon bursitis is associated with gout or rheumatoid arthritis it will usually respond to treatment of the underlying disease process. Where it reflects repetitive trauma then individuals should be advised to avoid exacerbating factors such as leaning on their elbows. There may be a response to NSAIDs. Aspiration and local injection of corticosteroid can be beneficial; however, the sac is very superficial and so hydrocortisone is preferable to depomedrone in order to minimise the risk of skin thinning and scarring over the site of injection. Very occasionally referral for surgical excision of the bursal sac may be appropriate.

6.7.3. *Iliopsoas Bursitis*

Anatomy and Aetiopathogenesis

The iliopsoas bursa is the largest bursa in the body and lies between the iliopsoas tendon and the lesser trochanter. In approximately 10% of individuals it communicates with the hip joint. Inflammation of this bursa usually occurs in association with significant arthritis of the hip or may occur in regular runners. Notably inflammatory changes around the iliopsoas tendon without true bursitis may present with similar clinical features.

Clinical Assessment

Patients experience pain that radiates from the groin down the anterior medial thigh towards the knee and they are often tender just below the inguinal ligament, just lateral to the femoral artery. On occasions the bursal swelling may be palpated in this area and may appear pulsatile due to the transmission of the femoral artery pulse. Often the clinical picture is not diagnostic and a US or MRI scan may be informative.

Management

If the condition is associated with regular running or other sporting activity then the patient should be advised to reduce levels of sporting activity. They may benefit from use of NSAIDs. Aspiration of fluid from the bursa with injection of corticosteroid may be beneficial.

6.7.4. *Trochanteric Bursitis*

Anatomy and Aetiopathogenesis

At least three bursae lie around the greater trochanter. The largest is the subgluteus maximus bursa which lies lateral to the greater trochanter and deep to the fibres of tensor fascia lata and gluteus maximus as they converge to form the iliotibial band. The subgluteus medius bursa lies beneath the gluteus medius muscle, superior and posterior to the greater trochanter. The subgluteus minimus bursa lies superior and anterior to the greater trochanter. There are variants in anatomy and other bursae may be present in some individuals. Trochanteric bursitis can affect any of these bursae. It is most commonly found in women in their 40s to 60s as well as in runners and dancers.

Clinical Assessment

Patients present with aching lateral hip pain and have tenderness around the greater trochanter. For the diagnosis to be made they should also describe radiation of the pain down the lateral aspect of the thigh or have pain at extremes of rotation, abduction or adduction or pain with resisted hip abduction. Even where these criteria are applied it is not possible to make a diagnosis of true trochanteric bursitis with a reasonable degree of specificity. MRI scanning and histopathology studies suggest that very few patients (possibly fewer than 10%) with the above clinical features actually have true inflammation of the relevant bursa although a significant proportion of the individuals have evidence of tendinosis or paratendinitis of the gluteus medius tendon. As a consequence the condition is increasingly being referred to as the 'greater trochanteric pain syndrome'.

Management

The 'greater trochanteric pain syndrome' may respond to NSAIDs and patients may also benefit from physiotherapy. The condition has conventionally been treated with a local injection of corticosteroid. Interestingly, studies do show a good outcome from this intervention despite the more recent work suggesting a lack of evidence of true bursitis. A US scan may be used to guide injection of corticosteroid more accurately to an affected bursa or to lie around the gluteus medius tendon at its insertion.

6.7.5. *Ischial Bursitis*

Anatomy and Aetiopathogenesis

The ischial bursa lies between the ischial tuberosity and the gluteus maximus. It may become inflamed in athletes, particularly marathon runners or footballers, and in the context of prolonged sitting ('weaver's bottom') or other local trauma.

Clinical Assessment

Pain is felt locally over the ischial tuberosity and radiates down the posterior aspect of the thigh. Local tenderness is helpful in distinguishing the condition from that due to nerve root compression within the lower lumbar spine. However, it may be difficult to distinguish clinically between injuries to the hamstring origin from the ischial tuberosity and local bursitis. A US or MRI scan can be helpful in this respect.

Management

Patients should be advised to avoid sitting on hard surfaces and may obtain symptomatic relief from NSAIDs. Injection of corticosteroid into the bursa may be beneficial.

6.7.6. *Prepatella, Infrapatella and Pes Anserine Bursitis*

Anatomy and Aetiopathogenesis

The prepatella bursa lies between the patella and the skin and may become inflamed in the context of frequent kneeling ('housemaid's knee'). These days this condition is most commonly seen in workmen such as carpet layers and may also be a problem for gardeners. The infrapatella bursae lie both superficial and deep to the patella tendon and the superficial one in particular may become inflamed on recurrent kneeling, particularly with an upright upper body posture ('clergyman's knee'). The pes anserine bursa lies between the lower fibres of sartorius, gracilis and semitendinosus and the tibial plateau and can extend posteromedially around the knee joint. It is particularly prone to inflammation in the context of osteoarthritis of the knee where there is a developing valgus deformity and the patient is obese.

Clinical Assessment

Patients present with local pain and swelling may be visible over the inferior pole of the patella (prepatella bursitis), inferior to the patella around the patella tendon (infrapatella bursitis) or over the superior medial or posteromedial aspect of the tibia (pes anserine bursitis). The superficiality of the prepatella bursa renders it very susceptible to infection and clinicians should have a low threshold for arranging aspiration of bursal fluid for microscopy and culture. There is rarely a need for imaging in diagnosis although if the diagnosis is in doubt then the bursal sacs can be easily seen on US or MRI scans.

Management

An infected bursa should be treated promptly with antibiotics as outlined in the introduction to this section. Patients should be advised to avoid kneeling in the case of prepatella and infrapatella bursitis and may respond to NSAIDs. Where conservative measures fail the bursal sacs may be aspirated and injected with corticosteroid.

6.7.7. *Calcaneal Bursitis*

Anatomy and Aetiopathogenesis

The superficial (subcutaneous) calcaneal bursa lies between the Achilles tendon and the skin and the deep retrocalcaneal bursa lies between the tendon and the calcaneum. Either bursa can become inflamed, particularly in the context of repetitive trauma or overuse. Inflammation can be aggravated by tight-fitting shoes and is more common in individuals with a prominent posterosuperior aspect of the calcaneum (Haglund's deformity).

Clinical Assessment

Tenderness and swelling may be apparent on the posterior aspect of the calcaneum. An X-ray may demonstrate an associated Haglund's deformity. Further imaging studies are not usually required.

Management

Patients should review their footwear in order to minimise recurrent trauma to the back of the heel. The symptoms may respond to NSAIDs. It is possible to inject the inflamed bursa but care must be taken to avoid damage to the Achilles tendon and this manoeuvre is only performed in resistant cases. A Haglund deformity may require resection.

6.7.8. *Intermetatarsal Bursitis*

Anatomy and Aetiopathogenesis

The intermetatarsal bursae lie superior to the deep transverse metatarsal ligament, between the interosseous tendons as they pass between the metatarsal heads. Inflammation of these bursae is most common in the 2/3 and 3/4 interspaces and is a common cause of forefoot pain.

Clinical assessment

The development of intermetatarsal bursitis is usually associated with pain across the forefoot particularly on standing. Tenderness affecting one of the interdigital spaces at the level of the metatarsal heads may be evident and squeezing across the metatarsal heads may reproduce the pain.

Management

The condition may be affected by inappropriate footwear and patients should be encouraged to use broader, low heeled shoes which are well cushioned. In resistant cases an injection of corticosteroid may be helpful; this is generally performed under US guidance. The presence of intermetatarsal bursitis may be associated with the development of a Morton's neuroma.

6.8. Morton's Neuroma

Anatomy and Aetiopathogenesis

Morton's neuroma is also known as interdigital neuroma or interdigital neuritis although it is not a true nerve tumour nor demonstrably inflammatory in aetiology. The interdigital nerves are derived from the medial and lateral plantar nerves, which are themselves derived from the tibial nerve. They pass between the metatarsal heads, below the intermetatarsal bursae, to supply the toes. At the level of the metatarsal heads they are susceptible to recurrent compression and stretching and it is thought that this mechanical irritation leads to perineural fibrosis and nerve damage. Histological findings include thickening of the perineurium with demyelination of the nerve fibres, hyalinisation of the walls of endoneural vessels and sclerosis of the endoneurium. The condition usually affects the 3rd or, less often, the 2nd, intermetatarsal spaces, which are relatively narrow. It very rarely involves the 1st or 4th space.

Clinical Assessment

Patients are usually women in their 50s and describe a sharp, shooting pain, often with an associated numbness or burning. On occasions they report a sensation of walking on a pebble. Examination shows local tenderness, usually most evident on the plantar aspect of the interdigital space. Squeezing of the forefoot may reproduce the pain or even produce a palpable click due to displacement of the neuroma. Similar localised tenderness affecting the forefoot may be seen with an intermetatarsal bursitis (see above) or even a stress fracture of the metatarsal. If there is doubt about the diagnosis then a US or MRI scan is helpful. However, it should be remembered that interdigital neuromas may represent an incidental finding on MRI scans and are not necessarily symptomatic.

Management

Patients often respond to conservative treatment with modification of their footwear to shoes that are broad, well cushioned, low heeled and worn with an additional neural pad to protect the tender area. NSAIDs may relieve the pain.

The condition does also often respond to local injection with corticosteroid. Rarely the symptoms persist despite these measures and may warrant referral for surgical excision.

6.9. Ganglions

Anatomy and Aetiopathogenesis

Ganglions are cysts that are usually connected to an underlying joint capsule or ligament or to a tendon sheath. The walls consist of collagen and the cysts are filled with viscous mucin containing hyaluronic acid as well as glucosamine and albumin. Their aetiology remains uncertain although they may develop as a consequence of a congenital defect or a local area of degeneration within a capsule, ligament or sheath.

Clinical Assessment

Ganglions affect women more than men and most commonly develop in the hand and wrist region. They are usually small (<2 cm in diameter) and solitary and often arise on the dorsal aspect of the wrist. Whilst most ganglions are asymptomatic some can present with local pain and with paraesthesia, presumably due to local nerve irritation.

Ganglions of the distal IP joints may occur in association with osteoarthritis and are termed mucous cysts. They tend to lie distal to the distal IP joints and can affect the nail plate, giving longitudinal grooving of the nail.

Management

In general there is no requirement to treat a ganglion. If the patient would like treatment then the cysts will generally respond to aspiration and injection with corticosteroid. In some instances aspiration itself will fail because of the very high viscosity of the ganglion contents; in these cases one should simply proceed to injection of corticosteroid. Aspiration and corticosteroid injection is, however, associated with a recurrence rate of approximately 50%. If necessary, patients may be referred to a surgeon for a ganglionectomy.

6.10. Overuse Syndromes

The term 'overuse syndrome' is broadly synonymous to that of 'cumulative trauma disorder' or 'repetitive strain injury'. When used to describe symptoms affecting the upper limb that may be occupation-related the term 'work-related upper limb disorder' is sometimes used. However, the condition may involve other parts of the body and may be associated with recreational or habitual rather than occupational activities.

Aetiopathogensis

'Overuse syndromes' are presumed to result from repetitive challenge to a tissue without allowing for sufficient recovery time. High forces, vibrations and malpositioning of limbs away from the neutral position all further increase the risk of developing an 'overuse syndrome'. Nerves are particularly vulnerable and muscles, tendons and ligaments are also frequently affected. Carpal tunnel syndrome, lateral elbow tendinopathy, stress fractures and Raynaud's phenomenon associated with vibration are all examples of conditions that may result from repetitive challenge.

Clinical Assessment

The term 'overuse syndrome' refers to a very wide array of different diagnoses including many discussed in this chapter. It is important to obtain a detailed history about the onset of symptoms and any exacerbating or relieving factors. It is also important to obtain comprehensive information about the possible culprit activity; this may involve discussion about workstations in work-related upper limb disorder or about training schedules in an athlete. The affected area should be examined in the usual way, initially using the 'look, feel, move' principle and proceeding to perform a neurological examination if appropriate. Blood tests are rarely helpful but imaging studies or neurophysiological investigations may be useful.

Management

The key to successful management is usually 'relative rest'. This term implies avoidance of the precipitating activity and may, for example, involve workstation modifications, a different training schedule for athletes or use of better equipment. Participation in a carefully planned programme of rehabilitation with supervised use of the injured area can be beneficial. NSAIDs and other analgesics, amitryptiline at night and local injections of corticosteroid may have a place in management of some cases.

6.11. Fibromyalgia

Anatomy and Aetiopathogenesis

Fibromyalgia is a poorly understood condition characterised by chronic widespread pain associated with fatigue and often with a variety of other somatic symptoms. The condition has a prevalence of around 2% and is much more common in women than men.

The aetiology is unclear although it is likely to be multifactorial. There may be a history of an emotionally traumatic childhood or stresses during adult life. There is some evidence for alterations in levels of neurotransmitters and regional blood flow within the brain, consistent with the idea that the condition is associated with an alteration in central processing of pain.

Clinical Assessment

Patients complain of severe pain, often of a burning nature, that tends to focus on the axial skeleton. They almost invariably experience a poor sleep pattern and constant fatigue. They may in addition report difficulties with memory and attention, dizziness, peripheral tingling, breathlessness, urinary frequency and urgency and may also have diagnoses of regional pain syndromes such as irritable bowel syndrome, atypical chest pain, jaw pain or chronic pelvic pain. They often have negative beliefs, a sense of helplessness and a tendency to heavy use of medical services. There is a significant overlap with depressive illness.

Examination will show heightened sensitivity to pain with very widespread tenderness.

The 1990 classification criteria for the disease, intended for research rather than clinical use, require patients to have widespread pain for more than four months and to experience pain at 11 of 18 defined sites when manual pressure of around 4 kg/cm^2 is applied as described in Chapter 2.

In the assessment of patients with possible fibromyalgia it is important to exclude other conditions as an early priority (Table 6.7). Blood tests to look for systemic causes of malaise, an inflammatory illness or endocrine disease are usually appropriate. Imaging studies to identify degenerative joint disease (usually within the lumbar spine) or bursitis (usually of the subacromial bursa) may also be indicated. It is not infrequent for inflammatory or local musculoskeletal conditions to coexist with fibromyalgia and both need to be treated appropriately.

Some individuals experience myofascial pain with a few focal trigger points, particularly within the trapezius and rhomboid musculature. This frequently

Table 6.7. Investigations to exclude other pathology in patients presenting with features of fibromyalgia.

Possible alternative disease process	Tests to be considered
Anaemia	FBC
Major organ failure	C&E, LFT
Inflammatory disease	ESR, CRP, RF, anti-CCP, ANA, CK
Metabolic disease	Calcium, Vitamin D
Endocrine disease	TSH
Regional pain affecting spine or shoulder	US scan shoulder Imaging of neck and spine

ANA anti-nuclear antibody, anti-CCP anti-cyclic citrullinated peptide, C&E creatine and electrolytes, CK creatine kinase, CRP C-reactive protein, ESR erythrocyte sedimentation rate, FBC full blood count, LFT liver function test, RF rheumatoid factor, TSH thyroid stimulating hormone.

occurs in association with cervical spondylosis or as a consequence of a poorly designed work station. In the absence of widespread, chronic pain and prominent fatigue such individuals should not be diagnosed as suffering from fibromyalgia.

Management

It is important to perform relevant investigations early and then not to persist with further unnecessary tests. All treatable causes of pain such as subacromial bursitis need to be managed properly. Depression should be treated actively. With respect to the fibromyalgia itself patients need to be given a clear diagnosis and information about the condition. The doctor needs both to acknowledge the reality of the patient's pain and to reassure them about the absence of sinister pathology. Patients may find it difficult to understand that the pain may not reflect a process that can be detected by blood tests or imaging studies and they often request multiple investigations. With appropriate explanation they may come to understand the broad idea that there is an abnormality in the process of sensing, transmitting and/or perceiving pain and that this is not something that can be easily measured. It is important to explain how social and behavioural factors can impact on pain perception and amplify the symptoms. The individual should be encouraged to address any factors that may be promoting stress and to self-manage their condition as far as possible. There is evidence that low dose tricyclics given at night can be helpful in management (amitryptyline 10 mg nocte increasing to 40 mg nocte as tolerated). More recent trials have suggested a role for the anti-convulsants gabapentin or pregabalin or the serotonin and noradrenaline re-uptake inhibitors such as venlafaxine in relieving symptoms. Injections of trigger points can be helpful as can massage although both promote dependence on other individuals that may be unhelpful in the longer term. Hot baths or saunas also provide some relief. A graded aerobic exercise programme is of proven benefit and patients should be strongly encouraged to pursue this.

Chapter 7
Paediatric Rheumatology

Editor: Sally Edmonds

Sally Edmonds, Anne Miller, Nick Wilkinson

7.1. Approach to the Assessment and Management of Children with Rheumatic Disease

Introduction

How does the assessment and management of children with rheumatic disease differ from that of adults? There are, of course, many aspects of the general management that differ little from that of adults. For example, the investigations requested are generally the same; many of the drugs that are used are the same for children and adults, and a multi-disciplinary team (MDT) approach is appropriate for patients of all ages. However, differences in how children present to rheumatologists, the fact that children cannot always tell you 'where it hurts' and the importance of involving the rest of the family, make paediatric rheumatology a specialty in its own right. Children frequently present to general practitioners with musculoskeletal symptoms and even juvenile idiopathic arthritis (JIA) itself has an incidence of approximately 1/1000; about the same as that for juvenile diabetes. In addition, chronic pain syndromes are becoming increasingly common in the younger population and it is therefore important that any doctor dealing with children has a working knowledge of the childhood rheumatic diseases.

Presentation

Children with rheumatic disease may present in a very similar way to an adult with a similar problem, for example, with pain and swelling in one or more joints. If this is the case, then making the diagnosis may be straightforward. Not uncommonly, however, the child will present with much vaguer symptoms; the parents have noticed that their toddler seems a bit reluctant to walk or an older child has complained of pain following a game of rugby. Developmental delay or failure to reach a particular milestone may also be the first sign that a child has a musculoskeletal problem. Symptoms may be dismissed both by parents and clinicians on the basis that this is unlikely to be anything serious in someone so young. Such symptoms can, and often do, settle spontaneously, but it is knowing when to simply give reassurance and when to investigate further that is key. Children with musculoskeletal disease may present with non-musculoskeletal symptoms; the child with systemic onset JIA may present with fever and a rash and the child with oligoarticular arthritis may have eye problems before any joint becomes troublesome. Clues to the diagnosis may be gained from the age of the child at the onset of symptoms and from whether the child is male or female. It is rare for rheumatic disease to present neonatally, although conditions such as neonatal lupus should not be forgotten. However, many of the childhood diseases have a peak age of onset and are more common in one or other gender. In a 13-year old boy presenting with pain in his heel, juvenile enthesitis related arthritis (ERA) would be an important differential diagnosis. On the other hand, a teenage girl presenting with arthritis would be more likely to have polyarticular juvenile arthritis, similar to adult rheumatoid arthritis. It should be remembered also that there are conditions that are specific to children such as oligoarthritis with uveitis, Kawasaki disease, periodic syndromes and skeletal dysplasias. It should never be forgotten that malignancy in children may present with sometimes very non-specific, musculoskeletal symptoms.

Children may be referred directly from their general practitioners but are also often referred from other paediatric specialties. Referrals are commonly made from orthopaedic surgeons, who have been asked to see a child with an 'irritable hip' type problem or an isolated swollen joint on the basis that this may represent septic arthritis. Whilst septic arthritis needs to be excluded, many paediatric rheumatologists would argue that they would prefer to see these patients first.

Examination and Investigation

When examining the child's musculoskeletal system it is often necessary to use play as part of the examination, depending on the age of the child. For example, observing how the child reaches out for a toy; does he/she use both hands equally or avoid using one hand altogether? For older children, the paediatric gait, arms, legs, spine (GALS) examination technique can be used and has been adapted from the adult version with some additions and amendments. For example, the child should be asked to walk on tiptoes and heels in addition to being observed walking. They should be asked to put their hands together and back to back to demonstrate wrist flexion and extension. The child can be asked to 'reach up to the sky' to check shoulder range of movement and 'open your mouth and put three of your fingers in your mouth' to check mouth opening and temporo–mandibular joint function. The investigation of children with rheumatic disease is fundamentally the same as that of adults in terms of which blood tests are done and which imaging techniques are used. It is important, however, not to over-investigate children, to keep blood tests to a minimum and to use non-invasive techniques whenever possible. The use of ultrasound (US) scanning to look for subtle synovitis in children presenting with joint pains has made investigation a much easier experience for the child and their parents. It may of course be necessary to perform more invasive procedures or procedures where the child has to keep very still, such as magnetic resonance imaging (MRI). In these cases, and particularly in younger children, a general anaesthetic may be required.

A Family-Centred Approach

Any child with chronic disease must be seen in the context of the family, not only parents, but siblings as well. It is important to recognise the pivotal role of the child and the family in the planning of care and to empower the family through education and support. It is inevitable that there is going to be a degree of parental anxiety when the diagnosis is first made and there will be a lot of questions to be answered. There may be feelings of guilt, that somehow they have passed this condition on to their child, or that they ignored or underplayed the child's symptoms. Parents may feel that there is a dichotomy between their role as 'carers' and their role as parents and they may feel frustrated that they are unable to do anything to help their child. All of this needs to be dealt with sensitively by members of the MDT who should be involved right from the start. It may not always be possible to provide an accurate diagnosis when the child is first seen, and great skill and patience are required to support the family in managing the child's problems in the face of diagnostic and prognostic uncertainties. Stress related to living with chronic illness affects every member of the family, including siblings. There may be a perception by the siblings that extra time and attention is being given to the affected child and it may be impossible, particularly for single parents, to provide adequately for the developmental needs of the siblings. It is important to evaluate the needs of siblings in caring for children with chronic illness and to help support their needs.

Management

The general principles of managing children with rheumatic diseases are the same as for adults: early diagnosis and early aggressive treatment. One of the main aims in adult rheumatology is to enable patients to carry on working; with children it is to keep them at school. It is vitally important that a child does not 'stand out' from his or her peers because they are unable to do certain activities. This includes academic lessons and, importantly, physical activity in the form of physical education at school as well as activities outside of school. There are very few situations which would lead to a child with arthritis not attending school. Schooling may of course be interrupted by hospital visits, but these should be kept to a minimum and when necessary, the team looking after the child needs to liaise with the child's teachers and other staff members.

Starting a child on treatments such as disease-modifying therapy for arthritis has significant implications not only for the child but for the rest of the family. The drugs may need to be given by injection, may cause unpleasant side effects (although children on the whole tolerate these drugs very well) and may require monitoring with blood tests. In addition these are drugs that the child is likely to be on for years rather than months and it is important therefore to gain the child's confidence and understanding from the start. In a way, the child's 'permission' needs to be sought before commencing drugs such as methotrexate and this can only be achieved through careful explanation and counselling from the members of the MDT. The nurse specialist in particular has an important role to play in this area, acting as a liaison between the rheumatologist, the child and their family and their general practitioner. The issue of childhood vaccinations also has to be considered as live vaccinations cannot be given to children on methotrexate or high-dose steroids. There may be a 'window of opportunity' to give a vaccination such as varicella to a child who has not had chickenpox before commencing methotrexate, but if they have already been started on steroids this may not be possible. The family then need to be made aware that they should report if the child comes into contact with chickenpox so that he/she can be given immunoglobulin.

Another issue that has to be considered when treating children with rheumatic disease that is not of such concern in adults is that of growth. Abnormalities of growth and development are not uncommon complications of chronic arthritis or its treatment, largely because these are occurring in the context of a growing skeleton. Generalised growth disturbances may occur as a result of severe active disease or as a result of treatment with glucocorticoids. The aim therefore is to keep the disease under as good control as possible with minimum use of steroids. Clearly there may be significant psychological consequences for any child whose growth is retarded enough for him or her to stand out from their peers. Localised growth disturbances may also occur. For example, in a knee where there has been prolonged active synovitis, overgrowth may lead to leg length discrepancies. Again the aim is to keep inflammation to a minimum and to use heel raises or orthotics as necessary on a temporary basis until the other leg 'catches up'.

The Multi-Disciplinary Team

It should already be clear that the MDT is essential for the optimal management of the child with rheumatic disease. The child should get to know all the members of the team early on: clinician, nurse specialist, occupational therapist, physiotherapist and, when necessary, clinical psychologist. Ideally, clinics should be run with all members of the MDT present as a 'one stop shop'. Perhaps the 'lynch pin' of the team is the clinical nurse specialist as it is he/she who provides the link between the rheumatologist, the child and their family and the family doctor. The clinical nurse specialist is likely to be the one who helps the child and their family come to terms with the diagnosis, gives general support and specifically gives information and help regarding the drugs that are prescribed. Physiotherapists and occupational therapists also have vital roles to play, not only in terms of their specific roles in relation to exercise and activities of daily living, but also to 'reinforce' everything that the doctors and specialist nurses have said. It is important that all members of the team are saying the same things and that there is no conflicting information or advice being given. The clinical psychologist does not necessarily need to be involved with every child's care but should be seen as part of the team from the beginning, so that it does not come as a surprise to the child or their family, if at a later date, psychological input is felt to be necessary. For example, it may be that a child develops a needle phobia which psychological input can help to overcome. Most children with a chronic pain syndrome will need psychological support from an early stage.

Summary

The approach therefore to assessing and managing children with rheumatic diseases has much in common with that of assessing and managing adults. There are some important differences, however, which those who deal with children should be aware of. The presentation may be subtle and a high index of suspicion is required if important diagnoses are not to be missed. In general, investigations in a child should be kept to a minimum and should be non-invasive whenever possible. A family-centred approach should be adopted by the MDT and this team working is a fundamental element of the child's care. A major underlying aim of treatment is to enable the child to continue with school, not just to attend academic lessons, but to participate fully in school life including physical education and extra-curricular activities. Finally, it is hoped that the child with arthritis will turn into an adult who may still have arthritis but who, to all intents and purposes, functions as though they did not.

7.2. Juvenile Idiopathic Arthritis

Juvenile idiopathic arthritis (JIA) is a chronic inflammatory disease affecting the joints and certain extra-articular tissues such as the eyes. By definition it begins before the sixteenth birthday and persists for at least six weeks, but treatment will begin before then. The prevalence in the United Kingdom is 65/100,000 and annual incidence is 10/100,000. JIA is a clinical diagnosis based on history and examination as there are no diagnostic tests.

Classification

Before reading about the conditions it is well worth understanding their classification, which will help organise one's approach to a child presenting with joint disease. It is important that standard classification and terminology is used in communication between health professionals and in the study of diseases and their management.

There have been various ways of classifying juvenile arthritis and this explains the use of the terms 'juvenile rheumatoid arthritis' and 'juvenile chronic arthritis', referring to the American College of Rheumatology and European League against Rheumatism criteria respectively. In current use is the International League of Associations for Rheumatology (ILAR) classification of JIA. Use of the term 'Still's disease' as an umbrella term for juvenile arthritis is unacceptable as it refers specifically to systemic onset JIA.

The ILAR classification is a useful framework but it should be borne in mind that it is flawed and under continuous review. Arthritis in children is different from that in adults both clinically and in pathogenesis and it is inappropriate to apply adult diagnostic criteria to the paediatric disease. It is recommended to spend some time studying Table 7.1 and to look again at each definition before reading the section dealing specifically with the disease. This will act as a guide to asking relevant questions when seeing a patient and making a diagnosis. The different types of JIA can occur in any age group but tend to peak at certain ages. For example oligoarticular JIA tends to occur in toddlers and is associated with inflammatory eye disease (uveitis). Enthesitis related JIA tends to occur in teenagers.

Table 7.1. ILAR classification of juvenile idiopathic arthritis.

Classification	Features	Exclusions
Systemic	Arthritis in any number of joints with fever of at least two weeks' duration, documented to be quotidian for at least three days, accompanied by one or more of the following: Evanescent rash Generalised lymphadenopathy Enlargement of liver or spleen Serositis	1, 2, 3, 5
Oligoarthritis	Arthritis in four or fewer joints during first six months of disease	1, 2, 3, 4, 5
Persistent	Never more than four affected joints	
Extended	More than four joints affected after first six months	
Polyarthritis *Rheumatoid factor positive*	Arthritis affecting more than four joints during first six months of disease	1, 2, 3, 4
Polyarthritis *Rheumatoid factor negative*	Arthritis affecting more than four joints during first six months of disease	1, 2, 3, 4, 5
Psoriatic arthritis	Arthritis and psoriasis	
	Or arthritis and at least two of the following: Dactylitis Nail pitting or onycholysis Family history of psoriasis in a first-degree relative	2, 3, 4, 5

(*Continued*)

Table 7.1. (*Continued*)

Classification	Features	Exclusions
Enthesitis related arthritis	Arthritis and enthesitis Or arthritis or enthesitis with at least two of the following: Sacroiliac joint tenderness and/or inflammatory joint pain Presence of HLA B27 Family history of HLA B27 associated disease Anterior uveitis Onset of arthritis in boy > eight years old	1, 4, 5
Undifferentiated arthritis *Fits no other category* *Fits more than one category*		

HLA human leukocyte antigen.
Exclusions

1. Psoriasis or a history of psoriasis in the patient or a first-degree relative.
2. Arthritis in HLA B27 positive male after the sixth birthday.
3. Ankylosing spondylitis, enthesitis related arthritis, sacroiliitis with inflammatory bowel disease, Reiter's syndrome, or acute anterior uveitis or a history of one of these disorders in a first-degree relative.
4. The presence of systemic JIA.
5. Presence of IgM rheumatoid factor on at least two occasions at least three months apart.

7.2.1. *Systemic Onset Juvenile Idiopathic Arthritis*

Aetiopathogenesis

Systemic onset JIA (SOJIA) accounts for 10% of cases of JIA and the disease occurs at any age. There is evidence for a genetic predisposition to the condition with a trigger by an unknown environmental agent such as an infection. Abnormal expression of cytokines has been demonstrated including high levels of interleukin (IL)-1 and IL-6, giving targets for treatment with biologic agents.

Clinical Features

The child with SOJIA presents with marked systemic features and arthritis may not be immediately evident. The presentation resembles a number of other serious conditions presenting in childhood, which should be excluded (Table 7.2).

Table 7.2. Differential diagnosis of SOJIA.

Other causes of pyrexia of unknown origin in a child
Infection
Malignancy — leukaemia, neuroblastoma
Inflammatory bowel disease
Periodic fever syndrome
Connective tissue diseases

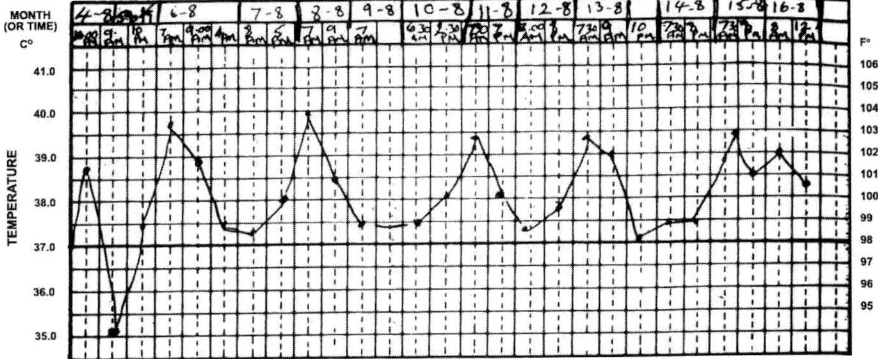

Fig. 7.1. The quotidian fever of systemic onset juvenile idiopathic arthritis.

Certain features are characteristic and help support the diagnosis. The quotidian fever is pyrexia occurring once or twice a day returning to the baseline at least once in 24 hours (Fig. 7.1). The rash is classically salmon pink, maculopapular and evanescent, meaning that it appears and disappears, but may also be urticarial and pruritic (Fig. 7.2). It is often concurrent with the pyrexia. Additional diagnostic features are lymphadenopathy, liver and/or spleen enlargement, and serositis, e.g. pericardial or pleural effusions. Joint disease may be very severe, affecting any number of joints, particularly knees, wrists and ankles and, characteristically, neck, hips and temporomandibular joints.

Approximately half the cases have a monophasic disease course with complete recovery. Others have a more protracted disease course and poor prognosis with the risk of severe disability if the disease is not brought under control.

Long-term complications include joint damage, growth retardation, amyloidosis and the side-effects of steroids including osteoporosis, infection, growth retardation and skin fragility. A more immediate complication occurring during the acute phase of the illness is macrophage activation syndrome (MAS). This is a rapid-onset life-threatening complication consisting of persistent fever, cytopenia,

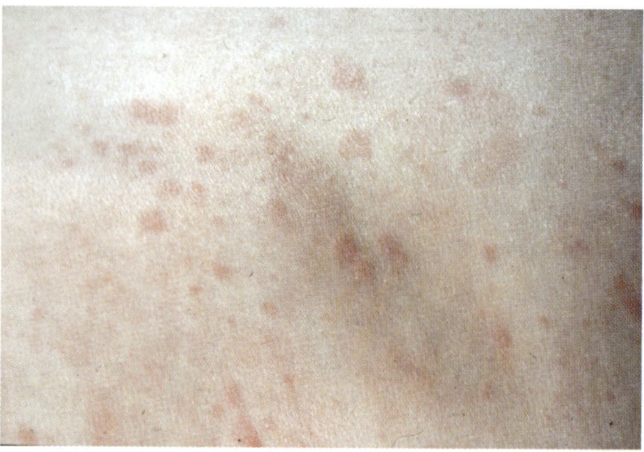

Fig. 7.2. The typical 'salmon pink' rash associated with systemic onset juvenile idiopathic arthritis.

Table 7.3. Characteristic laboratory features of SOJIA and MAS.

	SOJIA	MAS
Haemoglobin	Low	Low
White cell count	High	Normal/Low
Platelets	High	Normal/Low
ESR	High	Normal
PT/PTT	Normal	High
CRP	High	High
ALT/AST/Alk phos	Normal	High
Ferritin	High	High
Albumin	Normal	Low
Triglycerides	Normal	High

ALT alanine transferase, AST aspartate transferase, Alk phos alkaline phosphatase, CRP C-reactive protein, ESR erythrocyte sedimentation rate, PT prothrombin time, PTT partial thromboplastin time.

liver dysfunction, intravascular coagulation and neurological involvement. Table 7.3 shows typical blood features of SOJIA compared with MAS.

Investigations

Investigations are aimed at considering and excluding other serious conditions (see Section 7.5 for details). Tests may include a full infection screen, full blood count (FBC), inflammatory markers, ferritin, triglycerides, liver and renal function, a blood film, spot urinary metadrenaline:creatinine ratio (to exclude neuroblastoma), blood film and bone marrow biopsy for leukaemia and MAS.

Management

SOJIA can be very difficult to treat and at onset often requires hospitalisation. Corticosteroids remain an important component of treatment along with bone protection such as calcium and vitamin D. Non-steroidal anti-inflammatory drugs (NSAIDs) and paracetamol are also helpful. Typically methotrexate is prescribed as either an oral or subcutaneous preparation, although it is less effective for this form of juvenile arthritis than for other forms. Anakinra (an IL-1 receptor antagonist) and tocilizumab (an anti IL-6 receptor monoclonal antibody) are now used for resistant disease. Other agents such as ciclosporin may be used by some centres. The role of autologous stem cell transplantation is unclear but may be considered for severe unremitting polyarthropathy.

7.2.2. *Oligoarticular Juvenile Idiopathic Arthritis*

A child has oligoarticular JIA if four or fewer joints are affected during the first six months of the disease. If the number of joints affected remains four or less, it is termed persistent oligoarticular JIA but if more joints are involved it is called extended oligoarticular JIA. The peak incidence is between two to four years and it is more common in girls than boys (female:male ratio is 3:1).

Aetiopathogenesis

The aetiology is unknown but thought to be the result of an environmental trigger, such as a virus, in a genetically susceptible individual. It can occur in siblings but this is very rare.

Clinical Features

The affected child may present with pain, delayed walking, abnormal gait or preferred handedness and on examination have a swollen joint with a reduced range of movement. Lower limb joints are more commonly involved than upper limb joints (Fig. 7.3). Leg length difference may result from increased bone growth around an affected knee relative to the normal side. Mid-foot and subtalar joint involvement may cause an everted foot posture. There may be

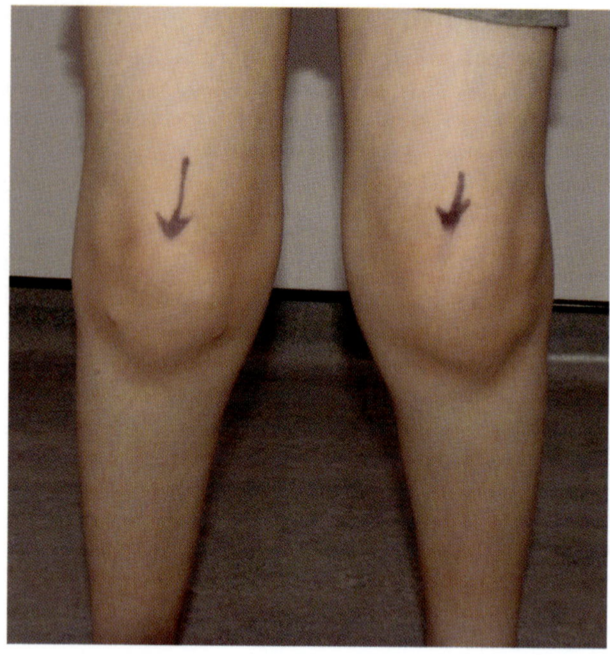

Fig. 7.3. Bilateral knee swelling in a child with oligoarticular juvenile idiopathic arthritis.

marked local muscle wasting. The child is usually systemically well and apyrexial.

Uveitis, caused by inflammation in the anterior chamber of the eye, occurs in up to 20% of children with oligoarticular JIA and is five times more common in girls than boys. It is asymptomatic until vision is severely impaired and can lead to cataract formation, intraocular adhesions and blindness. Neither the young child nor parent will know of its presence and for this reason screening by an ophthalmologist familiar with paediatric uveitis is mandatory.

Investigations

Investigations include blood tests for a FBC and anti-nuclear antibody (ANA) and imaging such as US or MRI scanning which confirm synovitis and exclude infection, haemophilia or malignancy. A positive ANA is a risk factor for developing uveitis. However, uveitis can occur in ANA-negative children and is more likely to be severe in this group. All children with oligoarticular JIA should be considered to be at risk of developing uveitis whether ANA-positive or -negative.

Management

The aim of management is to bring synovitis under control, restore muscle strength and encourage normal growth and use of the limb. This is achieved with a combination of medication, physiotherapy, occupational therapy, orthotics and increased physical activity with effective pain control. NSAIDs such as ibuprofen provide symptomatic relief; they have a more significant anti-inflammatory action when given regularly at the appropriate dosing interval for periods of at least two to four weeks. Most children are initially treated with intra-articular steroid injection, usually triamcinolone, into each affected joint. In young children this is done under a general anaesthetic. If joints require more than three injections, long-term treatment with methotrexate is prescribed. If unsuccessful, consideration may be given to treatment with biologics such as the anti-tumour necrosis factor (TNF)-α agents, etanercept and adalimumab.

Similarly, uveitis is managed with steroid eye drops with progression to methotrexate and then either mycophenolate or adalimumab, depending on extent of joint involvement. Etanercept is considered ineffective for JIA-associated uveitis. Eye disease may also be managed with ciclosporin.

7.2.3. *Polyarticular Juvenile Idiopathic Arthritis*

Aetiopathogenesis

In polyarticular JIA, five or more joints are affected during the first six months of disease. As in other forms of JIA, there is likely to be genetic predisposition with triggering by an undefined environmental event. The disease is further classified by the presence or absence of rheumatoid factor (RF). Inflammatory cytokines including TNF-α play a key role in the process which involves chronic inflammatory cell infiltration of the synovium, destruction of cartilage and erosion of the joint.

Clinical Features

The child will have multiple swollen and tender joints with joint restriction, morning joint stiffness and may have marked disability (Fig. 7.4). There is more likely to be systemic illness than in oligoarticular JIA, including fatigue, anaemia, high inflammatory markers and effects on growth but not a rash or pyrexia.

RF-positive polyarticular JIA typically affects girls older than 12 years, is severe and symmetrical with involvement of the small joints of the hands. There

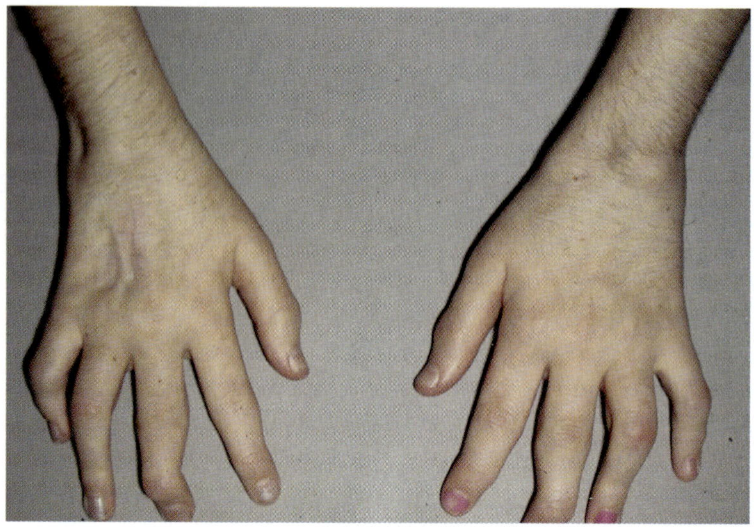

Fig. 7.4. The hands of a child with polyarticular juvenile idiopathic arthritis. Note the involvement of wrists, metacarpophalangeal and interphalangeal joints and the subcutaneous fat atrophy on the dorsum of the right hand where a steroid injection has been administered.

is more likely to be erosive disease but only rarely rheumatoid nodules or vasculitis.

Investigations

Blood tests may show raised erythrocyte sedimentation rate (ESR) and C-reactive protein (CRP), anaemia, raised platelets and a positive or negative value for RF. The ANA should be checked as systemic lupus erythematosus (SLE) may initially present with polyarticular arthritis. Anti-cyclic citrullinated peptide (CCP) antibodies may be present in RF-positive JIA but are currently not part of routine investigations. US may be useful in demonstrating synovitis and early erosions in affected joints if the diagnosis is uncertain. X-rays may demonstrate erosions and joint damage later in the course of the disease.

Management

The prognosis depends on the number of joints affected, the presence of RF, the presence of high inflammatory markers and duration of uncontrolled disease. Untreated polyarticular JIA can cause significant erosive joint damage and functional impairment. Hip disease may be particularly severe in this group of children and young adults. Growth may be affected generally, with growth retardation, and locally: for example, damage to the temporomandibular joints results in abnormal jaw development (micrognathia). The outlook for well-controlled disease is good, with normal height and joint development. Therefore an aggressive approach should be taken to bring the disease under control as quickly as possible. This is with the usual combination of medication, physiotherapy, occupational therapy and physical activity. The child and family may need a great deal of support in the initial stages and in the longer term.

Methotrexate should be started at 15–20 mg/m^2 subcutaneously for long-term control. Since this can take up to two months to take effect, oral or intravenous corticosteroids may be required in the initial stages and during subsequent flares. NSAIDs provide initial symptomatic treatment for pain and stiffness.

If methotrexate does not achieve disease control, early consideration should be given to the addition of an anti-TNF-α agent; etanercept is effective and adalimumab has been approved for use in older children. Abatacept, a biological agent that inhibits T cell activation, also has efficacy in this condition.

Patients with arthritis should not be advised to rest and stop sport but should be encouraged to be as active as possible, pain permitting. Treatment with physiotherapy and occupational therapy is particularly important to encourage joint movement and maintenance of range of movement. Therapists should work with the family and school to maximise participation in all school activities including sport.

7.2.4. *Juvenile Psoriatic Arthritis*

Juvenile psoriatic arthritis (JPsA) is arthritis in a child with psoriasis. JPsA is also defined as arthritis occurring with a family history of psoriasis in a first-degree relative, with dactylitis or with nail pitting, and may therefore occur in a child without psoriasis. At least half of the children with JPsA have arthritis before developing psoriasis.

Aetiopathogenesis

The cause of JPsA is unknown and there is no explanation as to why psoriasis predisposes to arthritis or to the asymmetrical nature of the disease. There is a strong genetic contribution to disease susceptibility. Angiogenesis has an important role in the pathogenesis of psoriasis and psoriatic arthritis as do activated CD8+ T cells and inflammatory cytokines such as TNF-α.

Clinical Features

JPsA may initially resemble oligoarticular JIA and has an asymmetrical distribution affecting large and small joints. Psoriasis is characterised by well-demarcated erythematous scaly lesions but may present as scattered macules (guttate psoriasis) or pustules or may only be evident as nail pits (Fig. 7.5). Dactylitis is a 'sausage-like' swelling of a finger or toe caused by arthritis with surrounding tendonitis and is characteristic of JPsA. There may be anterior uveitis and eye screening is important.

Investigations

There are no characteristic laboratory tests for JPsA but there may be raised inflammatory markers, chronic anaemia and thrombocytosis. RF is absent by definition but the ANA may be positive. X-ray, US or MRI scans may demonstrate erosive changes.

Management

There are fewer studies on the management of JPsA than on the oligo-, poly- and systemic onset forms of JIA but the principles are the same. Synovitis is brought

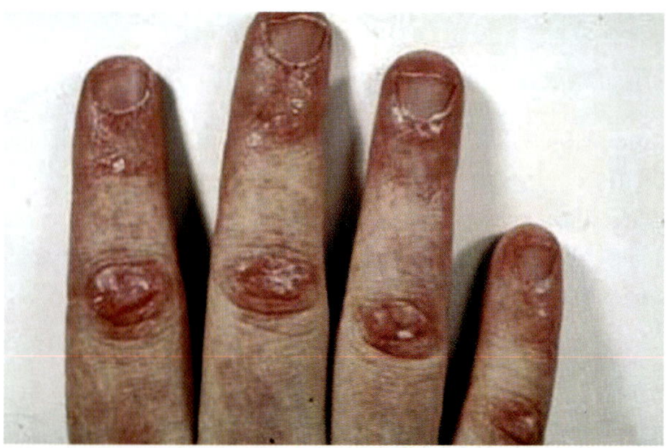

Fig. 7.5. The hands of a child with psoriatic arthritis. Note the nail pitting and psoriasis affecting the skin overlying the interphalangeal joints.

under control with a combination of intra-articular injections, NSAIDs and methotrexate. Trials of leflunomide in adults with psoriatic arthritis have been encouraging and this medication can also be successful in controlling JPsA. Methotrexate and leflunomide may contribute to controlling cutaneous psoriasis, which can also be helped with topical application of emollients, keratolytics and steroids. Use of TNF-α antagonists for management of joints and skin may be necessary. Involvement of the physiotherapist and occupational therapist as well as ophthalmologist and dermatologist is integral to care.

7.2.5. *Enthesitis Related Arthritis*

Enthesitis related arthritis includes the spondyloarthropathies exemplified by juvenile ankylosing spondylitis (JAS), but takes into account the early stages of the disease in children which often presents as oligoarthritis or enthesitis with no, or late, development of axial disease. This differentiates it from the adult form of ankylosing spondylitis (AS) where axial disease predominates. Seronegative enthesitis and arthritis (SEA) is another useful way of describing the onset of this disorder in the under-16 population.

ERA is diagnosed if there is arthritis and enthesitis or either of these with at least two other features of the following: inflammation of the sacroiliac joints, human leukocyte antigen (HLA) B27 positivity, arthritis developing in a boy after the age of eight, and a relevant family history. It is excluded by the presence of psoriasis, which classifies the disease as JPsA even if other features of ERA are present. The ILAR classification excludes reactive arthritis and inflammatory bowel arthritis although these may be HLA B27 related diseases.

Aetiopathogenesis

There is a genetic association with HLA B27 although the mechanism by which it is involved in disease pathogenesis remains unclear. There is infiltration of T cells and macrophages with increased production of TNF-α in the synovium and at entheses.

Clinical features

Clinical features include arthritis, enthesitis and axial disease. The pattern of arthritis is initially unilateral or asymmetric mono- or oligoarthritis affecting the lower limbs and may be similar to oligoarticular JIA. Enthesitis is a more discriminatory feature, involving inflammation of tendon, ligament, joint capsule or fascia insertion into bone. This occurs classically at the pole of the patella, insertion of the Achilles tendon and insertion of the plantar fascia, making walking very painful. JAS involves spinal and sacroiliac arthritis and enthesitis and may present five to ten years after the development of the SEA syndrome. In the longer term, patients with JAS tend to have less severe axial involvement than adult onset AS but more severe hip disease. Extra-articular manifestations include acute uveitis, non-specific inflammatory bowel disease, cardiac conduction disturbances and lung abnormalities.

Investigations

Blood tests may show anaemia of chronic disease. Inflammatory markers may be normal and if very high suggest the presence of inflammatory bowel disease. HLA B27 is not a diagnostic test but indicates risk. It is present in 90% of children with JAS and approximately 8% of the Caucasian population. Imaging with MRI may demonstrate enthesitis and is useful in confirming inflammatory spinal disease.

Management

NSAIDs are important in pain management and patients should have on-going physiotherapy. Orthotics may help relieve the pain of enthesitis, particularly plantar fasciitis. TNF-α antagonists have been very successful in reducing inflammation in spinal disease in adult AS and have been reported to be useful in JAS.

7.3. Reactive Arthritis

7.3.1. *HLA B27 Associated Reactive Arthritis*

Reactive arthritis is a form of arthritis appearing after an infection. Although it may follow viral, bacterial or parasitic infections, the term is usually reserved for HLA B27 associated reactive arthritis triggered by certain bacteria such as Salmonella, Yersinia, Campylobacter, Shigella and Chlamydia. Extra-articular features of reactive arthritis include apthous stomatitis, conjunctivitis, erythema nodosum, balanitis, keratoderma blenorrhagica, anterior uveitis, urethritis, cervicitis, aortic insufficiency, myocarditis and pericarditis. Reiter's syndrome refers to a form of reactive arthritis with prominent extra-articular features including conjunctivitis, urethritis or cervicitis.

The presence of HLA B27 in the patient or a family history of spondyloarthropathy increases the risk of developing an arthritis that is more severe and prolonged.

Investigations are as for inflammatory arthritis, and an infective screen as clinically indicated, which may include stool cultures and a genitourinary screen.

The arthritis is treated with NSAIDs, intra-articular and oral steroids as clinically indicated and eradication of any on-going infection, particularly Chlamydia in a sexually active adolescent. Prolonged arthritis may need a second line agent such as sulphasalazine or methotrexate.

7.3.2. *Post-Streptococcal Arthritis*

Arthritis may occur as a complication of upper respiratory tract infection with Group A β-haemolytic streptococcal infection either as an isolated post-streptococcal reactive arthritis (PSRA) or in the context of rheumatic fever. Whether PSRA and rheumatic fever are part of the same disease spectrum or are distinct in terms of pathogenesis is controversial. PSRA usually presents as an oligo- or polyarthritis with tenosynovitis, is non-migratory, very painful and often accompanied by systemic features. It may persist for some months. Arthritis as a manifestation of rheumatic fever tends to be migratory and involves large joints such as knees, ankles, elbows and wrists. It generally lasts two to three days in each joint and two to three weeks in total.

Patients may have anaemia, neutrophilia, high inflammatory markers and a positive throat swab culture for Group A Streptococcus. Elevated titres of anti-streptolysin O (ASOT) on two separate occasions confirm invasive infection but may be negative. If PSRA or rheumatic fever is clinically evident where the ASOT is negative, anti-hyaluronidase, anti-deoxyribonuclease B or anti-streptokinase antibodies should be tested. Cardiac features of rheumatic fever should be sought with electrocardiograph (ECG) and echocardiogram, and an MRI scan of the brain performed if features of chorea are present.

Treatment of arthritis is with NSAIDs, and oral steroids if severe. Streptococcus should be eradicated with a 10-day course of penicillin.

7.3.3. *Other Forms of Reactive Arthritis*

Other forms of reactive arthritis are defined by the precipitating infectious organism. Viral arthritis is known to be triggered by rubella, parvovirus, measles, mumps, varicella and hepatitis. Vaccinations may also cause a short-lived reactive arthritis. Joint involvement in Lyme disease occurs weeks to months after infection with the spirochete *Borrelia burgdorferi*. There may be migratory joint pain in the early stages of disseminated infection and chronic arthritis and enthesopathy in the late stages.

7.4. Chronic Recurrent Multifocal Osteomyelitis

Sterile bone inflammation is described in a number of diseases and may occur as isolated lesions or at multiple sites. Chronic non-bacterial osteomyelitis (CNO) is an umbrella term for inflammatory bone lesions which may be single or multiple in number and isolated, continuous or recurrent in timing. At the severe end of the spectrum, chronic recurrent multifocal osteomyelitis (CRMO) describes a syndrome of recurrent episodes of osteitis, which may be at a number of sites, causing bone pain and local soft tissue swelling. It shares a number of clinical features with a similar disease in adults referred to as the SAPHO syndrome (synovitis, acne, pustulosis, hyperostosis and osteitis).

Aetiopathogenesis

There is localised bone inflammation with increased osteoclast activity and bone resorption. Increased levels of TNF-α have been demonstrated.

Clinical Features

The child presents with bone pain which may be severe and may have localised soft tissue swelling. General health is otherwise good with no pyrexia, fatigue or weight loss. The disease may be associated with psoriasis and chronic bowel disease. Pathological bone fractures may occur, particularly in the vertebrae.

Investigations

Blood counts tend to be normal and there may be raised inflammatory markers. X-rays may show osteolytic or sclerotic lesions with periostial reactions, hyperostosis or pathological bone fractures. MRI scans demonstrate inflammatory lesions and are useful in the initial diagnosis, at further presentation of pain to confirm new lesions and to demonstrate healing. Isolated lesions should undergo biopsy in order to exclude malignancy and bone infection. Histological examination of osteitis will demonstrate non-specific inflammation, which may resemble infection. Samples should be cultured to exclude atypical infections.

Management

Many patients will have been treated for suspected bone infection with antibiotics but there is no evidence that they have any role to play in the management of this condition. Treatment should be started with full dose NSAIDs. If this is unsuccessful, treatment with pamidronate, oral or systemic steroids and anti-TNF-α medication such as infliximab have been used with varying success.

7.5. Multi-System Inflammatory Disorders in Childhood

Diagnosis of these rare conditions requires a high level of suspicion because many of the presenting features of disorders such as SLE, juvenile dermatomyositis (JDM) and the periodic fevers overlap with common paediatric infections. Non-specific constitutional features such as malaise, low-grade fever, fatigue and unexplained weight loss should raise suspicion if they persist. Rashes may provide specific clues and multi-organ involvement in the absence of sepsis or neoplasia should stimulate a thorough paediatric rheumatology review.

Leukaemia, lymphoma and neuroblastoma may also present with fever, constitutional disturbance and multi-system involvement. They require consideration, and sometimes exclusion, prior to establishing an inflammatory diagnosis. A blood count and film discussed with a haematologist will help when considering leukaemia, the commonest childhood malignancy to result in musculoskeletal pain, but a bone marrow aspirate is definitive. In those patients less than five years of age, urinary metadrenalin levels will help rule out neuroblastoma whereas radiological assessment of chest and abdomen may be required for lymphoma.

Reactive inflammatory or post-infectious conditions may also present with a multi-system presentation. In the acute setting, Kawasaki disease and Henoch–Schönlein purpura (HSP) should be considered. Contact with cats, ticks and infectious diseases such as tuberculosis are important points of enquiry and a travel history essential.

In order to facilitate further consideration here, the multi-system inflammatory disorders in children have been differentiated by the predominant feature of either fever (Table 7.4) or rash (Table 7.5). However, overlap in presentation is common and the true diagnosis may not be immediately apparent. Indeed the diagnostic label may change with time, based on surveillance of all organs including eyes, ears, nose and throat at each follow-up. Such evaluation will also monitor the extent and severity of inflammation to guide intervention, which is often similar to that in adults.

Owing to many similarities with adult disease the reader is directed to the relevant chapters and only specific paediatric concerns will be discussed here.

Table 7.4. Pyrexial presentation of multi-system inflammatory disease in childhood.

Diagnosis	Characteristic features
Kawasaki disease	High spiking fever (39–40°C) > five days plus four of five criteria (see text). Coronary artery aneurysms if untreated
Reactive illnesses	Arthritis following infection
• Arthritis & eye disease	Preceding enteric infection, often stool culture positive
• Rheumatic fever	Jones criteria, positive throat swab, ASOT and/or antiDNAse b
• Lyme disease	Rash & arthritis following a tick bite, positive ELISA for *Borrelia burgdorferi*
Chronic vasculitides • Polyarteritis nodosa • Wegener's granulomatosis • Microscopic polyangiitis	Fever, weight loss, fatigue, plus vasculitic rash, myositis, arthritis, focal neurological deficit, nephritis and hypertension. Diagnostic tests include biopsy, renal angiography, MRI & MRA, ANCA
SOJIA	Quotidian fever and evanescent rash may precede polyarthritis by months Serositis, hepatosplenomegaly, lymphadenopathy
Periodic fever syndromes	60% of periodic fevers are unclassifiable but genetic analysis helpful
• Familial Mediterranean Fever	One to three days of fever, peritoneal/pleuropericardial pain, arthritis
• Hyper-IgD Syndrome	Three to seven days of fever, erythema, aggressive arthritis, raised IgD, MVK mutation
• TRAPS	> Seven days of fever and ocular signs, diagnosis with TNF-α receptor studies
• Muckle–Wells syndrome	Prolonged fever, urticaria and deafness
• PFAPA	**P**eriodic **F**ever, **A**pthous ulcer, **P**haryngitis, **A**denitis
Macrophage activation syndrome (also known as haemophagocytic lymphohistiocytosis)	Life-threatening complication of SOJIA, SLE, viral infection. Persistent fever, lymphadenopathy, hepatic failure and purpura, with sudden fall in ESR and platelet count and marked rise in LFTs and ferritin.
Neoplasia (leukaemia, lymphoma, neuroblastoma)	Consider if indeterminate multisystem disease and in presence of thrombocytopenia with high ESR. Request blood film, bone marrow aspirate, abdominal US/CT

ANCA anti-neutrophil cytoplasmic antibody, ASOT anti-streptolysin O titre, CT computed tomography, ELISA enzyme-linked immunosorbent assay, ESR erythrocyte sedimentation rate, LFTs liver function tests, MRA magnetic resonance angiography, MRI magnetic resonance imaging, SLE systemic lupus erythematosus, SOJIA systemic onset juvenile idiopathic arthritis, US ultrasound.

Table 7.5. Skin presentation of multi-system inflammatory disease in childhood.

Diagnosis	Characteristic features
Post-streptococcal vasculitis (cutaneous polyarteritis)	Palpable nodules or purpura with livido; may be associated with arthritis and transient neuropathy. Request throat swab, ASOT, anti DNAse b.
Henoch–Schönlein purpura	Palpable purpura of classic distribution. Possible intussusception, arthralgia, nephritis (monitor urinalysis and blood pressure).
Juvenile dermatomyositis	Violaceous heliotrope rash on upper eyelids, Gottron's papules, periungual erythema and proximal inflammatory myopathy confirmed by MRI/US of thighs. May also have synovitis, peptic ulceration, pulmonary fibrosis, neurological disease.
Systemic lupus erythematosus	Similar to adult onset disease but often more severe. Rash in 75% of patients, malar rash in 50% of patients. Lupus nephritis and neurological disease determine outcome.
Juvenile sarcoidosis	'Sago' rash, boggy arthritis, eye disease. Diagnosed by biopsy rather than ACE level.
Scleroderma	Linear scleroderma describes long narrow plaque of waxy thickened skin that results in limb deformity. Oval plaques of morphea may occur. Systemic sclerosis very rare. Skin and blood vessels assessed using thermography and capillaroscopy.
Mixed connective tissue disease	Raynaud's phenomenon and arthropathy with positive anti-RNP antibody.
CINCA (chronic infantile neurological, cutaneous and articular syndrome)	Onset in infancy of triad of rash, symmetric arthropathy & chronic meningitis.
Neonatal lupus erythematosus	Inflammation of skin with liver and haematological complications. Heart block evaluated using ECG and echocardiogram.

ACE angiotensin converting enzyme, ASOT anti-streptolysin O titre, ECG electrocardiogram, MRI magnetic resonance imaging, RNP ribonucleoprotein, US ultrasound.

7.5.1. *Pyrexial Presentation of Multisystem Inflammatory Disorders*

Five days of high spiking fever should always raise suspicion of Kawasaki disease to ensure early use of immunoglobulin and aspirin and avert life-threatening coronary aneurysms. Four of five other features are diagnostic: conjunctivitis, oral mucosal changes, polymorphic rash, lymphadenopathy >1.5 cm and palmar erythema. The criteria are often incomplete in infants but suspicion increases with inconsolable irritability in the absence of meningitis.

Streptococcal illnesses overlap with Kawasaki disease including involvement of the heart, although rheumatic fever typically affects the valves rather than the coronary vessels. A vasculitic rash may indicate post-streptococcal vasculitis and a throat swab should be mandatory. Other forms of vasculitis also occur in childhood and, excepting giant cell arteritis, the spectrum of chronic vasculitis is similar to that of adult disease.

SOJIA has a characteristic quotidian fever; spikes to >39°C once or twice a day and a return to normal in between. The associated rash may be subtle, urticarial or even vasculitic in appearance and both features may precede the polyarthritis by months.

Periodic fever syndromes, also called auto-inflammatory disorders, have characteristic recurrences of fever. These are inherited disorders of the immune system with defects in the genes that control cytokine expression. Familial Mediterranean Fever, the most common variant, has attacks lasting one to three days associated with serositis and arthritis. The other periodic fevers are summarised in Table 7.4. Tissue damage may arise with recurrences, but the development of amyloidosis is the major long-term concern. Cytokine therapies, including use of IL-1 receptor antagonist and TNF-α blockade, appear effective in some of these syndromes.

Fever, abnormalities of liver function and a rapid fall in blood cell counts and ESR may indicate a life-threatening complication of SOJIA, SLE and the other multi-system inflammatory disorders. This is MAS, already discussed. Methylprednisolone, given as intravenous 'pulses,' is the first line of treatment.

7.5.2. *Skin Presentation of Multisystem Inflammatory Disorders*

Autoimmune conditions in childhood associated with a characteristic rash include post-streptococcal vasculitis, HSP and JDM. HSP has a diagnostic purpura over the backs of the calves and buttocks and may be accompanied by arthritis, scrotal swelling or intussusception. HSP is typically self-limiting although haematuria and blood pressure need monitoring as 4% of patients may go on to end stage renal failure.

JDM is characterised by raised red lesions on the knuckles, knees and elbows called Gottron's papules and a purplish hue to the upper eyelids called heliotrope. Ulceration of the skin is a sign of severe disease. Muscle pain and weakness affects the proximal muscles and confirmation of myositis is with an MRI scan of the thighs rather than biopsy or electromyography. Corticosteroids are the mainstay of JDM treatment facilitated by the use of methotrexate or, in severe disease, cyclophosphamide.

The malar rash of SLE is less common in the paediatric population. SLE begins before the age of 17 years in 20% of SLE patients and tends to be more aggressive with renal and cerebral involvement in many.

Juvenile sarcoidosis, distinct from sarcoidosis in adolescents and adults, has a sago rash accompanied by fever, boggy joint swelling and eye involvement.

Localised scleroderma may result in thickened patches of skin on the trunk or may migrate down a single limb. The inflammation and fibrosis of the subcutaneous layers affect muscle development and growth (Fig. 7.6).

Inflammatory illnesses peculiar to the first few months of life that may manifest with a rash include chronic infantile neurological cutaneous and articular

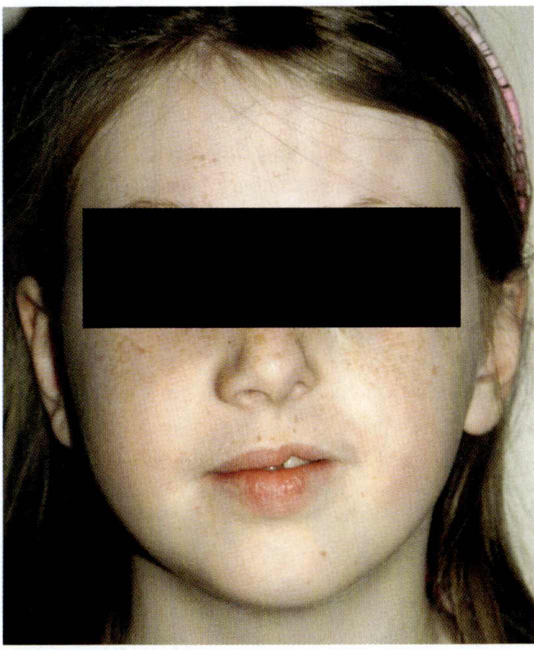

Fig. 7.6. A child with localised scleroderma causing asymmetry of her face.

syndrome (CINCA) which is one of the periodic fever syndromes, and neonatal lupus, attributable to transplacental passage of maternal autoantibodies. Although neonatal lupus is typically self-limiting the occurrence of heart block is permanent.

7.6. Non-Inflammatory Musculoskeletal Pain Disorders

Up to 10% of paediatric consultations in general practice are for assessment of musculoskeletal pain (Table 7.6). The conditions include anterior knee pain (a third), non-specific ankle, wrist or heel pain (a third) and soft tissue pain (a fifth). The high prevalence of benign conditions may contribute to the delayed diagnosis of neoplasia, arthritis or other conditions associated with significant disability or morbidity. Careful evaluation and timely X-ray will ensure this significant minority will not be overlooked.

7.6.1. *Neoplasia*

Osteosarcoma and Ewing's sarcoma typically present with focal bone pain and are often diagnosed with a plain X-ray. They account for 5–10% of childhood malignant neoplasms and are high grade with early metastasis, especially to the lungs. In order to avoid spread and improve the survival rate (currently 60–70%), persistent bone pain for longer than two weeks should be screened with an X-ray.

Osteosarcoma, arising principally in the metaphases of the femur and tibia and proximal metaphysis of the humerus, has a 'moth-eaten' appearance on X-ray with cortical destruction and periosteal elevations. Ewing's sarcoma shows as an elongated lytic lesion within the diaphysis of long bones, axial skeleton or flat bone, with disruption of the cortex and periostium (described as an 'onion skin' or 'sun burst' appearance).

The pain of leukaemia is typically more intense than that of JIA and localises to the metaphysis. In addition, constitutional upset, a disproportionately high ESR and low platelet count should raise suspicion. Spinal pain in children under five years may indicate neuroblastoma.

7.6.2. *Back Pain*

Although non-specific back pain is increasingly prevalent in adolescents, persistent back pain in children is more likely to be associated with an underlying pathology than in adults. Pathologies include bone tumour, infection (osteomyelitis and discitis) and structural changes such as spondylolisthesis,

Table 7.6. Non-inflammatory musculoskeletal pain in childhood by site.

Site	Diagnoses (not exclusive)
Upper limb	
Shoulder	Osteosarcoma Rotator cuff instability (from over-use or deconditioning)
Elbow	Osteochondritis dissecans of the elbow Apophysitis affecting medial or lateral epicondyle
Wrist and hands	Hypermobility Poor writing posture Chilblains, erythromelalgia, Raynaud's phenomenon
Back	*See text*
Ribs	Costochondritis/Tietze's syndrome Slipping rib syndrome
Lower limb	
Hip and pelvis	Osteosarcoma Perthes' disease (femoral head) Slipped upper femoral epiphysis Acute idiopathic chondrolysis of the hip Pelvic apophysitis
Knee	Patellofemoral pain — usually secondary to biomechanical disturbance including hypermobility Osgood–Schlatter disease (tibial tubercle)/ Sinding-Larsen–Johansson syndrome (inferior pole patella) Osteochondritis dissecans of the knee Recurrent patella dislocation Osteosarcoma
Shin	Ewing's sarcoma Growing pains Medial tibial stress syndrome
Feet	Sever's disease (calcaneal)/Köhler's disease (tarso-navicular)/Freiberg's disease (2nd metatarsal) Plantar fasciitis Tarsal coalition

Scheuermann's disease (a form of osteochondrosis) and disc injuries. Back pain may also be inflammatory (juvenile spondyloarthropathy) or referred from abdominal pathology. Key features that indicate possible serious pathology are shown in Table 7.7.

Table 7.7. Key feature of serious pathology.

Features of serious pathology
Age less than four years
Persistent back pain of longer than four weeks (especially if deteriorating)
Loss of function
Fever and weight loss
Neurological features
Recent onset scoliosis
Morning stiffness

7.6.3. *Limp*

The majority of children who present with a limp have a benign and transient condition. Of 243 patients seen in an Accident and Emergency department, 30% had no specific final diagnosis and made a complete recovery without intervention. An additional 40% had a diagnosis of irritable hip or transient synovitis. In the presence of a fever, septic arthritis, especially of the hip, should be considered. Other hip-specific causes include Perthes' disease in children aged three to ten years and slipped upper femoral epiphysis in early adolescence. Although relatively rare, this last diagnosis should always be considered as, untreated, it may produce catastrophic consequences. Hip X-ray with 'frogs legs' view is usually diagnostic but a MRI scan may be required.

7.6.4. *Non-Accidental Injury*

Repeat presentation with musculoskeletal pain of indeterminate origin may be a cry for help. Suspicion is paramount and even if abuse in whatever form (emotional, neglect, physical or sexual) cannot be confirmed, ongoing support or surveillance through effective communication with primary care will help in the long term.

7.6.5. *Growing Pains*

Growth is not painful, but the prevalence (10–20% of school-aged children) and the level of distress attributed to 'growing pains' are sufficiently high to justify mention here. There are two typical age groups.

Between the ages of three to eleven years, the pain occurs at night and responds to massage and reassurance over 20 to 30 minutes. Simple pain relief may help. Symptoms disappear by morning, there is no associated limp and activity levels are normal. A positive diagnosis and explanation that there is no ongoing damage or inflammation reassures most parents.

Lower limb pains in the adolescent age group are commonly associated with biomechanical abnormalities, especially tight hamstrings, quadriceps and calves. Reassurance should be given along with a home exercise plan.

7.6.6. *Sport Associated Limb Pain*

Younger athletes suffer many of the same injuries as their adult counterparts. However, owing to anatomical and developmental differences there are additional injuries attributable to traction apophysitis, metaphyseal stress fractures and avulsion fractures and osteochondritis dissecans, a presumed form of intra-articular avascular necrosis attributed to recurrent microtrauma. These diagnoses largely result from overuse, with the knee being most commonly affected.

Osteochondroses such as Sever's disease, Kohler's disease, Freiberg's disease and Perthes' disease may also present as pain associated with exercise. These conditions reflect focal disturbances of endochondral ossification. They can affect many different sites including the knees, hips and feet and are self-limiting with symptoms lasting up to two years. Management is based on thorough assessment of biomechanical abnormalities that contribute to discomfort. Activity modification will reduce pain, but there is no evidence that this, or complete rest, accelerates the healing. NSAIDs and ice packs may also be helpful in addition to an explanation and reassurance.

7.6.7. *Benign Joint Hypermobility*

Hypermobility, or laxity, of the joints, whether widespread or localised, may be associated with non-inflammatory musculoskeletal pain. Benign hypermobility (in the absence of conditions such as Ehlers–Danlos or Marfan syndrome) is common, affecting between 8% and 20% of white populations with a higher prevalence amongst Asians and West Africans, but only a small proportion complain of long-term pain. Children aged three to ten years are more commonly affected. The pain typically occurs towards the end of the day and is often provoked by increased levels of physical activity.

It is debatable whether hypermobility itself is the cause of chronic pain. The prevailing view is that hypermobility results in biomechanical imbalances and these need to be addressed by physiotherapy-led home exercises. Reassurance that there is no inflammation and tissue damage is important.

7.6.8. *Chronic Pain or Pain Amplification Syndromes*

Chronic pain of uncertain aetiology may occur in children with or without an associated disease. Pain as a normal sensation becomes disabling when it persists and is associated with suffering and loss of quality of life. The spectrum of pain disorders is similar to that in adults and includes diffuse pain similar to fibromyalgia and complex regional pain such as reflex sympathetic dystrophy. However, the aetiological factors are different and the outcome is much more favourable, especially the response to exercise therapy.

Epidemiology

This condition has been under-recognised and results in a spectrum of disability that has complicated epidemiological assessment. In a school-based study 31% of children and adolescents identified that they had had a pain for over six months of which 64% was due to musculoskeletal pain. Approximately 8% of adolescents have pain that affects their quality of life. Only a minority of these present to secondary care due to significant disability including school absence, but presentation is increasing. Between 5% and 25% of new referrals to a paediatric rheumatology unit are for assessment of amplified musculoskeletal pain.

Aetiopathogenesis

These syndromes are causally related to injury, illness and psychological distress. In complex regional pain there is often an episode of minor trauma cited as the trigger for ongoing difficulties. Illnesses such as arthritis or leukaemia may be associated with amplified pain. Psychological distress, including maladaptation to life events, is reported to be important in several case series, but is not present in all patients.

Family history and the role of the family have an important impact on paediatric chronic pain. Up to 71% of children with chronic pain have a parent with fibromyalgia or other chronic pain disorder and 28% of mothers with fibromyalgia have been observed to have a child who develops similar symptoms. Genetic risk factors have yet to be determined, but it is clear that psychosocial maintenance factors include those within the home and at school. Consultations with parents or carers are required to understand and reduce their role in the experience of pain and to develop coping strategies for the whole family. Furthermore, in one case series, 9% of patients admitted to having been sexually abused.

Clinical Assessment

The character of the pain and any associated features should be mapped over time. In addition, level of disability, sleep patterns, pre-morbid personality, coping strategies, goals of the patient as well as family history of pain should be assessed. Alteration in sensation may be apparent on examination. Abnormalities in biomechanics should be detected and corrected.

Pain syndromes have been considered as diagnoses of exclusion (see Table 7.6 for differential diagnosis of non-inflammatory pain), but there are positive diagnostic features to assist early diagnosis and avoid over-investigation and medicalisation (Table 7.8).

The complications of chronic pain are far-reaching and need to be fully assessed. Typically, chronic pain affects concentration and is often associated with fatigue. School performance may be affected leading to school absence. There is reduced social contact and a loss of sporting activity. Family life is frequently affected with loss of family outings and support for siblings. Subsequent enmeshment of adult carers may become an unacknowledged problem and

Table 7.8. Positive diagnostic features of pain syndromes.

Features of pain syndromes
Absence of tissue damage or inflammation to reasonably explain the symptoms
Pain that persists
for longer than one month in one limb for localised idiopathic pain
for longer than three months at three sites for diffuse idiopathic pain
Pain that fails to respond to appropriate levels of analgesia
Allodynia (the sensation of pain to non-noxious stimuli) and hyperaesthesia (abnormal sensitivity to touch) with shifting margins of distribution that are not in keeping with a peripheral nerve or dermatome.
Disability in marked excess to that expected from the clinical findings (in the absence of enthesopathy)
Fear of movement and touch — excessive avoidance behaviour
The presence of cool, mottled and sometimes swollen areas of skin
Abnormal perception of temperature
An emotional detachment to the level of pain and disability described ('la belle indifference')

motivating factor. Some patients become non-weight bearing and rely upon crutches, wheelchairs or even become bed-bound.

Management

These patients not only present a diagnostic challenge, but also a management challenge owing to the level of disability and a disengagement of the patient and family with medical services. Prolonged periods without a confirmed diagnosis and ineffective reassurance with inadequate explanation by previous clinicians may result in patients and families feeling that they are not being heard or, worse, not being believed.

Trust is essential to effective treatment. This begins with a therapeutic assessment that demonstrates that the clinician understands the situation fully. There should be clear acknowledgement of the pain; it must not be asserted that the pain is only in the head as it will alienate the patient and family. The positive diagnosis of chronic pain syndrome should be made using the above criteria and an explanation given that the pain experienced is not generated by tissue damage or inflammation. Most children and parents envisage pain as a warning signal so time spent discussing pain pathways and abnormalities that may arise is always helpful.

If there is a sleep abnormality this should be managed first because tiredness amplifies pain and the fear of pain. Tiredness also reduces engagement with the rehabilitation programme. Advice should be given to improve sleep hygiene and the chance of restorative sleep. Amitriptyline may be used to regulate sleep and control anxiety. In paediatric chronic pain this is the only medication used other than simple NSAIDs. There is no evidence that gabapentin and other drugs used in adult practice have a role in paediatric chronic pain. This is supported by the experience of many services including that of the author.

The mainstay of management is cognitive behavioural therapy conducted through a MDT with shared roles. This team includes a clinical psychologist, physiotherapist, occupational therapist and nurse specialist. The focus is on a return to normal activities and improvement of quality of life. Coping strategies for pain are developed to facilitate this but there is no direct treatment of the pain itself. In addition, relaxation techniques are given and the impact of psychological stressors reduced. A goal-orientated approach directs a return to normal activity. Only with time will the pain improve and the patient and family need to understand this.

Some services offer transcutaneous electrical nerve stimulation (TENS) and sympathetic blocks, but it is the author's experience that these have little value in management of paediatric pain amplification. Instead it has been shown that children respond well to graded increase in exercise associated with skin desensitisation for allodynia through rubbing or massage exercises.

Outcome

With effective support, complex regional pain or reflex sympathetic dystrophy typically resolves within four to six weeks; however, this is dependent on patients and parents being fully engaged in rehabilitation. Diffuse pain is more difficult to treat but the outcome is improved compared to adults. The improvements are seen in quality of life rather than pain which may ease months or years later. Relapses are common but the patients are taught a new set of skills that help them to cope and recommence treatment independently.

7.7. Osteoporosis in Children and Adolescents

In children, primary forms of osteoporosis such as juvenile idiopathic osteoporosis and osteogenesis imperfecta are rare but should be considered. On the other hand, the frequency of secondary osteoporosis (including that due to neuromuscular disorders, childhood cancer, endocrine disorders and inborn errors of metabolism) is increasing. The diagnosis of osteoporosis in children can be problematic as the relationship between bone mineral density (BMD) and bone fragility is incompletely understood. In children BMD is converted into a Z-score by comparison to paediatric normative data. A child is considered to have 'low bone density for chronologic age' if the Z-score is below –2.0 standard deviations (SD) from the mean score. However, the diagnosis of osteoporosis requires the presence of a clinically significant fracture history as well as low bone mass. Therapeutic interventions start with calcium and vitamin D supplementation and ensuring adequate protein intake. Physical activity is encouraged to increase BMD. Effective control of the underlying disease (e.g. coeliac disease) is the best first-line approach to prevent secondary osteoporosis. Growth retardation, pubertal delay or hypogonadism must be corrected with appropriate hormonal therapy. In severe osteoporosis bisphosphonates have been used successfully.

Chapter 8

Local Injections in Rheumatology Practice

Editor: Nick Shenker

CYH See, Maliha Shaikh, Nick Shenker

8.1. Introduction

Local injections are a very important tool in the management of rheumatic conditions. They are useful for diagnostic purposes as well as for treatment of inflammatory and painful local conditions. The decision to inject, however, may not be clearly evidence-based and outcomes for some injections do not greatly differ from dry needling or placebo injections. This does not mean that injections are not of great help, rather that an injection is a complex intervention composed of several parts (patient expectation, needle, injectate) with soft outcome measures (pain, functioning) that have not been adequately understood nor controlled for in relatively small randomised controlled trials. Different study paradigms and outcome measures are required to advance our understanding of the role of injections in the management of rheumatic conditions.

This chapter is limited to common joint and soft tissue injections but it is helpful to remember that there are other interventions that may be beneficial in relieving pain. These include regional nerve blockades, botulinum toxin and dry needling techniques. In all patients, injections form only one strand of the management plan that should also include pharmacological, environmental, biophysical, psychosocial and surgical interventions.

Making a Decision to Aspirate or Inject

Although common in rheumatology practice, it is important to remember that joint aspirations and injections are not risk-free and any decision to aspirate or inject must evaluate the risks and benefits. Joint aspiration to obtain a sample of synovial fluid is a crucial part of investigation of patients with suspected septic arthritis and should be undertaken promptly. In other conditions, drug treatment and conservative measures including physiotherapy and use of orthoses may obviate the need for injection and be more appropriate initial treatment. Indications for injection include chronic injuries refractory to such measures or pain improvement to aid rehabilitation. In patients with monoarthritis, oligoarthritis or single soft tissue lesions, intra-articular or intralesional injections may avoid systemic immunosuppressive treatment or supplement existing therapy. Important contraindications to corticosteroid injections include active infection (local or systemic) and tendon tears. A relative contraindication is the presence of a coagulopathy (including warfarin therapy) due to the risk of iatrogenic haemarthrosis. Local steroid injections should be avoided as far as possible in younger patients. Patients should be informed of the potential adverse effects of local corticosteroid injections (Table 8.1).

In a review of the literature, most of these complications were found to be rare. The rates of infection following intra-articular injection were estimated at 1/14,000 to 1/50,000 injections. Tendon rupture, subcutaneous fat necrosis or tissue atrophy and osteonecrosis were all very unusual, occurring in <0.1% of cases. Acute self-limiting synovitis occurred in up to 2% of people.

Corticosteroids

Corticosteroids are the mainstay of injection therapy and may be used with or without local anaesthetics. Inflammatory arthritis results in a very vascular synovium so

Table 8.1. Adverse effects of local corticosteroid injections.

Potential adverse effect
Worrying (occur in < 0.1% of cases)
Local or systemic infection
Tissue atrophy
Tendon rupture
Osteonecrosis or steroid arthropathy
Systemic hypersensitivity
Troubling
Symptom flare following injection
Facial flushing
Abnormal menstrual bleeding

molecules injected intra-articularly leave the joint very quickly. This is more pronounced with smaller molecules such as methotrexate while steroids, being slightly larger and less soluble, remain for slightly longer. This systemic absorption from intra-articular steroid injections is not insignificant as reflected by a marked depression in plasma cortisol levels within 24–48 hours. It is suggested that 48 hours of bed rest after steroid injections to weight-bearing joints may reduce side-effects and the risk of steroid arthropathy.

In soft tissue lesions corticosteroids are used primarily for their anti-inflammatory effects but may also modify non-inflammatory sources of pain although this is poorly understood. Inflammation occurs with bursitis and in early capsulitis whereas most chronic tendon lesions (apart from some cases of tenosynovitis) display alterations in the cellular and extracellular components of the tendon or its sheath. *In vitro* and *in vivo* studies have shown that tendons produce prostaglandin E 2 (PGE2) following repetitive mechanical stress. In animal models, prolonged exposure to this results in degenerative changes although this has not been demonstrated in humans. Tendon pain may also be caused by neurotransmitters such as substance P and biochemical irritants such as chondroitin sulphate released by damaged tendons as well as irritation of mechanoreceptors by vibration, traction or shear forces. The effects of corticosteroid on such processes are not known.

Various steroids may be used intra-articularly, with some available as different salts, each having its own properties and efficacy (Table 8.2). Of these, hydrocortisone most closely resembles the activity of the endogenous steroid cortisol. The hydrocortisone preparations are usually used for superficial soft

Table 8.2. Corticosteroids for injection and their equivalence rates.

Preparation	Relative dose needed for equivalent pharmacological effect
Hydrocortisone acetate	× 6.25
Hydrocortisone t-butyl acetate	× 6.25
Prednisolone acetate	× 5
Prednisolone t-butyl acetate	× 5
Methylprednisolone acetate	× 5
Dexamethasone acetate	1
Dexamethasone t-butyl acetate	1
Triamcinolone diacetonide	× 5
Triamcinolone acetonide	× 5
Triamcinolone hexacetonide	× 5

tissue injections and injections to the smaller joints. Prednisolone preparations are most appropriate for larger joints and may also be used for deeper soft tissue injections such as those performed around the greater trochanter. Although triamcinolone has the longest duration of action, it is also associated with an increased risk of complications, especially tissue necrosis if not injected into a joint cavity. It should not therefore be used for soft tissue injections and many operators only use this compound if using radiological guidance to ensure correct placement.

The minimum interval between injections should usually be at least six weeks. Generally a maximum of three injections should be used at one site. If the condition has not responded or has recurred after these three injections then alternative management strategies should be considered.

Anaesthetic

Practice with respect to use of anaesthetics during joint and soft tissue injections performed in adults varies widely. Insertion of the needle through the skin and injection into soft tissues is often painful due to the thick density of nociceptive fibres in the dermal tissues and small volume capacity of the tissues that are being injected. In contrast, joints themselves are relatively insensate. Most patients rate an adequately placed joint injection performed with no local anaesthetic as between two to three on the 10-point pain Visual Analogue Score (VAS) whereas a soft tissue injection is usually rated as seven to eight.

There are several techniques that can be used to reduce pain associated with passing the needle through the skin. Vapocoolant sprays (sprayed for less than 10 seconds), topical anaesthetics, entonox and distraction techniques such as the 'cough trick' can all be helpful in this respect.

Where a joint is being aspirated or injected then many operators like to enter the joint using a syringe that contains some anaesthetic (~2–5 ml of 2% lignocaine). This allows for local tissue anaesthesia in the event that entry into the joint is not straightforward. Injection of the remainder of the anaesthetic into the joint prior to performing an aspiration often makes the latter procedure more comfortable. The needle is left in place and the syringes switched in order to proceed to corticosteroid injection. If very small joints, such as interphalangeal joints, are being injected then a two-step procedure is not appropriate. In these cases it is more appropriate to mix the corticosteroid with a small volume of anaesthetic; the small volume of fluid that can be injected into the joints will preclude use of more than a very small amount of anaesthetic (~0.1–0.2 mls 2% lignocaine) in these cases.

In the case of soft tissue injections many operators will mix the corticosteroid preparation with a small volume of anaesthetic (~0.5 ml of 2% lignocaine) to make the procedure more comfortable.

If a local anaesthetic has been injected, it is important to warn the patient of early post-injection local anaesthesia to avoid concern and initial overuse.

8.2. Procedural Checklist

A clear decision must be made about the procedure that needs to be undertaken and particularly whether aspiration as well as injection will be attempted. The clinician must have knowledge of local anatomy and suitable experience. The patient should be as relaxed as possible; muscle contraction associated with tension may make entry to the knee joint or subacromial space more difficult.

Initial Checks

- Check number of prior injections and time elapsed since last injection.
- Check routine blood tests including platelets and coagulation screen if relevant.
- Check for allergies, including sticking plaster.
- Obtain informed consent, explaining risks, benefits and post-injection management.

Preparations for Injection

- Assemble equipment, including gloves, cleaning agent such as mediswabs or iodine solution, vapocoolant spray, hypodermic needles, syringe(s), local anaesthetic, corticosteroid, sharps bin, specimen pot, gauze or cottonwool, tape or sticking plaster.
- Select needles with larger diameters for aspiration (19 or 21 gauge (G)). For injections without aspiration then use the smallest diameter needle that will reach the relevant site (21–27G). Note that the higher the gauge size, the smaller the needle diameter.
- Mark a spot for the proposed injection. This is sometimes best done by making a small indentation in the skin using a thumbnail. Marks made with pens will disappear with the cleansing procedure.
- Wash hands thoroughly and open equipment, being very careful not to touch any areas that will come into contact with the injectate or patient.
- Put on gloves and draw up the medication. Use a sterile swab to wipe the tops of any vials that have a rubber barrier requiring piercing, prior to inserting

the needle. Anaesthetic, if used, may be drawn up in a separate syringe or mixed with the corticosteroid depending on the procedure.

- Change the needle on the syringe to be used for initial injection.
- Clean the patient's skin thoroughly using the cleaning agent, working away from the proposed site of injection.
- Employ a 'no touch' technique from this point onward; i.e. do not touch the cleansed area again but rely on the marking already made.

Soft Tissue Injection

- Use a syringe containing corticosteroid, with or without anaesthetic.
- Insert needle smoothly through the skin and direct the tip to the relevant structure. In the case of tendinopathies (e.g. 'tennis elbow', 'golfer's elbow') aim to direct the tip into the peritendinous area, avoiding the actual tendon as well as nerves and blood vessels. Moving a tendon may allow detection of needle insertion into the tendon, in which case the needle tip should be re-sited.
- Slowly inject the corticosteroid. It may be beneficial to perform partial withdrawals and reinsertions of the needle in a fan shaped pattern to increase the area of tissue infiltrated with corticosteroid. Attempt aspiration after each reinsertion to ensure the needle tip is not within a blood vessel. Never inject against resistance.
- Withdraw the needle and syringe and apply firm pressure to the injection site with gauze, securing with tape or sticking plaster.

Joint Injection

- Use a syringe containing corticosteroid, with or without anaesthetic.
- Insert needle smoothly through the skin and direct the tip into the joint, avoiding tendons, nerves and blood vessels.
- Slowly inject the corticosteroid. Do not inject against resistance.
- Withdraw the needle and syringe and apply firm pressure to the injection site with gauze, securing with tape or sticking plaster.

Aspiration and Injection of a Joint, Bursa, Ganglion or Tenosynovitis

- If aspirating, use the syringe containing anaesthetic only or the empty syringe if performing the procedure without local anaesthesia. Enter the skin smoothly, using distraction techniques as necessary and aim to direct the needle tip into the relevant space, avoiding tendons, nerves and blood vessels. If necessary inject anaesthetic to the soft tissues as you advance. Where injection of a superficial ganglion or bursa is being performed it is advisable to use a 'Z' track for needle entry to the structure as this may reduce risk of subsequent infection.

- Aspirate as the needle is advanced to confirm entry into the relevant space. In the case of joint injections patients may find the remainder of the procedure more comfortable if a small volume of the anaesthetic in the syringe is injected into the joint prior to withdrawing synovial fluid.
- Exchange syringes as many times as required, leaving the needle in place, to allow aspiration to dryness.
- Leave needle in place and replace the syringe with one containing corticosteroid. Slowly inject the preparation. Do not inject against resistance.
- Withdraw the needle and syringe and apply firm pressure to the injection site with gauze, securing with tape or sticking plaster.

Post-Procedure

- Dispose of sharps safely in a sharps bin.
- Where a joint has been injected, advise the patient to rest the joint for the next few days.
- Advise the patient to seek medical advice if any signs of infection or other significant adverse effects develop.
- Document the injection method and medication in the notes.

8.3. Specific Injection Techniques

Although the following details the commonly used methods of injecting, it is important to stress that these pictures are only a guide and not a substitute for the supervision required to gain expertise in injecting joints. It is important not to inject against resistance as this suggests that material is being injected into the tissues rather than tissue spaces. When the needle passes through the joint capsule, it will be felt as a slight 'give' in the tissues. Once in the joint, avoid moving the needle as this can lead to damage of the articular cartilage.

8.3.1. *Glenohumeral Joint and Subacromial Space*

Glenohumeral Joint

In cases of inflammatory arthritis with an effusion, injection of the glenohumoral joint is often simple. However, with degenerative joint disease and adhesive capsulitis it is often difficult to inject into the shoulder joint itself. The posterior approach is easier than the anterior approach and is associated with a lower risk of damage to surrounding neurovascular structures (Figs. 8.1 and 8.2).

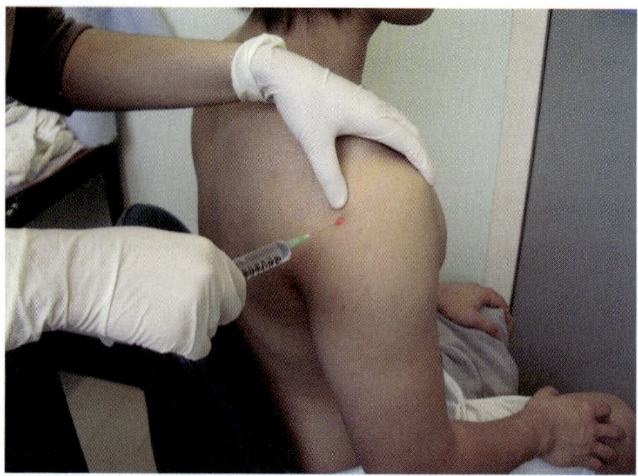

Fig. 8.1. Injection of the glenohumeral joint via a posterior approach. The posterior margin of the acromion is palpated and a point is marked 1 cm below and 1 cm medial to the posterior angle. In slight individuals, the joint line can be felt by holding the humeral head and moving the arm. A 21G needle is directed from this point towards the coracoid process which is palpated anteriorly. Injection of 40–80 mg methylprednisolone with lignocaine to make up to 5 ml is usually appropriate.

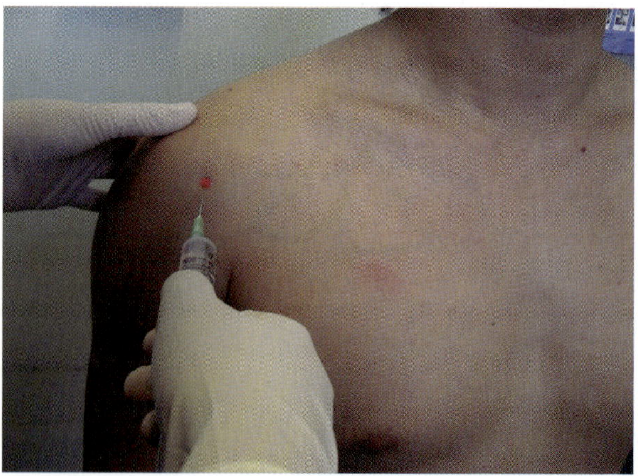

Fig. 8.2. Injection of the glenohumeral joint via an anterior approach. The anterior approach is more difficult and it is important to ensure injection is occurring in the correct space. The arm is placed in internal rotation with the forearm resting on the abdomen or lap. The coracoid process and the joint line are located and the needle is inserted just lateral and inferior to the coracoid process, aiming towards the joint line.

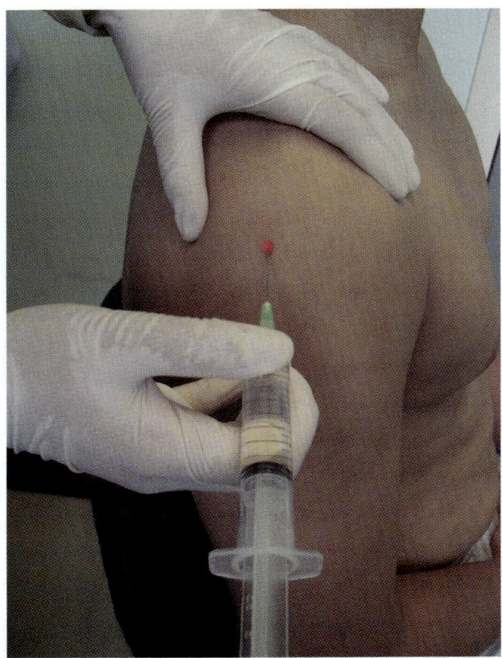

Fig. 8.3. Injection of the subacromial bursa. Sufficient muscle relaxation is important in opening the space between the acromion and head of the humerus. The skin is marked at the level of this space and the needle is aimed medially to pass through deltoid and into the subacromial space. 2–3 ml of a mixture of 40 mg methylprednisolone and local anaesthetic is usually injected using a 21 or 23G needle.

Subacromial Space

Injection of corticosteroid to the subacromial space may be indicated as part of management of rotator cuff tendonitis, impingement syndrome or subacromial bursitis (Fig. 8.3).

8.3.2. *Elbow Joint and Surrounding Tissues*

Elbow Joint

Injection of the elbow joint may be indicated in patients with inflammatory arthritis. There are several possible routes. The posterior approach is commonly used although care must be taken to avoid the ulnar nerve (Fig. 8.4). An alternative approach is to enter the joint laterally, midway between the olecranon and the lateral epicondyle, with the elbow flexed to 90°.

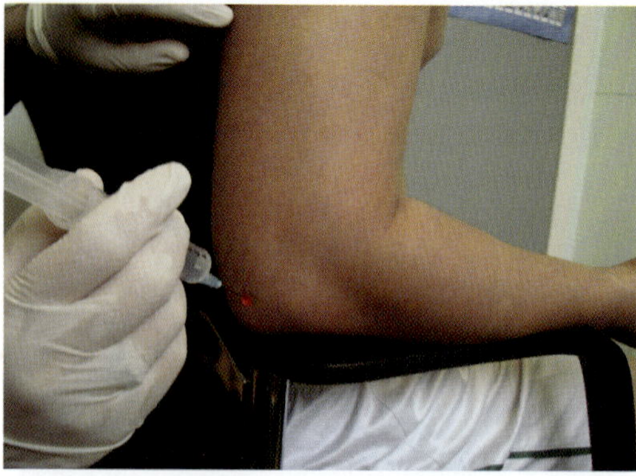

Fig. 8.4. Posterior approach to the elbow joint. The elbow is flexed to 90° with the hand supine, resting on the arm of a chair. The two halves of the triceps tendon are palpated posteriorly and the needle (23–25G) is passed just above the olecranon, angled slightly downwards and medially behind the triceps tendon. The ulnar nerve passes on the medial aspect of the elbow and should be avoided.

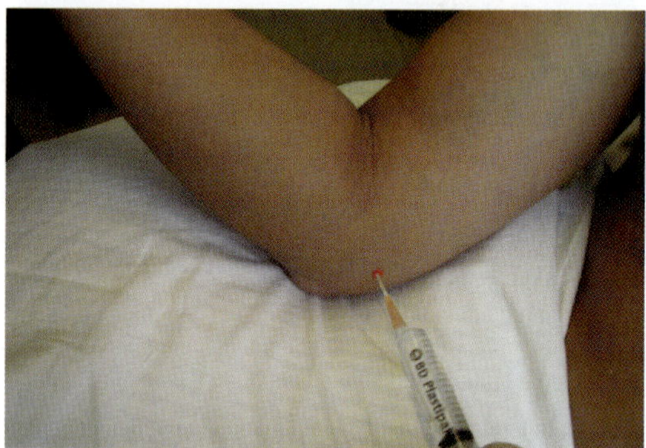

Fig. 8.5. Injection in medial epicondylitis. This is a soft tissue injection and the area is palpated for maximal tenderness with the elbow flexed at 90°. This is normally slightly lateral to the medial epicondyle but is variable. A 25G needle is used and the steroid with local anaesthetic is injected in a fan shape with partial withdrawal and reinsertion. Care must be taken to avoid the ulnar nerve in the groove just posterior to the medial epicondyle. Typically 25 mg hydrocortisone or 10 mg of methylprednisolone is used.

Medial and Lateral Epicondyles

Soft tissue injections around the medial and lateral epicondyles may be indicated as part of management of medial and lateral elbow tendinopathies ('golfer's' and 'tennis elbow' respectively, sometimes termed epicondylitis) (Figs. 8.5 and 8.6).

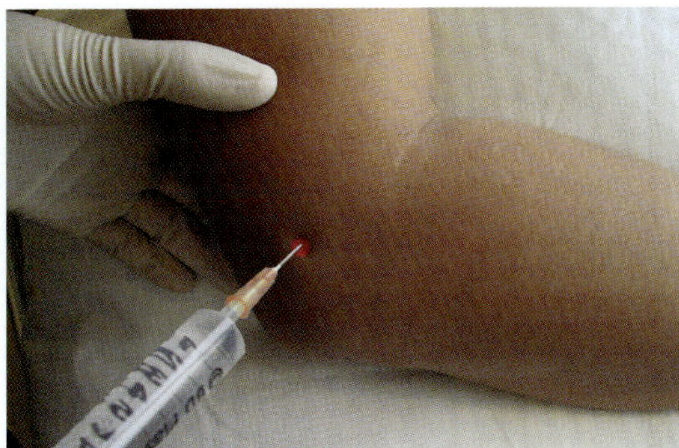

Fig. 8.6. Injection in lateral epicondylitis. This is performed similarly to that for medial epicondylitis. The elbow is flexed to 90° with the forearm supinated. The tender site around the lateral epicondyle is injected.

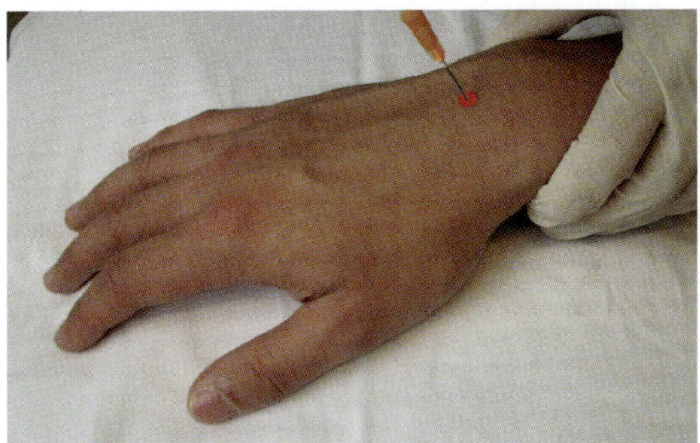

Fig. 8.7. Injection of the radiocarpal joint. The joint is entered from the dorsoradial side. The wrist is placed in slight palmar flexion and the point of injection, which lies to the ulnar side of the extensor pollicis longus tendon, is marked. The needle (25G) is inserted perpendicularly to 1–2 cm in depth and 25 mg hydrocortisone or 20 mg methylprednisolone is usually injected. All the important neurovascular structures are on the volar surface of the wrist but it is important to avoid the extensor tendons.

Care must be taken when injecting around the medial epicondyle as the ulnar nerve lies in the groove just posterior to the medial epicondyle.

8.3.3. *Wrist*

Radiocarpal Joint

Inflammatory arthritis of the wrist may respond well to corticosteroid injection of the radiocarpal joint (Fig. 8.7). This is commonly performed for patients with

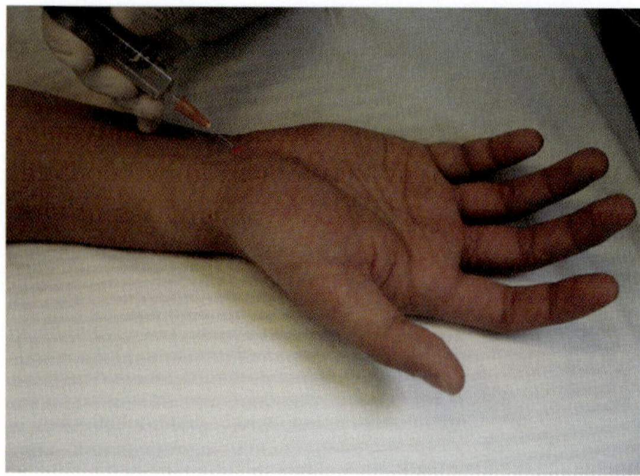

Fig. 8.8. Carpal tunnel injection. The flexor tendon of palmaris longus is identified. The needle (25G) is inserted to the ulnar side of the palmaris longus tendon at an angle of 45° with the wrist joint slightly extended. Many operators place the needle in the tunnel with use of local anaesthetic and then exchange the syringe, leaving the needle in place, to inject the carpal tunnel with 25 mg hydrocortisone.

rheumatoid arthritis and is also very effective in management of pseudogout which often involves the wrist.

Carpal Tunnel

Injection of corticosteroid into the carpal tunnel may provide effective, albeit often temporary, relief from symptoms of median nerve compression (carpal tunnel syndrome) where the condition is graded as mild-to-moderate by nerve conduction studies (Fig. 8.8). Patients with severe carpal tunnel syndrome should be referred for consideration of carpal tunnel decompression.

8.3.4. *Small Joints of the Hand*

Metacarpophalangeal and Interphalangeal Joints

The metacarpophalangeal and interphalangeal joints are commonly inflamed in rheumatoid or psoriatic arthritis and can be injected through either a dorsoradial or dorsoulnar approach (Fig. 8.9). As the joints are so small, aspiration is usually not possible. If the injection is placed correctly, the joint will distend symmetrically.

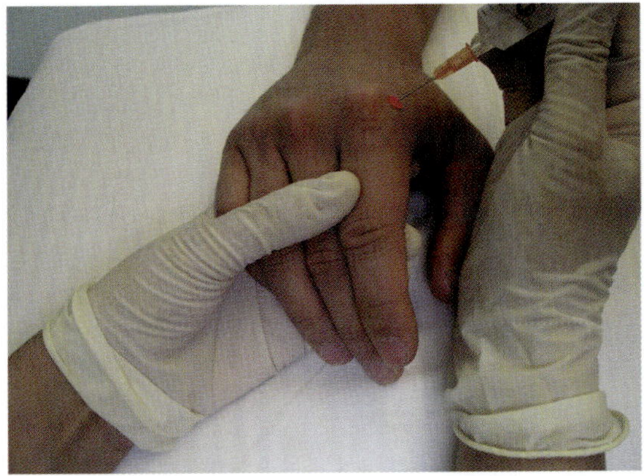

Fig. 8.9. Metacarpophalangeal joint injection via dorsoradial approach. The needle (25G) is inserted through the joint capsule and 10–15 mg hydrocortisone with a small volume of local anaesthetic (< 0.2 ml) is gently injected.

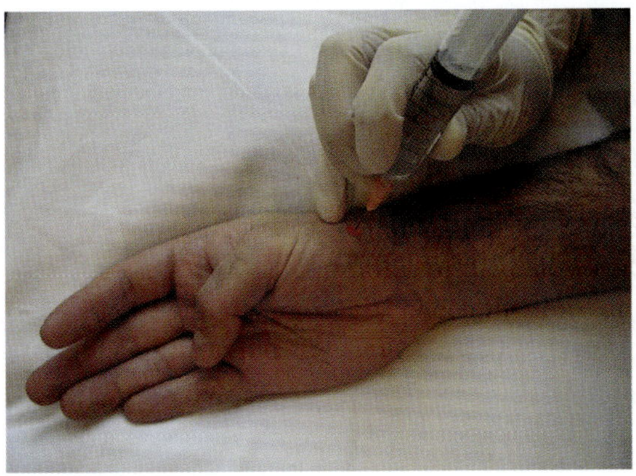

Fig. 8.10. Injection of the first carpometacarpal joint. The hand is supported and the thumb is flexed across the palm. The joint can be readily palpated at the base of the first metacarpal. The needle (25G) is inserted perpendicular to the skin to a depth of 2–4 mm and the joint is injected with 10–20 mg hydrocortisone.

First Carpometacarpal Joint

Injection of the first carpometacarpal joint may provide relief from symptoms of inflammatory arthritis or osteoarthritis (Fig. 8.10).

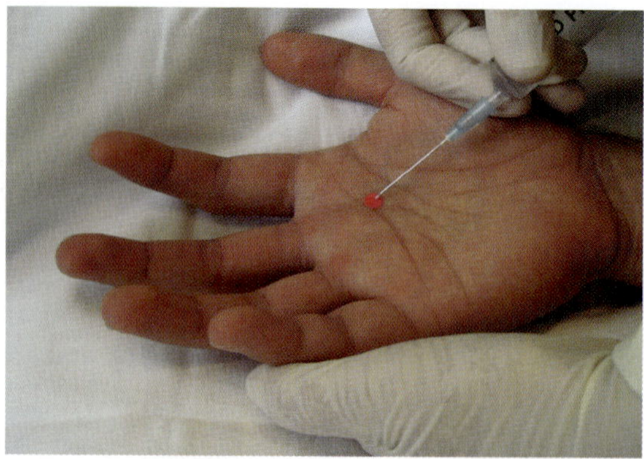

Fig. 8.11. Injection of flexor tendon sheath for 'trigger finger'. A 25–27G needle is inserted into the tendon sheath opposite the volar surface of the metacarpal head. The needle is advanced until the tip rubs against the surface of the tendon, evidenced by a crepitus-like sensation. This can sometimes be more easily felt if the patient is asked to slowly flex and extend the relevant finger. The needle is then withdrawn 1 mm before injecting the steroid, usually 15–25 mg hydrocortisone.

Thumb and Finger Flexor Tendon Sheaths

Injections into flexor tendon sheaths are performed for 'trigger' fingers or thumbs and are a very successful approach to management of these conditions. The tendon sheath is approached by inserting the needle at the level of the metacarpophalangeal joint and directing the needle tip distally (Fig. 8.11). Some operators prefer to insert the needle more distally and to direct the tip proximally as this allows easier positioning of the patient and operator. The tip of the needle needs to be carefully placed so that it lies just outside the tendon and within the sheath.

8.3.5. *Hip Joint and Surrounding Tissues*

Hip Joint

The hip joint should ideally be injected under fluoroscopic or ultrasound guidance. The patient is put in the supine position with the hip slightly flexed (place a cushion under the patient's knee) and internally rotated. The needle is inserted at the intersection between a vertical line from the anterior superior iliac spine and a horizontal line from the greater trochanter. The femoral vessels should be palpable 1–2 cm medial to the needle insertion point and must

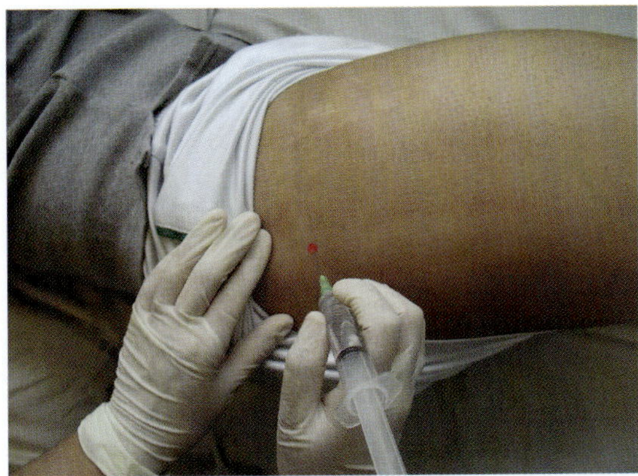

Fig. 8.12. Injection to soft tissue around the greater trochanter. The patient is positioned lying on the non-tender side. The point of maximum tenderness around the greater trochanter is palpated. Usually this is in a slightly posterior and superior position. The needle (21G) is inserted vertically almost to the bone. The injection is applied in a fan shape with partial withdrawal and reinsertion. In obese individuals, a 19G needle may need to be used to gain appropriate depth. 40 mg of methylprednisolone made up to 5 ml with 1% lignocaine is usually sufficient.

be avoided. The needle is angled slightly upward and medially until it passes through the capsule.

Trochanteric Bursa

A soft tissue injection into the area around the greater trochanter may provide pain relief in individuals with a trochanteric pain syndrome due to bursitis or, more commonly, a gluteus medius paratendonitis (Fig. 8.12).

8.3.6. *Knee Joint and Surrounding Tissue*

Knee Joint

The knee joint is involved in a wide range of rheumatic conditions; it is the most common site for a septic arthritis and frequently becomes inflamed in rheumatoid arthritis, the spondyloarthropathies and crystal arthritis. Aspiration of synovial fluid from the knee joint may be crucial for diagnosis of septic arthritis or crystal arthritis. Intra-articular injection with corticosteroid is beneficial in inflammatory arthritis and may also provide some pain relief in patients with osteoarthritis. The

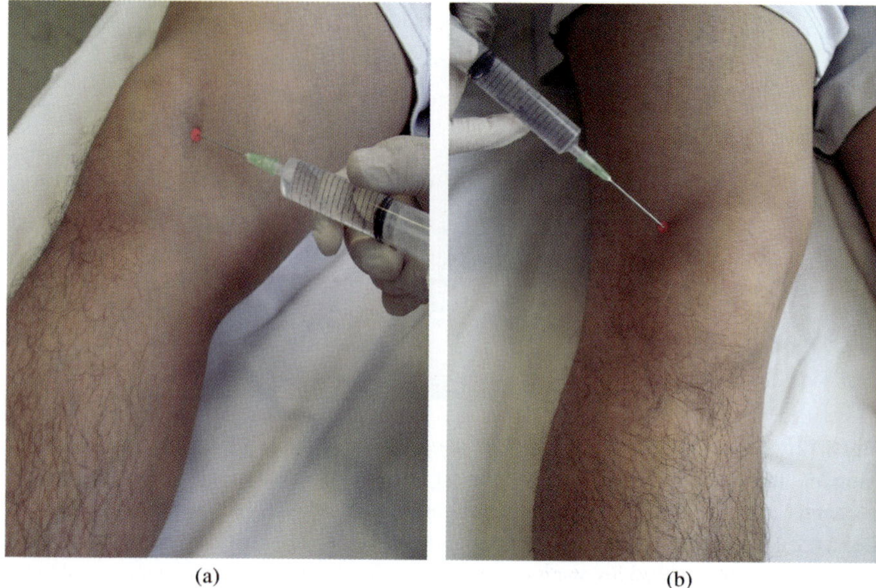

(a) (b)

Figs 8.13a and b. Injection of the knee joint. The patient lies supine on a couch with the knee extended or slightly flexed with a cushion underneath the joint. The needle is placed either (a) medially or (b) laterally at the border of the upper third and lower two thirds of the patella and inserted perpendicular to the skin so that the tip is directed underneath the patella into the knee joint. A 19–21G needle is used and up to 80 mg of methylprednisolone made up to 5 ml with 1% lignocaine can be injected.

knee is the easiest joint to aspirate and inject and may be approached medially or laterally (Figs. 8.13a and 8.13b).

Pes Anserine Bursa

The pes anserine insertion with its associated bursa lies inferomedial to the knee joint and is a common site of pain. Symptomatic relief may be gained by local injection of corticosteroid (Fig. 8.14).

8.3.7. *Ankle Joint*

The ankle joint is commonly involved in gout and is also often affected in rheumatoid arthritis. Aspiration and injection of the joint may be undertaken, most commonly using an anteriomedial approach (Fig. 8.15).

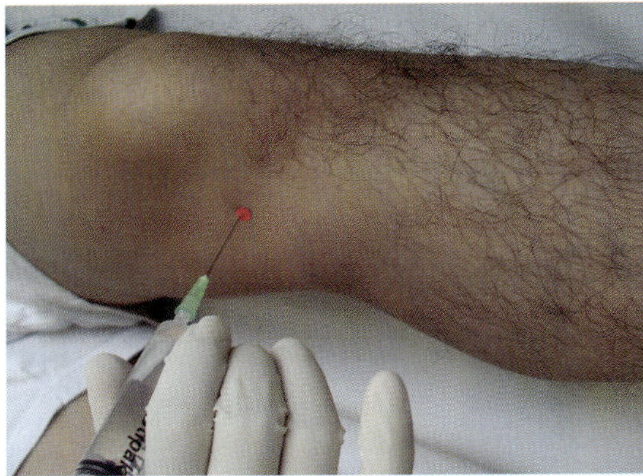

Fig. 8.14. Injection to the anserine bursa and around the pes anserine insertion. The needle (21–25G) is inserted perpendicular to the tibia at the point of maximal tenderness. If significant bursitis is present it may be possible to aspirate fluid although this is unusual. The steroid (usually 25 mg hydrocortisone) with local anaesthetic is injected into the bursa and in a fan shape around the tendon insertion.

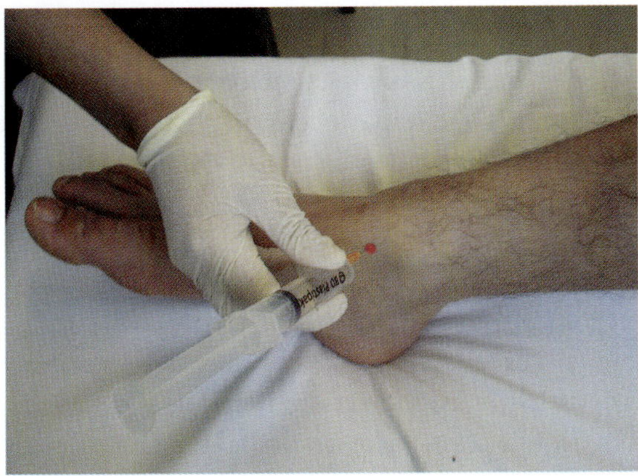

Fig. 8.15. Injection of the ankle. The joint is plantar flexed. The needle is inserted just medial to the tibialis anterior tendon distal to the lower margin of the tibia. It is angled posteriorly and laterally and inserted to a depth of about 1–2 cm. Usually a 23 or 25G needle is appropriate. However, a 21G needle will be required if aspiration is being performed. The ankle joint is normally injected with 40 mg methylprednisolone.

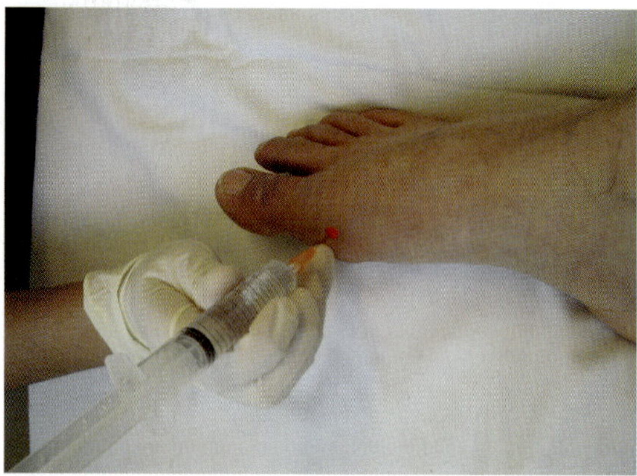

Fig. 8.16. Injection of the first metatarsophalangeal joint. A dorsomedial or dorsolateral approach may be used. The joint line can be easily palpated and the needle (25G) is inserted medial to the extensor tendon to a depth of 2–4 mm and 10–20 mgs hydrocortisone is injected. The interphalangeal joints of the toes may also be injected in a similar way.

8.3.8. *Feet*

Small Joints of the Feet

The first metatarsophalangeal joint is commonly involved with osteoarthritis, gout or rheumatoid arthritis and it may occasionally be appropriate to inject local corticosteroid (Fig. 8.16). The interphalangeal joints of the toes may also be injected using a small gauge needle.

Morton's Neuroma

This is an interdigital nerve entrapment, typically between the third and fourth metatarsals. The nerve is trapped under the transverse metatarsal ligament causing perineural fibrosis. It is often the result of chronic foot strain or biomechanical problems. The condition may respond to corticosteroid injection (Fig. 8.17). However if it recurs following injection then it is usually more appropriate to refer to an orthopaedic surgeon for excision.

Plantar Fasciitis

Plantar fasciitis often responds well to local corticosteroid injection, given in conjunction with use of an orthosis and physiotherapy. The steroid should be infiltrated around the insertion of the plantar fascia to the medial calcaneum (Fig. 8.18).

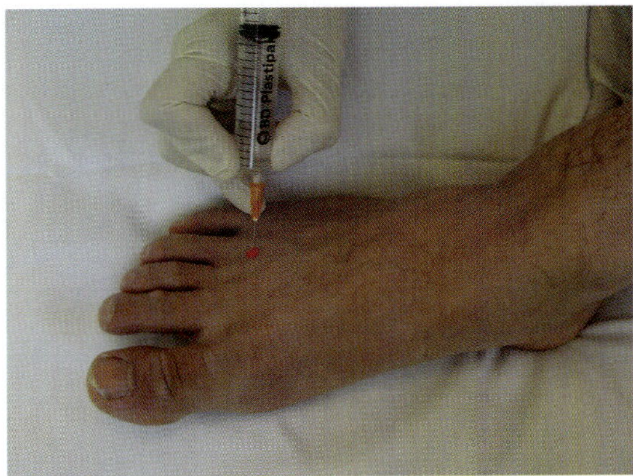

Fig. 8.17. Interdigital neuroma injection. A 25G needle is inserted into the intermetatarsal space, perpendicular to the skin and to a depth of 2–4 mm. Corticosteroid is injected to the area around the neuroma. Ultrasound imaging allows for accurate placing of the needle.

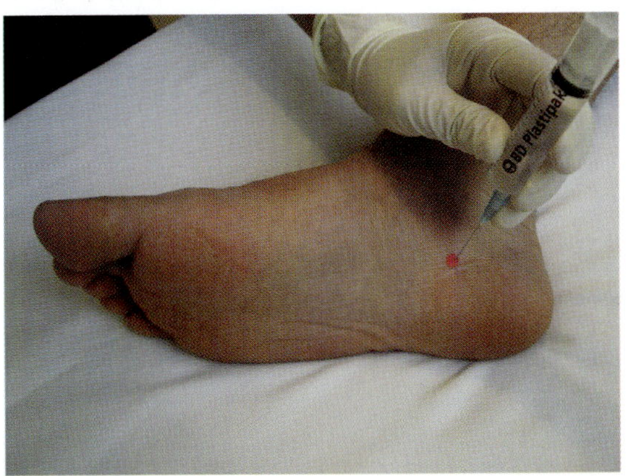

Fig. 8.18. Injection for plantar fasciitis. The injection is given from the medial side of the foot. The needle (23G) is advanced in a lateral direction, angled slightly upward so that its tip is positioned above the point of maximum tenderness on the heel. The injection, either of 25 mg hydrocortisone or 20 mg methylprednisolone, is made as close as possible to the plantar surface of the calcaneus.

8.4. Concluding Comments

There are many different factors that need to be considered prior to injecting a joint or soft tissue structure. This chapter is intended as a guide only and it is not a substitute for practical experience. If there are any concerns, the clinician should always seek advice before proceeding in order to minimise the risk to the patient.

Chapter 9

Drugs Used in Management of Rheumatic Disease

Editor: Suzanne Donnelly

Maha Azeez, Suzanne Donnelly, Paul MacMullan, Bryan Whelan

9.1. Introduction

A relatively limited number of drugs are commonly used in rheumatology practice. Simple analgesics are widely prescribed in medicine and are not further discussed here. Non-steroidal anti-inflammatory drugs (NSAIDs) may provide symptomatic benefit in a wide range of rheumatic conditions. Corticosteroids are important anti-inflammatory and immunosuppressive drugs but are associated with serious side effects that limit their use. The disease-modifying anti-rheumatic drugs (DMARDs) provide the mainstay of management of patients with rheumatoid arthritis (RA) and psoriatic arthritis (PsA). Drugs with potent cytotoxic or anti-proliferative properties have long been used for management of connective tissue diseases and vasculitides. Other immunosuppressive agents with varying degrees of specificity for individual immune mediators have been introduced more recently for management of RA; some of these also have a role in management of other rheumatic conditions. Drugs that block the production or excretion of uric acid are used in management of gout and those that interfere with bone turnover are used in management of the metabolic bone diseases (Table 9.1). An up-to-date British National Formulary will provide definitive prescribing advice for these medications.

9.2. Non-Steroidal Anti-Inflammatory Drugs

Non-steroidal anti-inflammatory drugs are effective anti-inflammatory and analgesic drugs. They are among the most widely used classes of medications in the developed

Table 9.1. Drugs commonly prescribed in rheumatology practice.

Group	Examples
Non-steroidal anti-inflammatory agents	Ibuprofen, diclofenac, etoricoxib
Corticosteroids	Prednisolone, hydrocortisone, methylprednisolone, triamcinolone, dexamethasone
Disease-modifying anti-rheumatic drugs	Methotrexate, hydroxychloroquine, sulphasalazine, leflunomide
Other immunosuppressive drugs with cytotoxic or anti-proliferative actions on immune cells	Azathioprine, mycophenolate mofetil, cyclophosphamide
Drugs targeting TNF-α or IL-6 receptor	Infliximab, etancercept, adalimumab, certolizumab, golimumab, tocilizumab
Drugs targeting B cells or T cells	Rituximab, abatacept,
Drugs used to treat gout	Allopurinol, febuxostat, sulphinpyrazone, colchicine
Drugs used in metabolic bone disease	Alendronate, risedronate, ibandronate, zoledronate, strontium ranelate, raloxifene, recombinant parathyroid hormone, teriparatide, denosumab

IL-6 interleukin 6, TNF-α tumour necrosis factor-alpha.

world and are routinely prescribed in a variety of inflammatory rheumatic conditions. Most NSAIDS are organic acids and all drugs within this class share a common mechanism of action although they differ in their selectivity, duration of action and pharmacokinetics. The discovery that aspirin mediated its effects through irreversible inhibition of the cyclooxygenase (COX) pathway led to the development of a range of reversible non-selective COX inhibitors. These include diclofenac, indomethacin, ibuprofen, ketoprofen and naproxen. The gastrointestinal toxicity (see below) associated with these agents led to the development of COX-2 selective inhibitors, sometimes termed 'coxibs', including celecoxib, etoricoxib and meloxicam, to preferentially target inflamed tissue. It is important to remember that the agents are only relatively selective for COX-2 versus COX-1 pathways and do exert some inhibitory effect on COX-1 pathways. Topical forms of NSAIDs are available as gels for local application over painful areas.

Indications and Dose

NSAIDs are widely prescribed in rheumatology practice for musculoskeletal pain, either inflammatory or degenerative. Long-term use of these agents should be avoided where possible; simple analgesics usually provide a safer alternative. Short-acting agents are most suitable for 'as needed' use and longer acting or slow release formulations are more appropriate for regular dosing.

Pharmacokinetics and Pharmacodynamics

Most NSAIDs are short-acting competitive COX inhibitors with a plasma half-life of less than four hours (e.g. ibuprofen, diclofenac and indomethacin), however, piroxicam and nabumetone continue to demonstrate pharmacological efficacy for more than 18 hours after a single dose. The availability of enteric-coated and slow-release formulations that allow for once or twice daily dosing is increasing. Almost all NSAIDs exhibit high protein binding *in vivo* (80–99% albumin bound) and this high affinity for binding sites on albumin results in a significant potential for drug interactions; NSAIDs may displace other drugs from protein thereby increasing the unbound concentration and toxicity of the other drugs. Furthermore, most NSAIDs are metabolised via the liver, further increasing potential drug interactions.

Mechanism of Action

Both the beneficial properties and unwanted side effects of NSAIDs are directly related to their pharmacological mode of action. Mechanistically, NSAIDS competitively inhibit prostaglandin synthesis via the COX-1 and COX-2 pathways. The COX-1 pathway is the main constitutive pathway of prostaglandin synthesis involved in gastroduodenal protection, renal perfusion and platelet activity. The COX-2 pathway is induced in damaged tissue and mediates inflammation, fever and pain and so is the true target for the drugs. However, the COX-2 pathway is also the constitutive pathway in the vascular endothelium.

Adverse Effects

Traditional or non-selective NSAIDs have long been associated with gastrointestinal bleeding due to COX-1 dependent prostaglandin depletion and subsequent mucosal injury. COX-2 inhibitors were developed specifically to reduce the incidence of such complications. However, several placebo-controlled trials of these agents have revealed an increased risk of myocardial infarction and other atherothrombotic events. Further studies show that these increased risks are also a feature of long-term use of most non-selective NSAIDs. The effect has been attributed to the reduction in prostacyclin bioavailability via COX-2 inhibition in vascular endothelial cells. Reduced prostacyclin enhances platelet activation and vasoconstriction thus creating a predisposition to thrombosis, hypertension and atherosclerosis.

In normal healthy individuals, direct renal toxicity is rare, however, the drugs are relatively contraindicated in renal impairment because of the dependence of renal parenchyma medullary interstitial cells on COX-mediated perfusion pathways.

9.3. Corticosteroids

Corticosteroids are sterol derivatives, naturally produced in the adrenal cortex as glucocorticoids or mineralocorticoids. The main natural mineralocorticoid is aldosterone and the main natural glucocorticoid is cortisol (hydrocortisone). The synthetic glucocorticoids have immunosuppressant and anti-inflammatory properties and have been used in the therapy of rheumatic diseases for over 50 years.

Synthetic glucocorticoids are available in long- and short-acting forms and are variably more potent than the natural hormones, a factor largely determined by their relative affinity for the cytosolic glucocorticoid receptor. The biologically inactive synthetic compounds have an 11-keto group (prednisone and cortisone) and require activation to the 11-hydroxy group (prednisolone, cortisol) in the liver before they can bind the cytosolic receptor. There are five commonly prescribed synthetic glucocorticoids of differing potency (Table 9.2).

Different glucocorticoid preparations are available for parenteral use. Esterified glucocorticoids (e.g. hexacetonide) are lipophilic and tend to persist for longer at the site of injection. They are therefore commonly used for intramuscular (im), intralesional and intra-articular (ia) injection but their use should be avoided in close proximity to nerves and tendons. Salts, such as succinates, are more water soluble and used intravenously (iv) or locally at sites close to neural or tendon tissue.

Table 9.2. Commonly prescribed glucocorticoids.

Drug	Dose equivalent	Relative potency	Duration (oral)
Short-acting			
Cortisol/Hydrocortisone	20 mg	1	24–30 h
Prednisolone	5 mg	4	24–30 h
Methylprednisolone	4 mg	5	24–30 h
Triamcinolone	4 mg	5	48–56 h
Long-acting			
Dexamethasone	0.75 mg	25	2.5 days

Indications and Dose

Glucocorticoids are indicated in the therapy of many rheumatic diseases. They may be used locally (topically for eyes, ia for joints, intralesionally for skin) or systemically via oral, im and iv routes. They may be the mainstay of therapy for steroid sensitive vasculitides such as giant cell arteritis or Takayasu's arteritis, or may be used as emergency or 'rescue' therapy for flares of systemic arthritis or autoimmune rheumatic diseases such as systemic lupus erythematosus (SLE). Evidence suggests that they possess disease-modifying properties when used in low dose in RA.

In general 'low dose' glucocorticoid therapy is agreed to be </= 7.5 mg/day of prednisolone or equivalent. 'High dose' glucocorticoid therapy is above 30 mg/day of prednisolone or equivalent and 'pulse' therapy refers to use of doses of >250 mg/day of prednisolone or equivalent (commonly as iv methylprednisolone) given on up to a total of three occasions at 24–48 hour intervals.

Glucocorticoids are now generally prescribed on a once daily dosing regimen. Where low doses of short-acting glucocorticoids are used then alternate day dosing may be associated with less adrenal suppression. However, patients frequently do not tolerate the poor symptom control on the second day. Alternate day regimens have no advantage when higher dose or longer acting glucocorticoids are used.

Pharmacokinetics and Pharmacodynamics

Glucocorticoids are available as oral, im or iv preparations for systemic use as noted above. Taken orally, they are absorbed from the gastrointestinal tract within 30 minutes with high bioavailability. Biologically inactive prednisone and cortisone are activated to prednisolone and cortisol in the liver. Prednisolone is highly protein bound (>90%) to corticosteroid-binding globulin (transcortin) and albumin. The 5–10% unbound fraction is biologically active. The other synthetic glucocorticoids are approximately 2:1 albumin bound:free. All synthetic glucocorticoids are metabolised in the liver via the cytochrome P450 isoenzyme 3A4 and excreted by the kidneys. Prednisolone half-life is prolonged in renal disease, liver cirrhosis, the elderly and African-Americans.

Mechanisms of Action

Glucocorticoids enter the cell and bind to the cytosolic glucocorticoid receptor with varying affinity. This complex migrates to the cell nucleus where it is hypothesised that one of two binding events drives the cellular response. Evidence is accumulating that if binding occurs between glucocorticoid receptor dimers and deoxyribonucleic acid (DNA), 'transactivation' leads to many of the metabolic/endocrine effects associated with steroid use. Alternatively, and purportedly via single glucocorticoid receptor binding to nuclear transcription and activation factors, 'transrepression' of genes induced and activated during the inflammatory response ensues. Hence, genes which may have been induced by pro-inflammatory cytokines are repressed, thus delivering the anti-inflammatory and immunosuppressant effects of the drug. Uncoupling of the beneficial 'transrepression' effects from the undesirable 'transactivation' events is a target of steroid drug development.

A multiplicity of effects of glucocorticoids on the immune system has been described. Glucocorticoids promote apoptosis of T and B cells and also have effects on cytokine, chemokine and adhesion molecule expression by lymphocytes. With respect to T cells an inhibition of Th1 cytokines and stimulation of Th2 cytokines has been reported. They also lead to a decrease in numbers and functional capacity of macrophages. Glucocorticoids inhibit adhesion molecule expression by neutrophils, thereby decreasing their capacity to adhere to endothelial cells and traffic to sites of infection; this results in an increase in the numbers of circulating neutrophils (Table 9.3).

Adverse Effects

Glucocorticoids have many unwelcome side-effects. While there is much interpersonal variation in thresholds for the development of these, most risk is dose and duration dependent, thus prudent prescribing is essential in order to minimise side effects.

An excess of naturally produced glucocorticoids gives rise to the clinical and biochemical features of Cushing's syndrome; excess of exogenous glucocorticoids

Table 9.3. Effect of glucocorticoids on immune leukocytes.

Cell	Effect of glucocorticoids
T cells	Decreased absolute numbers, reduced activation, trafficking and cytokine secretion.
B cells	Decreased absolute numbers, reduced activation, trafficking and cytokine secretion.
Monocytes and macrophages	Decreased absolute numbers, reduced trafficking, phagocytosis and COX-2 induction.
Neutrophils	Increased absolute numbers, decreased trafficking, inhibition of adhesion to endothelium.

results in iatrogenic Cushing's syndrome. Other endocrine effects include impaired glucose tolerance and frank diabetes mellitus, lipid profile alterations and weight gain. Cardiovascular effects include fluid retention, hypertension, ischaemic events and arrhythmias. Musculoskeletal effects include osteoporosis, avascular necrosis and steroid-induced myopathy. Glucocorticoids also predispose to glaucoma, cataract formation, gastritis and gastrointestinal ulceration, pancreatitis, impaired wound healing, infection, emotional instability, insomnia, agitation and frank psychosis. Abrupt withdrawal can lead to an Addisonian crisis with hypotension, hyponatraemia and hyperkalaemia. Careful management should help to reduce morbidity associated with side effects (Table 9.4).

Table 9.4. Minimising side effects due to corticosteroids.

Adverse effect	Comments
Osteoporosis	Consider calcium and vitamin D supplementation daily. Use bisphosphonates for significant osteopenia or established osteoporosis.
Osteonecrosis	Occurs with high dose or pulse therapy. Early diagnosis improves outcome; MRI detects earliest change.
Glucose intolerance/ diabetes mellitus	Highest risk for higher doses and other risk factors e.g. obesity, family history. Initiate anti-hyperglycaemic therapy if required.
Gastric irritation	Avoid concomitant NSAID/aspirin if possible. Add PPI for duration if NSAID combination treatment or other additional risk.
Alertness/insomnia	Morning dosing to preserve natural cortisol biorhythm.
Iatrogenic Cushing's syndrome	Aim to prescribe lowest effective dose for shortest period. Consider adding alternate immunosuppression (e.g. azathioprine).
Addisonian crisis	Taper dose carefully. Instruct patient to present to a doctor if unable to swallow or hold down daily maintenance therapy (e.g. vomiting).
Susceptibility to infection	Oral candida common. <10 mg prednisolone daily carries minimal excess risk of other infections. >10 mg prednisolone daily increases risk of infection.
Cardiovascular effects	Screen for and manage other risk factors for cardiovascular disease.

MRI magnetic resonance imaging, PPI proton pump inhibitor.

9.4. Disease-Modifying Anti-Rheumatic Drugs

Disease-modifying anti-rheumatic drugs form the cornerstone of management of RA and are also used in some other forms of inflammatory arthritis. Drugs are often prescribed in combination; methotrexate and hydroxychloroquine, with or without sulphasalazine, are commonly used together.

9.4.1. *Methotrexate*

Methotrexate is a folate analogue with a pteridine ring structure linked to para-aminobenzoic acid with a terminal glutamic acid residue. Methotrexate has several substitutions that render it inactive as a co-factor for folate dependent cellular reactions, accounting for its 'anti-folate' effects within the cell.

Indications and Dose

Methotrexate has been used in the therapy of RA for 30 years and has beneficial effects on all major outcomes in this disease. It is also widely used in management of juvenile idiopathic arthritis (JIA), PsA and peripheral arthritis in the other spondyloarthritides (SpA). It is increasingly used in the 'second line' therapy of other autoimmune and inflammatory conditions such as systemic vasculitis or polymyositis, either in induction or maintenance of disease remission alongside glucocorticoids. All rheumatology indications require once weekly dosing with 10–25 mg methotrexate whereas up to 5 g per week is standard in oncology practice. Methotrexate is available in oral, im and subcutaneous (sc) preparations. Due to differences in bioavailability, the equivalent effective dose of the parenteral preparations is approximately 10–20% less than that of oral preparations.

Pharmacokinetics and Pharmacodynamics

Following low dose oral administration, methotrexate is absorbed from the small intestine via folate receptors, in competition with folinic acid. This competition between folinic acid and methotrexate is used to advantage in managing toxicity; administration of folinic acid prevents further methotrexate uptake by cells. Under certain conditions active diffusion of methotrexate may be mediated by the reduced folate carrier, which usually transports dietary folic acid. There is considerable variability in the intestinal uptake of methotrexate, likely due to polymorphisms in the receptor and carrier genes.

Within cells, methotrexate undergoes polyglutamation, a reaction of importance in the efficacy and dosing schedule of this drug. Polyglutamated methotrexate has a prolonged half-life of seven days, may exert more potent intracellular effects than the parent compound and, importantly, is not a substrate for transmembrane pumps which actively efflux methotrexate from the cell.

Elimination is mainly via the kidneys with a small amount secreted through the biliary tract. Elimination is prolonged by tubular re-absorption and enterohepatic circulation and may be decreased in renal impairment. Dose reduction in moderate to severe renal impairment is advisable to avoid toxicity.

Mechanism of Action

Methotrexate has been shown, *in vitro* and *in vivo*, to have a wide range of anti-proliferative and anti-inflammatory effects, including effects on the innate immune system as well as on B and T cells. The underlying mechanisms of its actions have yet to be completely elucidated. Methotrexate is an inhibitor of dihydrofolate reductase, an enzyme required for purine synthesis. Both adenine and guanine, nucleobases required for DNA and ribonucleic acid (RNA), are purines; methotrexate thereby inhibits DNA and RNA synthesis and cell proliferation. Methotrexate also interferes with DNA synthesis by inhibiting thymidylate synthetase which converts the nucleotide dUMP to dTMP. Methotrexate inhibits the intracellular enzyme 5-aminoimidazole-4-carboxamide ribonucleotide transformylase which is involved in purine metabolism. One consequence of this last interaction is the accumulation of the nucleoside adenosine. Adenosine has well-documented anti-inflammatory properties including regulation of cell trafficking, suppression of IL-12 production from monocytes/macrophages and promotion of a shift from a T helper (Th)1 to a Th2 response. Furthermore, methotrexate prevents the transmethylation of polyamines such as spermidine and spermine, the pro-inflammatory toxic metabolites of which are reported to be up-regulated in RA.

Adverse Effects

Methotrexate toxicity arises when intracellular concentrations rise above the accepted therapeutic levels and is mediated at least partly through its anti-proliferative effect. Some of the complications develop in a sub-clinical fashion; hence methotrexate treatment requires ongoing toxicity monitoring. Patients who develop acute life-threatening consequences of methotrexate toxicity, sometimes as a result of inadvertent overdose, must stop the drug and should receive folinic acid rescue as well as supportive therapy.

Methotrexate induced hepatotoxicity

Use of high-dose methotrexate in childhood leukaemia was found to be associated with development of hepatic fibrosis. This condition was also found in up to 25% of patients treated for psoriasis in dermatological practice in the 1980s, leading to recommendations for surveillance liver biopsy at specific cumulative dose in dermatological practice worldwide. Review of the literature has led to a relaxing of this practice, as many early longitudinal studies did not screen for contributory factors such as hepatitis and alcohol consumption. The risk of hepatic fibrosis is increased in any pre-existing liver disease, the elderly, those in whom methotrexate clearance is impaired, those who consume >15 g of alcohol per day (one to two drinks), type II diabetes, the obese and those with non-alcoholic steatohepatitis. Additionally, risk may be greater for those with psoriasis. Risk is considerably reduced at doses of 15 mg or less weekly and all patients should have regular monitoring of liver function while on treatment. The role of serial biopsy based on cumulative dose is controversial and is not recommended by the American College of Rheumatology. Serious clinical consequences of methotrexate hepatotoxicity are now rarely seen as guidelines for prevention are widely implemented.

The use of liver biochemical monitoring is recommended. Persistent or recurrent elevation in serum transaminases, any decrease in the serum albumin level or the development of hepatomegaly warrants investigation. The pro-collagen type III peptide assay which was considered to indicate progressive hepatic fibrosis has not been proven sufficiently accurate to be of use in methotrexate monitoring.

Bone marrow suppression

The anti-proliferative effects of methotrexate may manifest as cytopenias, particularly neutropenias. Routine haematological monitoring of patients on methotrexate is strongly recommended. Reduced cell counts will usually rise again following cessation of methotrexate treatment; treatment can often subsequently be reinstated using lower doses. Where severe bone marrow suppression occurs, supportive treatment including use of granulocyte colony stimulating factor (GCSF) and broad spectrum antibiotics for neutropenic sepsis may be required.

Methotrexate pneumonitis

This is a rare complication of therapy, with an incidence of 1 per 100 patient years. Acute pneumonitis presents with a 'flu-like' illness, fever and sudden, progressive breathlessness. Chest X-ray may show diffuse interstitial or mixed interstitial and alveolar infiltrates, generally in the lower lung fields. Pulmonary function tests show a restrictive pattern with diminished diffusion capacity. If performed, lung biopsy may show cellular interstitial infiltrates or diffuse alveolar damage with perivascular inflammation. None of these findings is individually diagnostic and the possibility of rheumatoid lung disease, infection or other drug toxicity should be carefully considered. If diagnosed, the drug is immediately withdrawn and high-dose oral prednisolone commenced, with supportive therapy for hypoxia as indicated.

Non-dose related adverse drug reactions

Patients find nausea, hair loss and oral ulceration to be troublesome side effects of methotrexate. Co-prescription of folic acid is now widely practised although there is no universally agreed dose or regimen of folic acid supplementation. Use of folic acid has been shown to reduce hepatic side effects and may also improve the mucocutaneous and gastrointestinal 'nuisance' effects of methotrexate. A single dose of 5 mg folic acid taken 24–48 hours following weekly methotrexate is a common choice. Patients with persistent nausea may find that a switch to sc or im route for methotrexate administration relieves this.

Monitoring requirements

All patients need to have baseline blood tests and chest X-ray prior to initiation of methotrexate therapy. During treatment, ongoing monitoring, particularly for bone marrow and hepatic toxicity, is required. Blood tests are recommended initially at two-weekly intervals although testing can be reduced to four-weekly and then 12-weekly if the results are satisfactory.

Teratogenicity

Methotrexate is teratogenic and both male and female patients should be advised not to conceive within three months of taking the drug.

9.4.2. *Sulphasalazine*

Sulphasalazine is a combination of 5-aminosalicylic acid (anti-inflammatory) and sulphapyridine (anti-bacterial) joined by an azo bond.

Indications and Dose

Sulphasalazine is available in regular and enteric-coated tablets of 500 mg and is used in the treatment of RA, PsA and other spondyloarthropathies. It is also used in JIA and inflammatory bowel disease. Adults with rheumatic disease are maintained on 1.5–3 g/day in divided doses. The starting dose is usually 500 mg–1g/day in order to avoid side effects and is increased in increments of 500 mg–1g/day at intervals of a week or longer.

Pharmacokinetics and Pharmacodynamics

Approximately 30% of sulphasalazine is absorbed in the small bowel but much of this undergoes enterohepatic circulation and is secreted unchanged back into the bowel. Thus approximately 90% of the ingested drug reaches the colon where the azo bond is reduced by colonic bacteria, thus 'activating' the drug to its two components, sulphapyridine and 5-aminosalicylic acid (5-ASA). More than 90% of sulphapyridine is then absorbed and appears in the plasma four to six hours after oral dosing, while most 5-ASA remains in the colon. This latter moiety is the active component in ulcerative colitis.

The plasma half-life of sulphasalazine is six to 17 hours and that of sulphapyridine is eight to 21 hours. Sulphasalazine is excreted in the urine. Sulphapyridine is metabolised in the liver via acetylation and glucuronidation with variability according to acetylator phenotype, then excreted in the urine. 5-ASA is excreted mainly in the faeces. The dose of sulphasalazine should be reduced in the elderly due to reduced acetylation and in renal insufficiency.

Mechanism of Action

The mechanism of action of sulphasalazine in rheumatic diseases has not been fully elucidated, however, it possesses both anti-inflammatory and immunosuppressive effects. At the time of synthesis of the drug, it was considered that 5-ASA would confer anti-inflammatory effects and sulphapyridine antibacterial effects. Much evidence contrary to this original premise has now accrued. The active moiety in inflammatory arthritis remains the subject of some debate, however, sulphasalazine itself seems to be the most biologically active component, with some contribution from sulphapyridine. Of note, activity is not related to measured serum drug levels.

The drug has an anti-inflammatory effect mediated by inhibition of 5-aminoimidazole-4-carboxamide ribonucleotide transformylase resulting in increased levels of adenosine; the latter has a range of anti-flammatory actions. A similar effect is seen with methotrexate. There is also evidence, primarily from *in vitro* studies, that sulphasalazine can inhibit activation of T cells, natural killer (NK) cells and B cells and reduce expression of interleukin (IL)-6 and tumour necrosis factor (TNF)-α by cells of the monocyte/macrophage lineage. Furthermore, angiogenesis and metalloproteinase synthesis, established key processes in synovitis, are suppressed by sulphasalazine.

Adverse Effects

Most side effects occur within the first three months of treatment; the risk of side effects thereafter diminishes with time. Patients commonly experience nausea, diarrhoea, abdominal pain and dyspepsia; these can usually be minimised by introducing the drugs at low dose (500 mg daily) and gradually increasing the dose at weekly intervals. Serious adverse reactions include bone marrow suppression, pneumonitis and drug-induced lupus. Incidence of leucopenia and neutropenia is reported at 1–5%. Rash secondary to the sulpha moiety occurs in <5% of patients and these patients should avoid other sulpha containing medications.

Monitoring requirements

It is recommended that baseline haematological, renal and liver function tests (LFTs) should be performed prior to commencing sulphasalazine and blood monitoring should be carried out every two to four weeks for three months and every three to six months thereafter.

9.4.3. *Leflunomide*

Leflunomide is an isoxazole immunomodulatory and anti-proliferative agent which inhibits *de novo* pyrimidine synthesis by direct antagonism of dihydroorotate dehydrogenase.

Indications and Dose

Leflunomide is available in 10 mg and 20 mg tablets and is taken orally. It is indicated in the treatment of moderate to severe RA for the reduction of inflammation and the inhibition of structural (radiological) damage. The recommended starting dose is a loading dose of 100 mg daily for three days (see Pharmacokinetics below) followed by a maintenance dose of 10–20 mg daily. Most clinicians do not use loading doses as the initial experience was one of increased gastrointestinal toxicity and subsequent poor compliance. The dose is usually decreased to 10 mg daily if toxicity occurs or when disease is controlled.

Pharmacokinetics and Pharmacodynamics

Leflunomide is a pro-drug, which is well absorbed orally and converted to its active metabolite, malononitrilamide, A77 1726. Leflunomide has a long half-life of approximately 14–18 days; hence initial loading is recommended to more rapidly attain steady state concentrations. Active metabolites undergo further metabolism and are considered to undergo biliary recycling. Metabolites are eliminated very slowly from plasma, and excreted in both urine and faeces. In instances of serious toxicity or where patients who have been treated with leflunomide wish to become pregnant, a drug elimination procedure is advised using either oral cholestyramine 8 g three times a day for 11 days or activated charcoal orally or via nasogastric tube in case of hypersensitivity.

Mechanism of Action

The exact mechanism of action of leflunomide is unclear. The immunomodulatory effect observed is a reduction in activation of T lymphocytes. Leflunomide selectively inhibits the enzyme dihydroorotate dehydrogenase, one of the key enzymes in the *de novo* pyrimidine synthesis pathway, which is essential for the activation of T cells. At higher concentrations, it is also thought to inhibit phosphorylation of tyrosine kinase, which plays a major role in cell growth and differentiation of activated cells and this is thought to be responsible for its antiproliferative effects. Leflunomide has also been shown to block the activation of nuclear factor κB, which plays a key role in inflammation.

Adverse Effects

The most common side effects are diarrhoea, hypertension, headache and alopecia. Recurrent infections may necessitate withdrawal of therapy. Opportunistic infections have been reported. Rare cases of severe liver injury, some fatal, have been reported, usually within the first six months of therapy or in those with multiple hepatic risks. Bone marrow suppression may occur particularly in patients on dual immunomodulatory therapy. Other side effects include weight loss, allergic reactions, flu-like symptoms, rashes including Stevens–Johnson syndrome, peripheral neuropathy, hypokalemia and diabetes mellitus. There are a number of reports of interstitial lung disease developing during therapy. Leflunomide is teratogenic and a wash out procedure (see above) must be performed if patients wish to conceive.

Monitoring requirements

Full blood count (FBC) and LFTs should be checked prior to commencing treatment and two- to eight-weekly thereafter.

9.4.4. *Hydroxychloroquine*

Hydroxychloroquine is an aminoquinolone anti-malarial.

Indications and Dose

Hydroxychloroquine is used in RA, frequently in combination therapy for moderate disease. It is indicated in SLE for constitutional, joint and skin manifestations and in 2007 was reported to be an independent predictor of survival in SLE. It is recommended as a maintenance therapy in 'quiet' SLE to prevent new flares. It has also been used in primary Sjögren's syndrome, in photosensitive skin disease, JIA and off-licence to treat calcium pyrophosphate crystal deposition disease. The recommended dose is 200 mg orally twice daily. The dose may be reduced to 200 mg once daily after six months in individuals weighing <60 kg.

Pharmacokinetics and Pharmacodynamics

Hydroxychloroquine is rapidly absorbed after oral administration. It is cleared from plasma and extensively distributed in tissues including liver, spleen, kidney, skin and retina. The large volume of distribution accounts for the extended half-life of 40–50 days and the fact that plasma levels can take three to four months to reach equilibrium. Most hydroxychloroquine is excreted unchanged in the urine.

Mechanism of Action

As a weak base, hydroxychloroquine may alter the pH in specific cellular compartments, resulting in interference with key subcellular reactions. This may confer immunomodulatory and anti-inflammatory effects in target cells including monocytes and macrophages in which antigen presentation and processing have been shown to be affected. Hydroxychloroquine has been demonstrated to inhibit the production of pro-inflammatory cytokines including IL-1, IL-6, and interferon (IFN)-γ production; an effect on TNF production is disputed. Other observed immunomodulatory effects of hydroxychloroquine include up-regulation of apoptosis accompanied by elimination of autoreactive lymphocytes, likely to be significant in SLE where defective apoptosis/clearance is considered important in the aetiopathogenesis of the disease.

Hydroxychloroquine has been shown to have additional benefits including inhibition of platelet aggregation, improvement in lipid profile and reduction in plasma glucose level, all of which would be expected to decrease the cardiovascular co-morbidity associated with rheumatic diseases.

Adverse Effects

Hydroxychloroquine is generally well tolerated and safe. In some individuals a mucocutaneous rash, photosensitivity and alopecia may occur and may be difficult to dissociate from underlying lupus activity. A minority of patients experience headaches and irritability or gastrointestinal side effects such as anorexia, nausea and diarrhoea. Ocular side effects are reported and include abnormal colour vision, retinal pigmentation, reduced visual acuity, corneal deposits and retinopathy. The classic retinopathy is described as 'bull's eye maculopathy', with central macular depigmentation presenting with visual loss, and is very rare.

Monitoring requirements

Visual acuity should be monitored on a yearly basis using a standard reading chart with referral to ophthalmology if there is a change in visual acuity or in vision. Abnormalities at baseline should be assessed by an optometrist with referral to ophthalmology as required. Patients on therapy for more than five years are at increased risk and may require more detailed testing; ophthalmology liaison is advised for these patients.

9.5. Drugs with Cytotoxic and Anti-Proliferative Effects on Immune Cells

Cytotoxic and anti-proliferative agents with some specificity for cells of the immune system are often used as an adjunct to corticosteroids in management of connective tissue diseases and vasculitis.

9.5.1. *Cyclophosphamide*

Cyclophosphamide is an alkylating agent that has immunosuppressive properties.

Indications and Dose

In rheumatology practice cyclophosphamide is used in the management of some forms of vasculitis, particularly microscopic polyarteritis, Wegener's granulomatosis and Churg–Strauss syndrome and for treatment of severe SLE, usually with renal or cerebral involvement. It may also be used for management of interstitial lung disease in other autoimmune rheumatic conditions such as systemic sclerosis. Historically cyclophosphamide was given as a daily oral dose for a period of up to two to four months. However, regimes using iv pulses of 500–1000 mg given at two- or four-weekly intervals for three to six months have been shown to be effective and are associated with lower total drug dose and thus reduced toxicity.

Pharmacokinetics and Pharmacodynamics

Cyclophosphamide is well absorbed if given orally. It is metabolised in the liver by cytochrome P450 dependent mixed function oxidases to 4-hydroxycyclophosphamide, its primary functional metabolite. The metabolites of cyclophosphamide are excreted via the kidneys. The dose of cyclophosphamide should be reduced in both hepatic and renal impairment.

Mechanism of Action

Active metabolites of cyclophosphamide add an alkyl group to the guanine base of DNA, thereby damaging DNA and causing cell death. Active metabolites of cyclophosphamide are cytotoxic to lymphocytes, although the effect is greater on B than on T cells as the latter recover better from alkylation. Cyclophosphamide likely also has more subtle effects on immune cell function although the mechanism for these is less well understood.

Adverse Effects

Cyclophosphamide causes myelosuppression and this may limit the dose of drug that can be used in rheumatology practice. Nausea, vomiting and hair thinning are also common. An active urinary metabolite of cyclophosphamide called acrolein can cause haemorrhagic cystitis; the risk of this is reduced by administration of mesna; this is recommended where high doses of cyclophosphamide are used iv. Gametogenesis is severely affected and there is a serious risk of subsequent infertility. Patients need to be counselled about this and offered sperm or egg banking if appropriate. Cyclophophosphamide is teratogenic and patients should not conceive whilst taking this drug. In the longer term, patients given high doses of cyclophosphamide are at risk of malignancy, particularly leukaemia and lymphoma.

Monitoring

The FBC should be checked once to twice weekly in patients on oral therapy and at 10 to 14 days after each iv pulse. Cyclophosphamide should be withheld if the patient is leukopenic or neutropenic until the bone marrow function has recovered and appropriate alterations made to subsequent doses.

9.5.2. *Azathioprine*

Azathioprine is a purine anti-metabolite and pro-drug of 6-mercaptopurine. It is a potent immunosuppressant used widely in the treatment of autoimmune disease, organ transplantation and malignancy.

Indications and Dose

Azathioprine has been used as a second line immunomodulatory agent in many rheumatic conditions including RA, SLE and the vasculitides. It is given orally; the usual starting dosage is 1 mg/kg daily, which can be increased as tolerated up to 2–2.5 mg/kg after two to four weeks. Azathioprine takes up to eight weeks to confer clinical benefit. Genetic polymorphisms in a clearance pathway of its active metabolites confer significant variability in intracellular levels and the potential for serious toxicity, particularly myelosuppression.

Pharmacokinetics and Pharmacodynamics

Azathioprine is well absorbed orally, and is rapidly converted to 6-mercaptopurine by the removal of an imidazole group by glutathione-S-transferase. After an oral dose of azathioprine, it takes one to three hours for 6-mercaptopurine to reach maximum concentration, and the half-life of 6-mercaptopurine is one to two hours. The parent drug and its metabolites are excreted by the kidneys and modest dose reduction is advised in renal impairment.

Inactivation of 6-mercaptopurine involves a thiopurine methyltransferase (TPMT) pathway. Genetically determined low levels and activity of TPMT result in the accumulation of active drug. Testing for TPMT genotype or phenotype should be performed prior to initiation of azathioprine treatment to identify those at risk of toxicity. Doses of azathioprine should be halved in heterozygotes and the drug should be avoided in homozygotes for low activity TPMT. Inactivation of 6-mercaptopurine also involves xanthine oxidase; the active drug therefore accumulates and may reach toxic levels if a xanthine oxidase inhibitor such as allopurinol is co-prescribed.

Mechanism of Action

Activation of 6-mercaptopurine occurs via hypoxanthine-guanine phosphoribosyltransferase (HGPRT) to form 6-thioguanine nucleotides (6-TGNs) as major metabolites. These metabolites are known to decrease *de novo* synthesis of purine nucleotides, thereby reducing cellular proliferation, and are also incorporated into nucleic acids of cells, thereby conferring cytotoxicity and an increased risk of neoplasia. Azathioprine and 6-mercaptopurine exhibit a range of immunomodulatory effects including suppression of lymphocyte proliferation, NK cell activity and inhibition of cell-mediated and humoral immunity.

Adverse Effects

Most common side effects are gastrointestinal, including nausea, vomiting and anorexia. Skin rashes may occur. An acute azathioprine hypersensitivity reaction is rare; it tends to present within four weeks of starting the drug with fever, shock and deranged liver function; rechallenge is dangerous and must be avoided. Bone marrow suppression is one of the important and common dose-related side effects and is predicted by low TPMT levels or activity. The risk of infection is also increased, especially in the setting of leucopenia.

While data from renal transplant cohorts clearly identify an increased risk of lymphoma with azathioprine use, the data from rheumatology studies are less conclusive, these patients already having a higher background incidence of lymphoma conferred by their disease.

Monitoring requirements

The FBC should be checked weekly for four to eight weeks and one to three monthly thereafter. Renal profile and LFT should also be monitored.

9.5.3. *Mycophenolate Mofetil*

Mycophenolate mofetil is an inhibitor of *de novo* purine synthesis and acts as an anti-proliferative immunosuppressive agent.

Indications and Dose

Mycophenolate mofetil is licensed for prophylaxis of acute rejection of transplanted organs. In rheumatology practice it is increasingly used as an alternative to either cyclophosphamide or azathioprine in management of SLE and is also used in Behçet's disease and other forms of vasculitis. In these patients it is usually prescribed orally at an initial dose of 250–500 mg bd gradually increasing to up to 1000 mg bd.

Pharmacokinetics and Pharmacodynamics

Mycophenolate mofetil is well absorbed from the gastrointestinal tract and is hydrolysed in the liver to mycophenolic acid, the active metabolite. It is subsequently glucuronidated to mycophenolic acid glucuronide, an inactive metabolite that is predominantly excreted in the urine. In rheumatology practice the dose of mycophenolate mofetil should be reduced in those with an estimated glomerular filtration rate (eGFR) <25 ml/min and care should be taken with those with hepatic impairment.

Mechanism of Action

Mycophenolic acid blocks inosine monophosphate dehydrogenase (IMPDH) and so blocks *de novo* guanosine nucleotide synthesis. It preferentially blocks the type II isoform of IMPDH which is the predominant form in lymphocytes. Furthermore, whilst purines may also be synthesised via the hypoxanthine–guanosine phosphoribosyltransferase pathway in most cells, lymphocytes lack this second pathway. Thus the drug has selective effects on T and B cells. Mycophenolic acid also prevents glycosylation of proteins involved in lymphocyte and monocyte adhesion to endothelial cells and so has potential to inhibit leukocyte migration.

Adverse Effects

Gastrointestinal upset with diarrhoea is frequent but can usually be minimized by introducing the drug at low dose with gradual subsequent dose increments. Leukopenia, pure red cell aplasia and hepatitis may all occur. Drug use is associated with increased risk of infection, particularly with *Candida albicans* and of re-activation of cytomegalovirus. Progressive multifocal leukoencephalopathy resulting from activation of John Cunningham Virus (JCV) has been reported. There is a small increased risk of lymphoma and cutaneous malignancies. Hypertension, headaches, breathlessness and oedema are also reported. Mycophenolate is teratogenic and patients must not conceive whilst taking, or for at least six weeks after stopping, the drug.

Monitoring requirements

The FBC should be monitored every week for the first four weeks; the time period between blood tests can then be gradually increased to monthly. Renal and liver function should be monitored every month.

9.6. Drugs Targeting the Cytokines TNF-α or IL-6

Research into the pathogenesis of inflammatory arthritis has identified TNF-α and IL-6 as important mediators of inflammation in inflammatory arthritis. Agents that block the action of these cytokines now play an important part in management of RA and some other rheumatic conditions. When used to treat RA these cytokine inhibitors are usually given in combination with methotrexate and/or other disease-modifying agents but should not be given in combination with each other.

9.6.1. *TNF-α Antagonists*

Infliximab, adalimumab, etanercept and the newer agents certolizumab and golimumab all inhibit the cytokine TNF-α. Infliximab is a chimaeric (part mouse sequence) antibody and adalimumab and golimumab are humanised (fully human sequence) antibodies. Certolizumab is pegylated and lacks the Fc region of the antibody so that it does not fix complement or cause antibody-dependent cell-mediated cytotoxicity. All four reagents are specific for TNF-α. Etanercept is a fusion protein comprising part of the TNF p75 receptor and the Fc portion of human immunoglobulin (Ig) G. It binds to both TNF-α and TNF-β (lymphotoxin). All agents are often termed TNF-α antagonists or blockers and are immunosuppressive agents.

Indication and Dose

TNF-α antagonists were developed for treatment of RA and are also used in JIA. They are effective in management of PsA and ankylosing spondylitis (AS) and are sometimes used in other inflammatory conditions including Behçet's disease. Infliximab and adalimumab are used by other disciplines including gastroenterology for management of some inflammatory diseases. Infliximab is given at a dose of 3–7.5 mg/kg iv; the initial dose is followed by further doses at two and six weeks and then at eight-weekly intervals. Adalimumab is given at a dose of 40 mg sc every two weeks. Etanercept is prescribed sc at a dose of 25 mg twice weekly or 50 mg once weekly. Certolizumab is recommended at a dose of 400 mg sc at weeks 0, 2, 4 followed by 200 mg every two weeks. Golimumab is prescribed as 50 mg sc every four weeks.

Pharmacokinetics and Pharmacodynamics

Infliximab is given by iv infusion and is cleared from serum with a half-life of seven to 10 days. Adalimumab is given as a sc injection; it is absorbed slowly, peaking in serum after five to six days and being cleared with a half-life of 15 to 19 days. For certolizumab, peak plasma concentrations are reached two to seven days after administration and the drug is cleared with a half-life of 14 days. Peak concentrations of golimumab are reached at two to six days with the half-life of the drug being approximately 11 days. Etanercept is absorbed to reach peak levels in serum at around one to two days and is cleared with a shorter half-life of three to five days.

Mechanism of Action

All five agents antagonise the action of TNF-α, a pro-inflammatory cytokine that is secreted predominantly by cells of the monocyte/macrophage lineage. TNF-α is a pivotal cytokine in the cytokine cascade that underpins inflammation in many forms of inflammatory arthritis. TNF-α inhibition results in reduction in synovitis and, in patients with PsA or RA, reduction in the extent of erosive damage.

Adverse Effects

TNF-α antagonism is associated with an increased risk of acute and chronic infection. Particular care needs to be taken with respect to patients who have had or are likely to have exposure to *Mycobacterium tuberculosis* (TB), hepatitis B

(HBV) and hepatitis C (HCV) and human immunodeficiency virus (HIV); active infection needs to be treated prior to initiation of a TNF-α antagonist. Live vaccines should be avoided. Concerns persist about the possibility of TNF-α blockers increasing the risk of development of malignancies in the longer term although initial studies are reassuring. The drugs are not usually recommended for individuals who have had a prior malignancy, particularly within the previous 10 years. They may exacerbate cardiac failure and should be avoided in those who already have significant cardiac failure. There have been reports of demyelination occurring in individuals treated with TNF-α antagonists and the drugs should be avoided in those with a prior history of demyelination. Neutropenia or even pancytopenias have been reported.

Monitoring

There is no consensus about requirement for monitoring but many rheumatologists check the FBC every three months.

9.6.2. *Tocilizumab*

Tocilizumab is a humanised antibody specific for the IL-6 receptor that prevents IL-6 from binding to and initiating signalling via the receptor.

Indications

Tocilizumab is effective in management of RA and can be effective in patients who have failed to respond to DMARDs or TNF-α antagonists.

Pharmacokinetics and Pharmacodynamics

Tocilizumab is given by iv infusion every four weeks. Steady state with respect to peak concentration of drug is reached after the first infusion and with respect to trough concentration of drug after 20 weeks. It is cleared from circulation in a concentration dependent manner. No adjustment is required for mild renal impairment, there are no data to inform practice in patients with severe renal impairment or hepatic impairment. Whilst tocilizumab itself does not affect the hepatic cytochrome P450 enzymes, IL-6 normally suppresses these enzymes. Hence administration of tocilizumab may result in a relative increase in cytochrome P450 enzyme activity and care needs to be taken with administration of other drugs dependent on this system such as warfarin and phenytoin.

Mechanism of Action

Tocilizumab binds specifically to both soluble and membrane-bound IL-6 receptors and inhibits signalling mediated via these molecules. IL-6 is produced by several different cell types including cells of the monocyte/macrophage lineage and both T and B lymphocytes. It serves to stimulate cells of the immune system, including subsets of T and B lymphocytes and promotes the generation of acute phase proteins by the liver. Tocilizumab therefore serves as an immunosuppressive agent and it has been shown to be effective in reducing synovitis and erosive damage in patients with RA.

Adverse Effects

Tocilizumab is associated with increased risk of acute infection and morbidity from chronic infections such as TB. All patients should be screened for latent TB infection prior to starting therapy and treated with antimycobacterials if appropriate. Patients should also be screened for infection with HBV and HCV. There are no data about possible increased risks of demyelination and malignancy but it is possible that risks may be increased. Abnormalities in liver function, neutropenia, thrombocytopenia and elevation in lipid levels have all been reported following tocilizumab infusions.

Monitoring

FBC and LFT should be checked every four to 12 weeks and a lipid profile requested four to eight weeks after the first infusion.

9.7. Drugs Targeting B Cells or T Cells

Both B cells and T cells have been implicated in pathogenesis of RA and agents that deplete B cells and reduce activation of T cells have now been shown to be effective in management of this condition. These drugs are usually used in patients who have failed to respond to both DMARDs and TNF-α antagonists. Rituximab or abatacept are generally prescribed with methotrexate but should not be prescribed with cytokine inhibitors or with each other. B cell depletion also has a therapeutic role in other rheumatic conditions, particularly SLE.

9.7.1. *Rituximab*

Rituximab is a chimaeric monoclonal antibody specific for CD20, an antigen expressed on mature B cells. It causes lysis of B cells and so acts as a specific cytotoxic agent that has immunosuppressive actions on one arm of the adaptive immune response.

Indications and Dose

Rituximab was originally licensed for treatment of lymphomas and is also used in management of other haematological diseases such as idiopathic thrombocytopenic purpura. In rheumatology practice rituximab is used for management of RA that has not responded to DMARDs or TNF-α antagonists. Two doses of 1000 mg rituximab are given iv two weeks apart approximately every six to nine months.

Pharmacokinetics and Pharmacodynamics

Following iv infusion rituximab is distributed with a half-life of approximately two days and cleared with a half-life of around 20 days. Administration results in effective B cell depletion that is present by week four and persists for many months in most patients. The beneficial clinical effects of rituximab are rarely apparent at four weeks and often only become manifest after two to three months.

Mechanism of Action

Rituximab binds to CD20 and causes lysis of mature B cells. Plasma cells do not express CD20 and so antibody secretion by plasma cells persists; overall levels of Igs remain stable at least after the first few infusions and specific immunity to previous encountered pathogens such as tetanus and pneumococcus is preserved. Levels of rheumatoid factor do, however, fall. Administration of rituximab is associated with reduction in B cells, macrophages and T cells within the synovium of patients with RA; this suggests that B cells play a role in orchestrating the cellular infiltration of the synovium and that rituximab may be effective by interfering with this process. The B cell compartment usually starts to be repopulated at approximately six months and patients need to be re-treated at this stage.

Adverse Effects

Infusion related reactions are commonly reported and most rheumatologists premedicate patients with iv corticosteroids. Patients given rituximab are at increased risk of infection although the persistence of previously generated plasma cells and antibodies provides some protection. There have been several reports of development of progressive multifocal leucoencephalopathy.

Monitoring

Some centres check lymphocyte subsets after six months in order to ascertain when a further infusion of rituximab should be administered. Other rheumatologists simply re-treat all their patients at six-monthly intervals or when their disease activity starts to increase.

9.7.2. *Abatacept*

Abatacept is a fusion protein comprising the extracellular domain of human cytotoxic T lymphocyte antigen 4 (CTLA4) and the Fc portion of human IgG. It is an immunosuppressive agent.

Indications

Abatacept is indicated for management of RA that has not responded to DMARDs or TNF-α antagonists. It is given by iv infusion at a dose of 500–1000 mg with repeat dosing two weeks and four weeks after the initial infusion and thereafter at four-weekly intervals. It should be used in combination with methotrexate.

Pharmacokinetics and Pharmacodynamics

Following iv administration abatacept is eliminated with a half-life of 12–23 days, justifying the four-weekly dosing schedule.

Mechanism of Action

CTLA4 binds to CD80 and CD86. Both CD80 and CD86 also serve as ligands for the co-stimulatory molecule CD28 which plays an important role in T cell activation. By binding to and thereby blocking the ligands of CD28, abatacept effectively reduces CD28-mediated T cell activation. There is a consequent reduction in secretion of IL-2. Inhibition of secretion of other cytokines including IL-6 and TNF-α occurs and inhibition of production of rheumatoid factor has been noted, all suggesting that reducing activation of T cells has indirect effects on function of other immune cell types.

Adverse Effects

Abatacept increases the risk of acute and chronic infection. Patients should be screened for exposure to HBV, HCV and TB and active infections treated as appropriate prior to starting abatacept. Acute infusion-related reactions may occur. Risks of malignancy may be increased although clear data are lacking.

Monitoring

Many rheumatologists check FBC every three months as neutropenia and thrombocytopenia have been reported in some patients.

9.8. Drugs Used in Management of Gout

Whilst NSAIDs are often highly effective in treating acute gouty arthritis, they are contraindicated in many patients. Colchicine or corticosteroids are effective alternatives. Drugs that inhibit synthesis of uric acid or promote its excretion in urine are effective in reducing plasma uric acid levels and preventing attacks of gout.

9.8.1. *Colchicine*

Colchicine is a plant alkaloid. Use of colchicine containing plant extracts for the treatment of acute gout dates back to the sixth century AD.

Indications and Dose

Colchicine is indicated for the treatment of acute gouty arthritis and its prophylaxis. It is reported to prevent both the frequency and severity of episodes. Colchicine also has a role in the treatment of acute pseudogout and other crystal arthropathies and has been used off label in the therapy of Behçet's disease, sarcoidosis, calcific tendonitis, amyloidosis and familial Mediterranean fever. In gouty arthritis, colchicine is generally given as a regular dose of 500 μg two or three times daily and may be continued following the acute attack on a prophylactic basis as a twice daily maintenance dose.

Pharmacokinetics and Pharmacodynamics

Colchicine is absorbed rapidly from the gastrointestinal tract; a process affected by multidrug resistant 1 P-glycoprotein (Pgp-170), an active efflux pump that is differentially expressed on gut mucosa. Oral bioavailability is very variable (likely related to Pgp-170 efflux activity) with peak plasma concentrations of 25–80% of administered dose found at two hours The plasma half-life of colchicine is four hours with elimination occurring mainly in the liver via the cytochrome P450 pathway. Excretion is in urine and faeces, following some enterohepatic recirculation. The half-life of colchicine is prolonged two- to ten-fold in hepatic and renal failure. Colchicine has a very narrow therapeutic index.

Mechanism of Action

Colchicine is anti-inflammatory, particularly in neutrophil driven inflammation, as it inhibits neutrophil adhesion to endothelium thus preventing neutrophil migration. It acts by binding to tubulin (a microtubular protein), disrupting many cellular functions such as motility and chemotaxis. Many anti-inflammatory effects have been described including inhibition of TNF-α, COX-2 activity and interference with NALp3 inflammasome activation.

Adverse Effects

Most common side effects include nausea, vomiting, abdominal pain and diarrhoea; the last is frequently dose limiting. Rare side effects include myopathy, agranulocytosis, aplastic anaemia, alopecia, rash and oligospermia which each occur in fewer than 1% of patients.

9.8.2. *Allopurinol*

Allopurinol is a purine analogue that acts as a xanthine oxidase inhibitor.

Indications and Dose

Allopurinol is used in the treatment of recurrent gout (primary hyperuricaemia), particularly where the serum urate or urinary uric acid excretion is high, renal function is impaired or where nephrolithiasis or tophi have occurred. It is also used in the treatment of conditions leading to secondary hyperuricaemia such as malignancies and chemotherapy.

Patients should initially be given 100 mg daily and the dose increased by 100 mg daily at approximately two-weekly intervals until the serum urate falls below 350 μmol/l. The most commonly required dose is 300 mg daily, however, higher doses may be required. Sudden changes in serum urate level can precipitate an acute attack of gout, therefore prophylactic treatment with colchicine or NSAIDS is recommended for a period of six months after the initiation of allopurinol treatment.

Allopurinol can also be used iv at a dose of 200–400 mg/m^2/day, in cases where oral medication is not tolerated, for example in patients receiving chemotherapy.

Pharmacokinetics and Pharmacodynamics

Allopurinol is fully absorbed with oral administration and metabolised in the liver. The main metabolite is alloxanthine (oxypurinol), which is also a xanthine oxidase inhibitor. The plasma half-life of allopurinol is short (two hours); however, the half-life of oxypurinol is long (15 hours). Oxypurinol is cleared by the kidneys and the dose of allopurinol should therefore be reduced in renal impairment.

Mechanism of Action

Allopurinol acts by competitively inhibiting xanthine oxidase, the enzyme which converts hypoxanthine to xanthine to uric acid.

Adverse Effects

The most common side effects include gastrointestinal upset and skin rash, which can occur even after months or years of chronic administration. Other side effects include fever, alopecia, bone marrow suppression and agranulocytosis. One of the more serious adverse effects is the allopurinol hypersensitivity syndrome, which presents with fever, rash, eosinophilia, hepatitis, renal impairment and may result in death. This condition is seen particularly in patients with pre-existing renal disease and patients on diuretics.

9.8.3. *Febuxostat*

Febuxostat is a non-purine inhibitor of xanthine oxidase.

Indications and Dose

Febuxostat is given orally at a dose of 80–120 mg daily for management of gout. It is usually used where patients are intolerant of allopurinol.

Pharmacokinetics and Pharmacodynamics

Febuxostat is rapidly absorbed and reaches peak plasma concentrations in around an hour. It is metabolised in the liver by glucuronidation and oxidation and the metabolites are eliminated partly via the liver and partly via the kidneys. Febuxostat can be used in mild/moderate renal or hepatic impairment.

Mechanism of Action

Xanthine oxidase is required for oxidation of hypoxanthine and xanthine to uric acid. Like allopurinol, febuxostat therefore prevents synthesis of uric acid.

Adverse Reaction

Nausea, diarrhoea and headaches may occur. There have been some reports of abnormalities of liver and renal function and thrombocytopenia developing with febuxostat use.

9.8.4. *Sulphinpyrazone*

Sulphinpyrazone is a uricosuric agent, meaning that it leads to increased excretion of uric acid in the urine. Probenecid and benzbromarone are further examples of uricosuric drugs although both are used less commonly than sulphinpyrazone.

Indications and Dose

Sulphinpyrazone may be used for prevention and management of gout; the latter usually where allopurinol has not been tolerated. It is given orally once daily, initially at a dose of 100–200 mg, increasing to 200–800 mg as needed. It is important that patients maintain a good intake of oral fluids.

Pharmacokinetics and Pharmacodynamics

Sulphinpyrazone is rapidly absorbed, reaches peak serum levels within two hours and has a half-life of four to six hours. It is metabolised by the liver to two active metabolites and is excreted in urine. Patients taking sulphinpyrazone should maintain a high fluid intake. The drug should be avoided in severe renal impairment.

Mechanism of Action

Sulphinpyrazone inhibits human urate anion transporter (hURAT1) and human organic anion transporter 4 (hOAT4). It thereby reduces uric acid resorption in the proximal tubules, allowing for increased excretion of uric acid in urine.

Adverse Effects

Sulphinpyrazone may cause nausea and vomiting. It can aggravate peptic ulceration and exacerbate cardiac failure. It may cause hepatitis or blood disorders.

Monitoring

FBC should be checked regularly.

9.9. Drugs Used in Management of Metabolic Bone Disease

Bone is remodelled throughout life with osteoclasts resorbing bone and osteoblasts laying down new bone. Drugs that inhibit osteoclasts and so reduce bone turnover may be used for management of osteoporosis and Paget's disease. Stimulation of osteoblast function is an alternative strategy for treating osteoporosis.

9.9.1. *Bisphosphonates*

There are two major classes of bisphosphonates: the basic bisphosphonates and the aminobisphosphonates. Both inhibit osteoclast activity and thereby act as 'anti-resorptive' drugs. However, bisphosphonates are also capable of inhibiting mineralisation of bone. For the basic bisphosphonate, etidronate, the dose required for the anti-mineralisation effect is only 10–100-fold higher than that required for the anti-resorptive effect. The new aminobisphosphonates, including alendronate, risedronate, ibandronate, pamidronate and zoledronate have more potent anti-resorptive effects and the dose required for the anti-mineralisation effect is very many orders of magnitude higher than that required for osteoclast inhibition, thereby creating a much better therapeutic margin.

Indications and Dose

Bisphosphonates are indicated for prevention and treatment of osteoporosis and are also used for management of Paget's disease. In oncology they play a role in management of bone metastases. Bisphosphonates can be given orally or iv and dosing schedules vary from daily to yearly. For management of osteoporosis daily oral bisphosphonates are now rarely used, alendronate and risedronate are prescribed orally weekly and ibandronate may be prescribed monthly as an oral dose or three-monthly if given iv. Zoledronate is given by annual iv infusion. Paget's disease can be managed using risedronate given as a daily oral dose for two months, pamidronate given as a weekly iv infusion for six weeks or, more commonly, with a single iv infusion of zoledronate.

Pharmacokinetics and Pharmacodynamics

The bisphosphonates are absorbed, stored and excreted in an unchanged form. All of the orally administered aminobisphosphonates are poorly absorbed and have a bioavailability of <1%. This figure is based on fasting administration; bioavailability is further reduced by 50–60% if the drugs are taken with food. Both basic bisphosphonates and aminobisphosphonates bind to hydroxyapatite in bone and are internalised by osteoclasts. The affinity of binding to hydroxyapatite varies considerably between the bisphosphonates with alendronate and zoledronate exhibiting particularly high affinity binding. The kinetics of bisphosphonate clearance reflect several different phases; initial clearance from blood, subsequent clearance following dissociation from bone surfaces and longer-term clearance of bisphosphonates incorporated into the skeleton or other tissues. The last is known as the terminal half-life; for a high affinity bisphosphonate such as alendronate it is as long as 10 years. Estimates for terminal half-life of ibandronate and risedronate are lower. Nevertheless the half-lives are such that long dosing intervals are possible. Bisphosphonates are excreted by the kidneys and should not be used where eGFRs are low.

Mechanism of Action

At the cellular level, the basic and aminobisphosphates differ in their mechanisms of action. The basic bisphosphonates form non-hydrolysable adenosine 5′-triphosphate

(ATP)-like metabolites which can inhibit ATP-dependent intracellular enzymes, thereby interfering with osteoclast function. The aminobisphosphonates inhibit farnesyl pyrophosphate synthase in the mevalonate biosynthetic pathway, disrupting the function of GTPases, and resulting in loss of osteoclastic activity.

Adverse Effects

The toxicity of the bisphosphonates varies between individual members of the drug class and route of administration. The most common adverse effect of oral bisphosphonates is oesophageal or gastric ulceration; the risk of this can be reduced by advising the patient to remain upright for at least 30 minutes after dosing. Impairment of renal function has been described following zoledronate infusions and a flu-like reaction may occur following use of any of the iv preparations due to cytokine release. The risks of osteonecrosis of the jaw and subtrochanteric fracture may be increased but these remain rare side-effects with doses of bisphosphonates used for management of osteoporosis.

9.9.2. *Raloxifene*

Raloxifene is a selective oestrogen receptor modulator (SERM). Whilst there are many SERMs available, raloxifene is the principal SERM used for the treatment of osteoporosis in postmenopausal women. Its efficacy in terms of fracture risk reduction is less than that of the bisphosphonates or strontium ranelate.

Indications and Dose

Raloxifene at a dose of 60 mg od may be used for prevention and treatment of osteoporosis in postmenopausal women.

Pharmacokinetics and Pharmacodynamics

Approximately 60% raloxifene is absorbed from the gastrointestinal tract; the majority undergoes first pass glucuronidation and only approximately 2% of the drug is therefore bioavailable. It is widely distributed within serum and tissues and is excreted predominantly in faeces.

Mechanism of Action

Individual SERMs differ in their effects on oestrogen receptors in different tissues. Most SERMs have a mixture of agonistic and antagonistic actions;

raloxifene has an agonistic effect on receptors in bone and an antagonistic effect on receptors in breast and uterus. This differential action may be due to the ratio of co-activator:co-repressor proteins in different tissues and the conformational change that occurs in the receptor following binding, in turn leading to greater recruitment of either co-stimulators or co-repressors. Its antagonistic effect on breast and uterine tissue is such that risks of breast and uterine cancer are not increased in individuals taking this drug. One effect of stimulating oestrogen receptors within bone is increased expression of osteoprotegrin, a soluble molecule that inhibits the stimulatory effect of the receptor activator for nuclear factor kappa β ligand (RANKL) on osteoclasts; the overall effect is therefore to reduce osteoclast function and bone turnover.

Adverse Effects

Hot flushes and leg cramping may reduce patient acceptability of raloxifene. The most serious adverse effect is the three-fold increased risk of venous thromboembolism.

9.9.3. *Strontium Ranelate*

Strontium ranelate comprises the salt of strontium and raneleic acid. It has some efficacy in stimulating osteoblasts and inhibiting osteoclasts and has been described as a 'dual acting bone agent'.

Indications and Dose

Strontium at a dose of 2 g daily can be used for treatment of osteoporosis.

Pharmacokinetics and Pharmacodynamics

Strontium ranelate is absorbed slowly, with approximately 25% becoming bioavailable. Absorption is much reduced by food or calcium rich drinks; strontium ranelate should therefore be taken at least two hours before/after meals or milky drinks. It has a high affinity for bone tissue. Strontium ranelate is cleared by the kidney and gastrointestinal tract. However, no dosage adjustment is required unless creatinine clearance is <30 ml/min. It may be used in patients with hepatic impairment.

Mechanism of Action

Strontium is chemically related to calcium and stimulates calcium sensing receptors on the surface of pre-osteoblasts. This leads to both the formation of increased numbers of osteoblasts and stimulation of these osteoblasts to produce osteoprotegerin, a protein which inhibits the formation of osteoclasts. Some strontium may also substitute for calcium in the apatite crystal of newly formed bone.

Adverse Effects

Strontium ranelate may cause headaches and diarrhoea, particularly when first introduced. A small increased risk of venous thromboembolism was noted in the initial clinical trials. A severe allergic reaction with drug rash, eosinophilia and systemic symptoms (known as DRESS) can rarely occur and may be fatal. All patients should therefore be told to stop taking the drug if they develop a rash.

9.9.4. *Teriparatide and Human Recombinant Parathyroid Hormone*

Teriparatide is a recombinant fragment of human parathyroid hormone (amino acids 1–34) that contains the parathyroid hormone receptor binding portion of the hormone. Full length recombinant parathyroid hormone (amino acids 1–84) is also available for management of osteoporosis.

Indications and Dose

Teriparatide is used for management of osteoporosis at a dose of 20 μg daily given subcutaneously. It is licensed for use for a two-year period and is usually followed by maintenance bisphosphonate therapy. Human recombinant parathyroid hormone is given at a dose of 100 μg subcutaneously daily, again for a maximum time period of two years.

Pharmacokinetics and Pharmacodynamics

Teriparatide is absorbed rapidly after sc injection with approximately 95% being bioavailable. The serum concentration peaks approximately 30 minutes after injection; it is cleared rapidly, becoming undetectable by three hours. Full length recombinant parathyroid hormone is likewise rapidly absorbed and then cleared. Non-specific proteolytic enzymes in the liver are thought to cleave the drugs into fragments which are then excreted via the kidneys. There is no requirement for dose adjustments in mild or moderate renal or hepatic failure.

Mechanism of Action

The effect of teriparatide and recombinant parathyroid hormone on the skeletal system is dependent on the dosing regime. Once daily sc dosing results in intermittent peaks of drug and favours a stimulatory effect on osteoblasts over a stimulatory effect on osteoclasts. Used in this way the drugs therefore have a potent anabolic agent.

Adverse Effects

In trials performed in rodents, use of teriparatide was associated with the development of sarcoma. For this reason teriparatide and full length recombinant parathyroid hormone may only be used for a maximum of two years and are contraindicated in patients with a history of osteogenic sarcoma, Paget's disease, a history of skeletal radiation exposure or age less than 18 years. There is a small risk of post-injection hypercalcaemia; the drug should be avoided in patients with hypercalcaemia and serum calcium should be checked every three months in patients using the full length recombinant parathyroid hormone. More common side effects include lightheadedness, dizziness or pain at the injection site.

9.9.5. *Denosumab*

Denosumab is a humanised monoclonal antibody specific for the receptor activator for nuclear factor kappa B ligand (RANKL).

Indications and Dose

Denosumab is effective in treatment of osteoporosis and is given at a dose of 60 mg every six months by sc injection.

Pharmacokinetics and Pharmacodynamics

Denosumab is absorbed rapidly following injection to reach a peak serum concentration at eight days. It is cleared with a half-life of approximately 25 days. It results in a rapid (within one day) and sustained suppression of bone turnover. In contrast with some other agents used for management of osteoporosis, there is no requirement to adjust dose in patients with renal impairment.

Mechanism of Action

In normal bone RANKL binds to the RANK receptor on osteoclasts and serves to promote their differentiation, function and survival. Denosumab binds to RANKL and prevents it from engaging with its receptor on osteoclasts, thereby decreasing osteoclast activity and reducing bone resorption.

Adverse Effects

The interaction between RANKL and RANK is important in regulation of immune responses and use of denosumab is associated with a small increased risk of infection. Osteonecrosis of the jaw has been reported rarely, affecting approximately 1/1000–1/10 000 patients receiving denosumab. Patients may develop a transient hypocalcaemia, particularly if they have renal impairment.

Chapter 10

Case Studies in Rheumatology

Editor: Simon Bowman

Simon Bowman, Alison Jordan, Sophia Khan

Case 1

A 24-year-old woman presented with a nine month history of low back pain and stiffness, with symptoms being most severe after rest. She complained of excessive fatigue and was missing long periods from work. She had failed to respond to several non-steroidal anti-inflammatory drugs (NSAIDS). Further enquiry revealed an attack of iritis 18 months previously. On examination, there was significant restriction of forward and lateral flexion of the lumbosacral spine and tenderness over the sacroiliac joints. There was also reduced chest expansion. Investigations showed a normal full blood count (FBC), erythrocyte sedimentation rate (ESR) 21 mm/h and C-reactive protein (CRP) 10 mg/dl. X-rays of the sacroiliac joints were normal.

1. What is the diagnosis?
2. What investigations are required?
3. What treatment may be appropriate?

1. Back pain is a common presentation to primary care; most episodes are mechanical and self-limiting. Low back pain due to inflammatory causes such as ankylosing spondylitis is often missed early in the disease process, especially in women. The features of low back pain and stiffness, prominent after periods of rest, together with decreased spinal mobility and sacroiliac joint tenderness and the extraskeletal manifestation of iritis, all suggest ankylosing spondylitis as a diagnosis. The lack of response to NSAIDs is atypical. Some patients with ankylosing spondylitis will develop a peripheral arthritis and enthesitis. Other possible

manifestations of established disease include aortic valvular disease, apical pulmonary fibrosis, amyloidosis, immunoglobulin (Ig)-A nephropathy, fractures of rigid segments of spine and cauda equina syndrome.

2. X-ray evidence of sacroiliitis may not be evident for several years and magnetic resonance imaging (MRI) has become the preferred modality for detection of early inflammation of the axial skeleton. Computed tomography (CT) scanning and bone scintigraphy have been used in the past. Whilst sacroilitis evident on X-rays is required for diagnosis of ankylosing spondylitis according to the modified New York criteria, patients with typical clinical features of inflammatory back pain and MRI evidence of inflammatory sacroiliitis but normal X-rays may be diagnosed as having an 'axial spondyloarthritis' or 'pre-radiographic ankylosing spondylitis'. The human leukocyte antigen (HLA) B27 is strongly associated with ankylosing spondylitis; 2% of HLA B27-positive individuals develop the condition, with the rate rising to 15–20% among HLA B27-positive individuals with an affected relative. Knowledge of HLA B27 status can therefore be helpful in assessing likelihood of ankylosing spondylitis where the X-rays are negative.

3. Physiotherapy is an essential part of the management of ankylosing spondylitis and patients need to perform a daily exercise programme to relieve pain and stiffness and improve posture and spinal movement. Hydrotherapy may be particularly beneficial. NSAIDs are used widely and some patients may need to try several before finding one that controls their symptoms. Simple analgesia can be used for additional pain relief. Disease-modifying anti-rheumatic drugs (DMARDs) such as sulphasalazine and methotrexate are used for peripheral arthritis but have no effect on spinal disease. Anti-tumour necrosis factor (TNF)-α therapy is effective for spinal and peripheral disease, irrespective of whether or not X-ray changes have developed.

Case 2

A 56-year-old executive was admitted with a hot, swollen left knee. He had experienced several short episodes of joint pain and swelling over 10 years but 12 weeks previously had developed persistent pain and swelling of both feet, which spread to involve the small joints of the hands, wrists and elbows. On admission, his temperature was 37.5°C, he was obese and hypertensive with a blood pressure of 160/95. He admitted to drinking six pints of beer per night and was a heavy smoker. He had a symmetrical polyarthritis and bilateral olecranon bursitis with nodular swelling. The left knee was hot, swollen and extremely tender with loss of extension and significantly reduced flexion. Investigations revealed ESR 91 mm/h, CRP 230 mg/dl, haemoglobin (HB) 12.5 g/dl, white cell count (WCC) 12.5 × 10^9/l, aspartate aminotransferase (AST) 84 U/l, glucose 9.2 mmol/l, urate 602 μmol/l, creatinine 113 μmol/l, rheumatoid factor (RF) 1:40, cholesterol 6.4 mmol/l, triglycerides 2.4 mmol/l. X-rays of his hands and feet showed erosions.

1. What is the differential diagnosis?
2. What investigations would you recommend?
3. What treatment should he have?

1. One needs to have a very high index of suspicion for septic arthritis in patients who present with a hot, swollen joint with restricted movement. Crystal arthritis and reactive arthritis are the two principal differentials for a hot, swollen joint. This acute episode has occurred on the background of an erosive polyarthritis. Rheumatoid arthritis is one possible cause of a polyarthritis with erosive damage. However, gout may be polyarticular in onset in about 10% of cases and tophaceous gout in particular can mimic rheumatoid arthritis. Tophi may be mistaken for rheumatoid nodules. Bony erosions can occur in gout although these are distinct from rheumatoid erosions in that they appear 'punched out' with sclerotic margins and overhanging edges.

2. This patient had a mild pyrexia, elevated inflammatory markers and high WCC and so required urgent joint aspiration. The fluid obtained from his left knee showed no organisms but crystals of monosodium urate confirming a diagnosis of gout. A biopsy of a nodule from the olecranon bursa confirmed tophus formation. The plasma urate was elevated in this case although it may be normal during an acute attack of gout.

3. Treatment of acute gout is with fast acting NSAIDs at maximum dose continued for one to two weeks, provided there are no contraindications. Colchicine is an effective alternative in renal impairment but works more slowly. Oral or intra-articular steroids are also effective and intramuscular methylprednisolone can be a useful alternative. Measures for long-term reduction of urate levels include xanthine oxidase inhibition with allopurinol and increased urate excretion with a uricosuric drug such as probenecid, sulphinpyrazone or benzbromarone. Newer agents include febuxostat, which is a non-purine selective inhibitor of xanthine oxidase, for use in people who do not tolerate allopurinol. Rasburicase can be used for refractory cases of tophaceous gout but is not approved for long-term use

and requires intravenous administration. Patients should be advised to avoid alcohol, particularly beer and spirits, and foods known to have high purine content. Gout is often associated with hypertension and hyperlipidaemia. This patient's risk of cardiovascular disease is significant and lifestyle alterations are essential. He needs to be advised to give up smoking and to lose weight. Treatment of hypertension can be difficult in gout and NSAIDs and diuretics need to be used with caution in patients with both these conditions.

Case 3

A 68-year-old woman presented with sudden onset of severe thoracic pain secondary to fractures at the fifth and seventh thoracic vertebral levels. She had pain on sitting and standing, relieved only when lying down. She had been fit and well with no apparent risk factors for osteoporosis. Blood tests were normal apart from a slightly elevated calcium level. Her phosphate was at the lower end of the normal range. X-rays of the spine showed widespread osteopenia and some degenerative change. On reviewing her old notes it became apparent that six years previously she had been seen in a medical clinic on several occasions with a mildly elevated calcium level. She was asymptomatic and, as she had only mild hypercalcaemia, no treatment was given and she was lost to follow-up.

1. What is the likely diagnosis?
2. What investigations are required?
3. How should this patient be managed?

1. Vertebral compression fractures in the context of hypercalcaemia suggest hyperparathyroidism, myeloma or malignancy. The chronicity of the hypercalcaemia here suggests a benign rather than a malignant process and the likely diagnosis is of hyperparathyroidism. Excess parathyroid hormone stimulates excessive calcium resorption and can result in osteoporosis. Bony fractures including vertebral compression fractures may occur in the long term if the condition is left untreated.

2. Individuals who present with vertebral compression fractures may have osteoporosis or other more local pathology such as malignancy or infection leading to bony fragility. A bone density scan will assess for osteoporosis and imaging studies will be helpful in excluding a local lesion. In this respect X-rays, MRI scans or isotope bone scans may each have a role. It is important to exclude myeloma

and so an immunoglobulin profile with electrophoretic strip and urinary Bence Jones proteins should all be requested. Other secondary causes of osteoporosis including chronic inflammatory conditions, hyperthyroidism, liver disease, malabsorption, vitamin D deficiency and hyperparathyroidism should all be considered. In this case the patient was found to have an inappropriately elevated parathyroid hormone concentration with high plasma calcium. In patients with hyperparathyroidism X-rays may show generalised or patchy osteopenia or evidence of bone resorption manifest as osteitis fibrosa et cystica (brown tumours) and subperiosteal resorption. In the skull, areas of decreased bone density are intermingled with more sclerotic areas, resulting in a classic appearance termed 'pepper-pot skull'.

3. Patients with vertebral fractures may experience very severe pain and need to be offered appropriate analgesics. Vertebroplasty or kyphoplasty can have a role where pain is persistent. Osteoporosis in the context of hyperparathyroidism can be managed using a bisphosphonate and either alendronate 70 mg weekly or risedronate 35 mg weekly would be appropriate. Vitamin D supplements may be required to maintain the vitamin D levels within the normal range but calcium supplements should not be given and the calcium needs to be carefully monitored. Definitive treatment of the hyperparathyroidism involves surgery although surveillance may be justified as an alternative in some patients whose calcium levels are only mildly elevated.

Case 4

A 52-year-old woman presented with a symmetrical polyarthritis affecting the small joints of both hands. She also complained of pain in both knees which was worse on climbing stairs. There was prolonged stiffness on sitting and her fingers were stiff in the morning for over an hour. She gave no history of eye problems, rash, bowel symptoms or preceding illness. There was a family history of osteoarthritis and she had an aunt with rheumatoid arthritis. Blood tests including FBC and renal and liver function were entirely normal and her ESR was 12 mm/h with a normal CRP. Her RF was also normal and X-rays of both knees showed narrowed joint space and osteophyte formation as well as patellofemoral osteoarthritis. X-rays of her hands were normal.

1. What is the likely diagnosis?
2. What other investigations might be helpful?
3. What treatment would be appropriate?

1. This patient has radiological evidence of osteoarthritis affecting both knees and it is tempting to assume that she also has osteoarthritis affecting the small joints of her hands. However, the story is more suggestive of an inflammatory form of arthritis with a distribution of joint involvement that is suggestive of rheumatoid arthritis. RF has a relatively poor sensitivity for the diagnosis of rheumatoid arthritis and X-rays are usually normal in early disease. Whilst inflammatory markers are often raised in rheumatoid arthritis they may be normal. The diagnosis of rheumatoid arthritis should not therefore be excluded on the basis of all these normal tests. Other conditions to consider in patients presenting with joint pain include the following:

- Viral arthritis (parvovirus, rubella, hepatitis B virus)
- Reactive arthritis (throat, gut, sexually acquired)
- Seronegative spondyloarthritis (including psoriatic arthritis)
- Connective tissue disorders
- Polymyalgia rheumatica
- Polyarticular gout
- Septic arthritis
- Fibromyalgia
- Lyme disease
- Medical conditions (thyroid disorders, sarcoidosis, diabetic cheiropathy, paraneoplastic sydrome, multiple myeloma, endocarditis, haemachromatosis).

2. Anti-cyclic citrullinated peptide (CCP) antibodies should be checked in people with suspected rheumatoid arthritis. Whilst this test has a similar sensitivity for the diagnosis of rheumatoid arthritis as the RF, it is much more specific and identifies a subpopulation of patients who are likely to develop erosive disease. Detailed imaging studies in the form of ultrasound (US) scans with Doppler or MRI are very helpful in identifying active synovitis and small erosions in the early phase of rheumatoid arthritis. Further blood tests to include uric acid levels, anti-nuclear antibody (ANA) and thyroid function tests (TFTs) can also be useful in helping to exclude the common differentials of gout, connective tissue disease and thyroid dysfunction.

This patient proved to be anti-CCP antibody positive and to have US scan evidence of active synovitis in the small joints of her hands.

3. All patients with early rheumatoid arthritis should have access to a range of health professionals including specialist physiotherapists, occupational therapists, podiatrists and orthotists, psychologists, social workers and dieticians. Treatment with a NSAID often gives good improvement but can falsely reassure

patient and general practitioner (GP) and lead to delay in initiating appropriate disease modifying therapy. All patients with a definite diagnosis of rheumatoid arthritis should be offered treatment with a DMARD as soon as the diagnosis is made. The conventional agents include methotrexate, sulphasalazine, hydroxychloroquine and leflunomide. The optimal sequencing of these drugs and whether to use combinations of therapies remains a source of debate although many clinicians do now use at least two DMARDs including methotrexate in the first instance. Gold, ciclosporin, D-penicillamine and azathioprine are used infrequently. Cyclophosphamide can be used to treat systemic vasculitis associated with rheumatoid arthritis. Systemic steroid therapy has an important early role in establishing control of synovitis and preventing early joint damage. Corticosteroids are also useful in managing flares of disease and providing bridging therapy when switching between DMARDs. The long-term use of corticosteroids is, however, not justified. Intra-articular steroid is a useful adjunct to drug therapy. Patients who fail to respond adequately to DMARDs should be offered treatment with anti-TNF-α therapy. Selection of an anti-TNF-α agent is usually based on patient preference and practical issues relating to drug administration and delivery. Rituximab, a chimeric anti-CD20 monoclonal antibody, used in combination with methotrexate, may be used where treatment with an anti-TNF-α agent has failed. Abatacept, which serves to block T cell co-stimulation, and tocilizumab, an antibody directed against the IL-6 receptor, are both also effective treatments for rheumatoid arthritis.

Case 5

A 29-year-old South Asian woman presented via the medical admissions unit with a two-month history of severe weight loss and loss of appetite. She had recently separated from an abusive husband and was profoundly depressed. She had a previous history of 'nocturnal epilepsy' treated with carbamazepine.

1. Why might this turn out to be a rheumatology patient?
2. What investigations are needed?
3. What treatment might be appropriate?

1. On the surface there is no obvious rheumatology link. A profoundly depressed patient may have loss of appetite, weight loss and malaise. General medical causes might include coeliac disease, bowel or brain or other tumours. In a South Asian female, tuberculosis (TB) should also always be excluded. However, the key rheumatic disease that should be considered in a South Asian female is systemic lupus

erythematosus (SLE). In this case the patient did not have classical clinical features of lupus such as mouth ulcers, hair loss, arthralgia, rashes, migraines, Raynaud's phenomenon or pleuritic chest pain at presentation. The previous 'epilepsy' may be relevant, particularly if the patient has an associated anti-phospholipid syndrome (APLS). It is always important to specifically enquire about the above SLE features as patients may not spontaneously volunteer the information.

2. The specific diagnostic tests for SLE are the ANA, anti-dsDNA antibodies and complement C3 and C4 proteins. Low or falling complement protein levels are a clue that lupus is particularly active. As well as an enzyme-linked immunosorbent assay (ELISA) test for dsDNA antibodies, the Crithidia test identifies highly specific dsDNA antibodies. This patient had a strongly positive ANA with a titre of 1:1600, dsDNA of 470 U/ml and low C3 and C4 of 0.37 g/l and 0.08 g/l respectively. She also had a neutropenia (0.5×10^9/ml), raised ESR of 57 mm/h and slightly raised CRP of 16 mg/l, although classically, in the absence of infection, the CRP is normal in SLE despite the high ESR. It is vital to dipstick the urine for blood and protein because this can indicate active nephritis and then to check a mid-stream urine sample and urinary albumin:creatinine ratio if the dipstick result is abnormal. An active urinary sediment may be the only sign of lupus nephritis; in some patients the serum creatinine and blood pressure may be normal in the early stages of disease. Other important tests are for antibodies to the extractable nuclear antigens (ENAs) (anti-Ro/La/Sm/RNP etc), anti-phospholipid antibodies (APLA) and lupus anti-coagulant. The FBC and liver function must also always be checked and will provide information about the presence of autoimmune cytopenias and hepatitis.

3. This patient received intravenous methylprednisolone and has been on oral prednisolone, azathioprine and subsequently mycophenolate mofetil. As she has not developed renal, pulmonary or other cerebral involvement she has not been given cyclophosphamide. She had one episode of pneumococcal sepsis. Since lupus patients are particularly susceptible to this it is worth evaluating pneumococcal titres in patients with moderate/severe disease activity and considering vaccination or prophylactic penicillin. Her condition has otherwise been under reasonable, but not perfect, control and has flared up intermittently.

Case 6

A 42-year-old previously fit man presented with a two-month history of weight loss, altered bowel habit and left iliac fossa pain. Colonoscopy showed resolving inflammation, a CT scan showed multiple small lymph nodes which on biopsy were reported as showing 'granulomatous change ?sarcoidosis, ?TB, ?toxoplasma'. He subsequently developed night sweats, a non-specific itchy rash on his back, chest and arms, polyarthralgia and morning headaches. His chest X-ray was normal, he had a raised neutrophil count of 11.5×10^9/l, raised ESR at 121 mm/h and CRP of 110 mg/l. Renal function and urine dipstick were normal.

1. What is the differential diagnosis?
2. What investigations would you recommend?
3. What treatment should he have?

1. There is clearly a systemic process. Typically the top three differentials are infection, haematological malignancy and an inflammatory disorder such as a vasculitis or connective tissue disorder.

2. The patient had a CT thorax and brain (normal), a lumbar puncture (borderline low glucose, one polymorph, otherwise normal), an echocardiogram (transthoracic was normal but a transoesophageal could still be considered in terms of excluding endocarditis), human immunodeficiency virus (HIV) and toxoplasma serology (both negative), ANA and anti-neutrophil cytoplasmic antibody (ANCA) (both negative). A serum angiotensin converting enzyme (ACE) level, however, was raised. In view of the possibility of TB, a TB-Elispot was performed which was reported as equivocal. At this point the patient and his wife were losing patience with all the investigations and the lack of a clear diagnosis.

3. The decision was to either consider a trial of anti-TB therapy blindly on the basis that this diagnosis could not be excluded or to start him on oral steroids for a presumptive diagnosis of either sarcoidosis (his serum ACE was raised) or a form of vasculitis such as giant cell arteritis (GCA). He interrupted this process by asking unexpectedly in clinic whether he might have syphilis as he had a friend who had developed a similar syndrome and been diagnosed with this. When tested for this, his VDRL/TPHA and IgM were all positive, suggestive of active/recent treponemal infection. Following antibiotic therapy his symptoms all resolved and inflammatory markers returned to normal. We informed the dermatologists who had performed a skin biopsy and this was subsequently reported as lymphoplasmacellular infiltrate with poorly formed granuloma suggestive of syphilis. Other features of secondary syphilis that he did not have include condyloma latum, hepatitis, glomerulonephritis, iritis and cranial neuropathy. In days gone by syphilis ('the great imitator') would have been high up on our differential when

considering a patient with arthralgias and a rash and it is still an important diagnosis to consider.

Case 7

A 20-year-old man was diagnosed with chlamydia urethritis and treated with doxycycline. At the time he had circinate balanitis and four weeks later developed a swollen warm right knee and tender toes. Two months later this had not settled and his knee was aspirated and injected with corticosteroids and he was started on sulphasalazine and, because of difficulty in working, oral prednisolone. His CRP was 113 mg/l, RF was negative. Two months later, despite increasing his prednisolone dose he still had active arthritis, his CRP was 150 mg/l, he had a keratoderma blennorrhagica rash and he was started on methotrexate. Five months later, there had been modest improvement although his CRP was still 68 mg/l, he was still requiring 20 mg prednisolone/day as well as the other medication and still had active arthritis. He did not feel that the methotrexate had any effect and therefore anti-TNF-α therapy was added in its place. Over the next six months his arthritis went into remission and his prednisolone dose is currently 5 mg/day with plans to reduce it further.

1. What is the diagnosis?
2. What is typical about this patient and what is unusual?
3. What is the long-term prognosis for patients who present with this condition?

1. This patient has a classic reactive arthritis with the associated extra-articular features of circinate balanitis and keratoderma blenorrhagica. In this case the patient gave a clear history of preceding infection. Typically this is of a sexually transmitted disease or gastrointestinal infection involving *Salmonella enteritica*, *Shigella* species, *Yersinia enterocolitica* or *Campylobacter jejuni*. Post-streptococcal reactive arthritis is also described and sometimes other infections such as a urinary tract or chest infection can lead to a reactive arthritis. Where appropriate, a formal assessment in a genitourinary clinic should be advised. Investigations to exclude other causes of inflammatory arthritis, an anti-streptolysin O titre (ASOT) test for streptococcus, stool culture and/or other serological tests for infections may be prudent. Some patients do not have a history of preceding infection and the diagnosis is suspected rather than proven. There is a suggestion that reactive arthritis is more common in patients with a history or family history of psoriasis, colitis or Crohn's disease.

2. The arthritis commonly involves a single joint, particularly the knee. A polyarthritic presentation is rare. Most patients will only have the inflammatory arthritis, some will have the 'triad' of arthritis, conjunctivitis and urethritis. Circinate balanitis and keratoderma blenorrhagica are extremely unusual. The CRP is usually elevated and is an important test; while it is raised the underlying process is still active and if the patient returns to normal levels of activity the condition will likely flare again.

3. The outcome from reactive arthritis ranges from complete recovery within a few weeks to a chronic severe form of inflammatory arthritis. In patients with a mild form of the disease, such as those with a single swollen knee, then one local corticosteroid injection may suffice as treatment. However, where inflammatory arthritis persists and, particularly where it is polyarticular, then corticosteroids and DMARDs will play a role. This patient reflects the more severe end of the spectrum of disease severity and chronicity.

Case 8

A 62-year-old woman was diagnosed with mild SLE 30 years previously. No major internal organ involvement was noted until 25 years later when a diagnosis of lymphoid pneumonia was made. On subsequent routine review she complained of increasing dryness affecting her mouth and said she had several chest infections over the past year. Examination showed persistent swelling of a parotid gland. Review of her investigations showed that she had a paraproteinaemia and a bone marrow biopsy showed 3% plasma cells, not sufficient to make a diagnosis of myeloma. She had a positive ANA at a titre of 1:640, was anti-Ro/La antibody positive, anti-dsDNA antibody negative and her C4 was low at 0.08 g/l. IgG was very high at 84.5 g/l but IgA and IgM were normal and functional antibodies were reduced. A US scan and an MRI scan of the parotid gland swelling had not been diagnostic. A CT chest, abdomen and pelvis showed a few enlarged lymph nodes only. She had a fine needle aspiration and then a tru-cut biopsy of the affected parotid but again with no diagnostic findings.

1. What is the diagnosis?
2. What investigations are required?
3. What treatment may be appropriate?

1. It can be difficult to decide whether a patient has SLE with secondary Sjögren's syndrome, a systemic form of primary Sjögren's syndrome (pSS) or a genuine

overlap of the two. A low complement C4 can occur in pSS. Occasionally patients with pSS can have a low positive anti-dsDNA antibody level. In this patient exact details of the scenario from 30 years ago are not known but the pattern of her disease at this presentation seems much closer to systemic pSS. The gold standard classification criteria for pSS are the American European Consensus Group Criteria, which require various combinations of symptomatic and objective dryness as well as focal periductal lymphocytic infiltrates on salivary gland biopsy or positive anti-Ro/La antibodies (or both). Lymphoid interstitial pneumonitis is often associated with connective tissue diseases but does not differentiate between SLE and pSS. Patients with pSS are at increased risk of lymphoma, particularly if they have a paraproteinaemia, low C4, vasculitis, neuropathy or cryoglobulinaemia. This patient had persistent parotid gland swelling and had a paraproteinaemia and low C4 and so a second diagnosis of lymphoma needs to be considered.

2. Unfortunately even a normal needle aspirate and tru-cut biopsy cannot fully exclude lymphoma. Eventually the patient underwent an open biopsy and a mucosal associated lymphoid tissue (MALT) lymphoma was identified.

3. Dry eyes are treated with regular use of a watery eye drop preparation such as hypromellose, moving to a more viscous preparation if required. Preservative free preparations are appropriate if frequent use is required. The ducts which drain tears from the eye can be blocked reversibly or permanently to help treat more severe cases. Treatment of oral dryness is less satisfactory although occasionally patients find oral sprays and gels helpful. A sugar-free pastille or chewing gum may be equally effective. Pilocarpine can be used where there is still some residual gland function. Good oral hygiene is important.

For mild systemic features, hydroxychloroquine or low-dose prednisolone can be prescribed empirically. For more severe disease, stronger immunosuppression may be given. Traditionally lymphoma has been treated with chemotherapy regimens and in recent years rituximab has been routinely incorporated into the regimens. Radiotherapy may also play a role in management.

Case 9

A 27-year-old woman presented five years previously with a left-sided stroke-like syndrome that partially recovered leaving some residual weakness such that she used a crutch to walk. At the time an MRI scan was abnormal with white matter lesions but the lumbar puncture showed normal pressures and fluid. The possibility of cerebral vasculitis was considered although she was not treated for this. She then presented with recurrent headaches and was noted to have a livedo reticularis rash. Blood tests showed a weakly positive ANA with a titre of 1:40, dsDNA antibodies were negative and complement levels were normal. She had a weak positive IgG anti-cardiolipin antibody result. Lupus anti-coagulant was negative. She had been taking aspirin at a dose of 75 mg od.

1. What is the diagnosis?
2. What investigations are required?
3. What treatment may be appropriate?

1. The history of a stroke-like syndrome and the presence of a livedo reticularis rash both point to the possibility of APLS. Whilst the lupus anti-coagulant test was negative, this patient did have one report of positive anti-cardiolipin antibodies (albeit weak) and this would be consistent with the diagnosis of APLS.

2. The diagnosis of APLS requires the presence of one clinical criterion (vascular thrombosis or pregnancy morbidity) and one laboratory criterion. In this patient it was considered that the stroke-like syndrome reflected vascular thrombosis. The laboratory criterion should be present on at least two occasions at least 12 weeks apart. Therefore the blood tests for anti-cardiolipin antibody were rechecked after an appropriate time interval and were found to be positive. It is important to note that, despite the current diagnostic criteria, some patients with clinical features suggestive of APLS have negative antibody results.

3. The treatment of patients who have not had a vascular thrombosis remains controversial; some rheumatologists prescribe low-dose aspirin or hydroxychloroquine to individuals with positive APLA, particularly in the presence of SLE. Treatment of patients who have had a thrombotic episode is with life-long warfarin because of the high risk of recurrent thrombosis. The decision in this case was not entirely straightforward. The patient's stroke had occurred five years previously and she had not had a further thrombotic event despite not receiving warfarin. Nevertheless she was commenced on warfarin and, as sometimes occurs with such patients, her headaches improved. The patient went on to have two children; she was converted to low molecular weight heparin for the duration of both pregnancies and did well.

Case 10

A 61-year-old man with a history of ischaemic heart disease had a cardiac arrest due to an episode of ventricular fibrillation and had an automatic defibrillator implanted. He subsequently had an unpleasant experience when the defibrillator discharged spontaneously. He then presented with difficulty in taking deep breaths, chest wall tenderness and a feeling of global muscle weakness. He was referred from neurology having been extensively evaluated with a chest CT scan, electromyography and nerve conduction studies, an echocardiogram and blood gases, all of which were normal. Lung function tests showed some reduction in lung volumes which was attributed to poor compliance with the investigation. Overall his symptoms were put down to anxiety, he was given diazepam and referred for psychological assessment. He was re-referred 14 months later and described worsening of his symptoms with discomfort on standing upright, jerking, weakness in the legs and painful muscle spasms precipitated by sudden noise. He had seen a different cardiologist for routine follow-up of his defibrillator who had suggested a specific diagnosis.

1. What is the diagnosis?
2. What investigations are required?
3. What treatment may be appropriate?

1. This case confused a neurologist, cardiologist, chest physician, psychiatrist and rheumatologist until a (very smart) cardiologist made the diagnosis based on their recollection of a similar case of 'stiff person syndrome' from when they were a medical student. The classic features are of truncal/lower limb muscle stiffness, often associated with muscle spasms or cerebellar ataxia. As the condition deteriorates patients may experience muscle tears and joint contractures. 'Stiff person syndrome' may be associated with other autoimmune diseases, particularly diabetes mellitus and thyroid disease. Patients may be referred to a rheumatology service because of the muscle pain and weakness and developing joint contractures.

2. Most patients have antibodies against glutamic acid decarboxylase (GAD). The electroymyogram should be repeated and is likely to have become abnormal by this stage with characteristic continuous motor unit activity. Because of the bizarre clinical features and worsening of the condition with stress, patients are often thought, as with this patient, to have psychiatric disease.

3. Treatment options are limited but benzodiazepines, baclofen, plasmapharesis and intravenous immunoglobulin have all been reported as providing benefit for some patients.

Case 11

A 62-year-old woman presented to the rheumatology clinic with a history of several months of intermittently experiencing cold, blue, painful fingertips and toes with development of areas of necrosis on some fingertips. She had also noticed tightening and puckering of the skin around her mouth and nose. On direct questioning she reported the recent development of shortness of breath and ankle swelling. On examination in clinic she was noted to have severe peripheral ischaemia of the fingers with several areas of ulceration, tight and shiny skin over hands, toes and face and telangectasia over her face. She had also been recently diagnosed as having a metastatic, malignant carcinoid tumour in the small bowel which had been treated with surgery and arterial embolisation.

1. What is the most likely diagnosis?
2. What investigations would be helpful?
3. What treatment would you recommend?

1. The story suggests severe Raynaud's phenomenon with development of ischaemia-related ulcers. This, together with the skin tightening and telangectasia, points to a diagnosis of systemic sclerosis. This is an uncommon connective tissue disease which affects approximately 2/100,000 individuals per year. Prevalence is approximately 65–265 per million worldwide. The term 'scleroderma' is derived from the Greek for 'hard skin' and emphasises the dermatological component of the disease. The term 'systemic sclerosis' emphasises the multi-system nature of the disease. The disease is classified as limited or diffuse, depending on the degree of skin involvement. Limited cutaneous systemic sclerosis used to be called CREST syndrome, an acronym for 'calcinosis, Raynaud's, oesophageal dysmotility, sclerodactyly and telangectasia'. In this form of disease skin involvement does not extend beyond the forearms, gastrointestinal involvement is usually limited to the oesophagus and calcinosis and telangectasia are common. Patients may, however, develop pulmonary hypertension, often late in the course of the disease. Anti-centromere antibodies are found in the majority of, but not all, patients. Diffuse cutaneous systemic sclerosis is characterised by skin involvement beyond the forearms, more widespread

gastrointestinal involvement with dysmotility and bacterial overgrowth and an increased risk of developing interstitial lung and renal disease. Anti-Scl70 antibodies are present in up to 40% of patients. Raynaud's phenomenon is a feature of both forms of the disease. Patients have a higher incidence of some malignancies, particularly lung, breast and haematological.

2. Blood should be sent for ANA, anti-Scl70 and anti-centromere antibodies. Some laboratories will offer testing for other autoantibodies associated with systemic sclerosis or overlap syndromes such as anti-RNA polymerase I/III, anti-U3RNP, anti-Pm/SCL. It is important to investigate the differential diagnoses of SLE and APLS by requesting anti-dsDNA, anti-ENA, APLA, anti-beta 2 microglobulin antibodies and a lupus anticoagulant. Cryoglobulinaemia may present with severe Raynaud's phenomenon; blood needs to be sent to the laboratory at 37°C for detection of cryoglobulins. The story of breathlessness and ankle swelling should prompt investigation of the respiratory and cardiovascular systems with chest X-ray, lung function tests, electrocardiogram (ECG) and echocardiogram in the first instance.

In this case the ANA was positive with a titre of 1:160 although all other more specific antibodies were negative. Cardiac investigations revealed that the right atrium and ventricle were dilated with severe tricuspid regurgitation and an estimated right ventricular systolic pressure that was high at 40 mmHg. The test results were consistent with a diagnosis of limited cutaneous systemic sclerosis with development of pulmonary hypertension.

3. There is no cure for systemic sclerosis and treatment is largely symptomatic. Heated gloves, calcium channel antagonists, angiotensin receptor antagonists and intravenous prostacyclin may be used to treat the Raynaud's phenomenon. Fluoxetine, alpha-adrenergic blockers such as moxisylyte and other vasodilating agents such as sildenafil have also been used in cases of moderate/severe Raynaud's, particularly when digital ulceration and/or ischaemia are present. Sympathectomy is another approach that can be considered. ACE inhibitors should be used in individuals with hypertension and as part of the management of associated renal disease. Immunosuppressive agents may be used for the interstitial lung disease. Endothelin antagonists (e.g. bosentan) improve morbidity and mortality in patients who develop pulmonary hypertension and also reduce new digital ulcer formation.

This patient was treated with intravenous iloprost for seven days; this led to significant improvement in the Raynaud's phenomenon and near complete healing of the ulcers. She was also given warfarin and diuretics in view of the pulmonary hypertension and right-sided heart failure and referred on to a specialist pulmonary hypertension unit. Additional chemotherapy was planned for treating the metastatic carcinoid tumour.

Case 12

A 35-year-old woman presented to the rheumatology clinic with a three month history of pain, stiffness and swelling in her wrists and knees. The symptoms were there all the time and were worse first thing in the mornings. She had consulted her GP who had put her on ibuprofen tablets and referred her to the local rheumatology department. She had also noticed a rash which had appeared on the soles of her feet and the palms of her hands over the last few months. Her past medical history included an episode of iritis. There was a family history of ulcerative colitis. When she was seen by the rheumatologist it was noted that she had synovitis in her right wrist with effusions in both knees. An erythematous, pustular rash suggestive of pustular psoriasis was present on the soles of both feet and palms of the hands. Examination was otherwise unremarkable.

1. What is the differential diagnosis?
2. What investigations should be requested?
3. What treatment options are available?

1. The clinical picture is of an inflammatory arthritis in an individual with psoriasis and the likely diagnosis is of psoriatic arthritis. It is, however, important to consider other forms of inflammatory arthritis when assessing an individual with psoriasis; patients are at increased risk of gout and some may have true rheumatoid arthritis.

About 40% of patients with psoriatic arthritis have a family history of psoriasis or psoriatic arthritis. Most patients develop psoriasis first but some develop the arthritis first, which can lead to diagnostic difficulties. There have been five patterns of joint involvement described: asymmetrical oligoarthritis (most common), symmetrical polyarthritis, distal interphalangeal joint arthritis, spondylitis and arthritis mutilans (least common). Nail changes, particularly onycholysis, nail pitting and transverse ridging are common.

2. There is no diagnostic test for psoriatic arthritis. The inflammatory markers may be raised, although this is not universally so, and it is important to check the FBC, renal and liver function as results may influence choice of drugs used in management. Diagnostic criteria for psoriatic arthritis include a negative RF and so this and an anti-CCP antibody test should be requested. Plain X-rays may show erosive damage or secondary degenerative changes; however, these changes are unlikely to be evident at initial diagnosis. US and MRI scans can show evidence of synovitis and effusions.

This patient had an acute phase response with a CRP of 65 and ESR of 50 with a platelet count that was elevated at 505. Tests for RF and anti-CCP were negative. Further haematological and biochemical studies were normal as were X-rays of hands, wrists and knees.

3. The aim of treatment is to control the inflammatory process and reduce the risk of joint damage. Symptomatic therapies such as NSAIDS are often used and intra-articular steroid injections can be helpful particularly in large joint oligoarthritis. Early use of DMARDs is recommended and the four main agents used are methotrexate, ciclosporin, sulphasalazine and leflunomide. If the patient fails to respond to an adequate trial of at least two out of these four drugs then it is appropriate to consider treatment with a TNF-α antagonist. The psoriatic skin rash may also respond to treatment with methotrexate, ciclosporin or a TNF-α antagonist and this may be an important consideration when selecting which therapy to use.

Case 13

A 50-year-old man presented to the casualty department with a four day history of fever, polyarthritis, tenosynovitis and a rash of the hands and feet. The arthritis was asymmetrical and involved the hands, wrists and ankles with extensor tenosynovitis. There was no other prior history reported by the patient and no eye, gastrointestinal nor genitourinary symptoms.

On examination he had a fever of 39°C, synovitis of his wrists and ankles and marked swelling around the extensor tendons of his fingers. He also had a widespread rash that looked vasculitic in appearance mainly on his hands and feet. The lesions were small, scanty in number, non-tender and non-blanching in nature. Initial blood tests showed a neutrophilia and a marked acute phase response with a CRP of 139 mg/l and ESR of 110 mm/h

1. What diagnoses should be considered?
2. What further investigations might be helpful?
3. How should he be treated?

1. This man presents with a short history of fever, rash and arthritis. Both infectious and non-infectious inflammatory disease need to be considered. Viral infections, including parvovirus, rubella, hepatitis B and alpha viruses, as well as infection with *Neisseria gonorrhoeae* and secondary syphilis can all present with this triad of features. Non-infectious causes include rheumatoid arthritis with

vasculitis, SLE, microscopic polyarteritis, Henoch–Schönlein purpura or other forms of small vessel vasculitides.

2. Blood cultures are mandatory and serological tests for specific viruses and syphilis should be sent. RhF, anti-CCP, ANA, ANCA and complement studies should all be requested.

In this individual the immunological tests proved negative but blood cultures grew *Neisseria gonorrhoeae* in one of two sets taken over the first two days of admission. Gonococcal arthritis is a relatively common cause of acute septic arthritis in young adults and should always be considered. It is caused by the Gram-negative diplococcus *Neisseria gonorrhoeae,* which is a highly infectious organism transmitted via mucosal surfaces during sexual contact. Initial infection may not cause symptoms but usually affects genitourinary, pharyngeal or rectal mucosa. Disseminated infection (haematogenous spread) is uncommon (less than 3% of cases). The two usual presentations of disseminated infection are with an arthritis–dermatitis syndrome or a localised septic arthritis although these two presentations frequently overlap. This patient presented with the classic triad of migratory arthritis, tenosynovitis and rash seen in the arthritis–dermatitis syndrome. The arthritis is described as usually being asymmetrical and affecting wrists and ankles. The rash occurs in 40–70% of patients and varies in nature. It is often ignored by patients and therefore goes undetected. Other sequelae of disseminated gonococcal infections include peri-hepatitis (Fitz-Hugh–Curtis syndrome), meningitis and endocarditis.

3. Initial treatment should be with parenteral ceftriaxone with further treatment being guided by antibiotic sensitivities. This patient was treated with intravenous ceftriaxone for five days followed by oral ciprofloxacin for seven days. The arthritis, tenosynovitis and skin rash all rapidly resolved and he was discharged home a few days later with follow-up from the genitourinary medicine department for contact tracing.

Case 14

A 47-year-old Caucasian man was brought to the casualty department in an acute confusional state, having been found wandering on the streets by a passer-by. He was known to have been an alcoholic in the past but, according to his daughter, had stopped drinking some years ago. His daughter also reported that, over the previous two months, his appetite had been poor and he had become increasingly confused, unsteady on his feet and generally weak but had refused to seek medical attention. On examination he had expressive dysphasia and a blood pressure of 200/140 mmHg. He had a widespread vasculitic skin rash on his arms and legs. Initial blood tests showed a normochromic normocytic anaemia, a lymphopenia, an elevated urea of 17.8 mmol/l and creatinine of 183 μmol/l, normal liver function and a CRP of 11 mg/l. Urinalysis revealed blood 2+ and protein 3+. A chest X-ray showed cardiomegaly and an ECG showed evidence of left ventricular hypertrophy. A renal US scan confirmed normal sized kidneys. An MRI scan of the brain showed diffuse high T2 signal in periventricular white matter, basal ganglia and cerebellum. Blood and urine cultures were negative.

1. What diagnoses should be considered?
2. Which further investigations might be helpful?
3. What treatment would you recommend?

1. This patient presents with neurological features, severe hypertension and renal impairment on a background of malaise and confusion. Whilst hypertension may lead to the development of cerebrovascular disease and renal impairment, the presence of a vasculitic skin rash should lead to the consideration of a connective tissue disease or vasculitis as an underlying diagnosis. This would also be more consistent with the presence of active urinary sediment and normal, rather than small, kidneys. The fact that the patient is a middle-aged man would make a vasculitic illness rather than a connective tissue disease such as SLE more likely. However, the relatively low CRP in the context of severe disease would be more in keeping with a diagnosis of SLE.

2. Immunological tests including ANA, dsDNA, ENAs, C3 and C4 complement levels, ANCA, RF and anti-CCP antibodies should be requested. Urinary protein excretion should be quantified and a renal biopsy performed.

In this case the ANCA was negative but the ANA and RF were positive at high titre. Anti-dsDNA antibodies were strongly positive. Testing for reactivity to ENA showed a positive anti-Sm and anti-RNP result. Both complement C3 and C4 levels were low. Urinary protein excretion was estimated to be 2.9 g/24 hours. A renal biopsy revealed a diffuse proliferative glomerulonephritis.

A diagnosis of acute SLE with lupus nephritis (World health organisation (WHO) class IV) and cerebral lupus was made. This patient fulfilled the American College of Rheumatology's criteria for diagnosis of SLE in that he had at least four of the stipulated features: renal involvement, neuropsychiatric involvement, haematological disorder, positive ANA and positive dsDNA and Sm antibodies.

Whilst SLE is much commoner in women and in certain racial groups such as people of African descent, Caucasian men do occasionally develop the disease.

3. Treatment for SLE is largely based on the degree of organ involvement. NSAIDS may be used for joint pains and anti-malarials such as hydroxychloroquine are commonly used to treat joint and skin disease. Systemic glucocorticoids are used in small doses for resistant cases of arthritis whilst larger doses are used in combination with other immunosuppressive agents to treat more significant organ involvement. Where there is severe renal or neuropsychiatric disease then cyclophosphamide may be used to induce remission, with an alternative agent such as azathioprine or mycophenolate mofetil being used to maintain disease control. New regimes using a combination of rituximab and mycophenolate mofetil as an alternative to cyclophosphamide and corticosteroids are under investigation.

This patient was initially treated with intravenous pulses of cyclophosphamide and methylprednisolone and responded well. His confusion and skin rash resolved and his renal function and proteinuria improved quickly. He was subsequently given maintenance therapy of oral prednisolone and azathioprine.

Poor prognostic factors in SLE include renal disease (particularly diffuse proliferative glomerulonephritis) hypertension, male sex, young age or older age at presentation, poor socio-economic status, black race, presence of APLA and high overall disease activity. This patient had several of these poor prognostic factors and will need to be monitored carefully in the long term.

Case 15

A 77-year-old man presented to his GP with pain in his right hip. The pain had been there for some months but had suddenly become more severe. In particular it was affecting him at night and keeping him awake. He also complained of increasing deafness affecting his right ear which was interfering with his social interactions. The GP arranged an X-ray of the pelvis which demonstrated widespread abnormalities in the lamellar bone with a pubic ramus fracture on the right. Blood tests showed a normal FBC, normal calcium and phosphate, elevated alkaline phosphatase of 750 U/l and normal vitamin D level.

1. What is the likely diagnosis and are there any further investigations that would be helpful?
2. What are the clinical features of this disease?
3. What treatment would you advise?

1. The most likely diagnosis is of Paget's disease of the bone (osteitis deformans) with involvement of the skull and pelvis and complicated by a fracture. The patient is an elderly individual, consistent with the observation that the incidence of Paget's disease increases with age. Whilst he did not have any relatives known to be affected by the condition, patients often do report a family history, reflecting a genetic predisposition to the disease. Paget's disease is a focal skeletal disorder characterised by an accelerated rate of bone turnover. It causes both excessive resorption and formation of bone, resulting in a 'mosaic' pattern of lamellar bone associated with increases in local bone blood flow and in fibrous tissue in adjacent marrow.

The abnormalities noted on the patient's X-ray are typical and fractures through Pagetic lesions are a well-recognised complication of disease. Hearing loss is a common feature of Paget's disease of the skull; a number of possible mechanisms have been proposed including obstruction of the external auditory meatus, ossicular fixation, obliteration of the labyrinth, cochlea damage and compressive damage to the auditory nerve. A skull X-ray would be helpful; in this case it confirmed Pagetic changes throughout. Isotope bone scans are a sensitive means of identifying the distribution of Pagetic lesions throughout the skeleton; these appear as 'hot spots' due to increased tracer uptake. If there is any doubt about the nature of the lesion then a bone biopsy should be considered. This patient had a typical biochemical profile; however, hypercalcaemia may be a feature in some less mobile patients. Urinary hydroxyproline is elevated in patients with Paget's disease although the lack of ready availability of this test precludes its use in many cases.

2. Most individuals with Paget's disease are asymptomatic and the diagnosis is often made when a biochemistry screen or an X-ray is done for another reason. Where the disease is symptomatic then the two main presenting features are local pain and deformity. The pelvis, spine, skull and long bones are the most common sites of involvement. The pain may arise directly from the Pagetic lesions or be secondary to fractures. It is typically worse on weight-bearing and at night. Skeletal deformities, particularly in the long bones may cause bowing and result in abnormal mechanical stresses, further exacerbating the pain. Neural compression, particularly involving the VIIIth cranial nerve but also involving nerve roots within the spine, may occur as a consequence of an increase in size of affected bones. Patients are at increased risk of developing bone tumours, especially osteosarcomas. The increased blood flow to involved bone can rarely lead to a state of high output cardiac failure.

3. Treatment with drug therapy is indicated if the patient has symptoms from their disease such as pain, hypercalcaemia or nerve compression. Some clinicians will also treat asymptomatic patients who have very high levels of alkaline phosphatase, extensive skull involvement or involvement of load-bearing areas of the skeleton. All drugs used suppress osteoclast activity and include bisphosphonates and calcitonin. Bisphosphonates such as risedronate or zoledronate are generally favoured because of increased efficacy compared to calicitonin and etidronate.

Case 16

A 64-year-old woman presented to her GP after waking one morning unable to turn over and get out of bed. She complained of pain in the upper arms, shoulders, back, thighs and buttocks and had noticed stiffness in the morning lasting between two and three hours. Examination confirmed that shoulder abduction was painful bilaterally but showed no other clear abnormalities.

1. What diagnoses should be considered?
2. Which further investigations might be helpful?
3. What treatment would you recommend?

1. This patient is describing upper and lower limb girdle pain and stiffness. The symptoms are of sudden onset, without any precipitating event. They are worse in the mornings suggesting they are inflammatory in nature. The most likely diagnosis is of polymyalgia rheumatica (PMR). However, alternative diagnoses including polymyalgic onset of rheumatoid arthritis or a paraneoplastic syndrome need to be considered. The patient should specifically be asked about features of GCA (temporal arteritis) such as headache, scalp tenderness, jaw claudication and visual disturbance as PMR and GCA constitute a spectrum of disease with the former sometimes being considered to be a 'mild' form of the latter. Ultrasound of the temporal arteries to demonstrate luminal irregularity and wall inflammation can also be helpful in supporting the clinical diagnosis.

2. Both the ESR and CRP are usually raised in patients with PMR. It is advisable to check RF, anti-CCP antibodies, TFTs, immunoglobulins with an electrophoretic strip and Bence Jones protein in all patients. If there are localising features to suggest a malignancy, then appropriate further studies should be taken forward. If there are any features of GCA then a temporal artery biopsy should be done.

Blood tests in this patient showed only modest elevation of the inflammatory markers with an ESR of 30 mm/h and CRP of 12 mg/l. All other investigations were normal.

3. Patients with PMR should receive treatment with prednisolone at an initial dose of 15 mg od and usually respond rapidly. When the symptoms have resolved and the inflammatory markers have normalised then the dose may be gradually decreased over approximately 18 months. Patients with GCA should be treated initially with higher doses of prednisolone (1 mg/kg up to 60 mg od) and should receive intravenous methylprednisolone if they develop concerning visual symptoms. Complications of long-term steroid treatment should be considered in all patients and include osteoporosis, gastric irritation, hypertension, diabetes, cataracts and infections. Appropriate gastroprotective and bone protective agents should be given. If either disease relapses as corticosteroids are withdrawn then consideration should be given to adding either azathioprine or methotrexate as a steroid sparing agent.

References for Diagnostic and Classification Criteria

American College of Rheumatology classification criteria for Churg–Strauss syndrome
The American College of Rheumatology 1990 criteria for the classification of Churg–Strauss syndrome (allergic granulomatosis and angiitis).
Masai AT, Hunder GG, Lie JT, *et al.*
Arthritis Rheum 1990 33:1094–100.

American College of Rheumatology classification criteria for Henoch–Schönlein purpura
The American College of Rheumatology 1990 criteria for the classification of Henoch–Schönlein purpura.
Mills JA, Michel BA, Bloch DA, *et al.*
Arthritis Rheum 1990 33:1114–21.

American College of Rheumatology classification criteria for polyarteritis nodosa
The American College of Rheumatology 1990 criteria for the classification of polyarteritis nodosa.
Lightfoot RW Jr, Michel BA, Bloch DA, *et al.*
Arthritis Rheum 1990 33:1088–93.

American College of Rheumatology classification criteria for Takayasu's arteritis

The American College of Rheumatology 1990 criteria for the classification of Takayasu arteritis.
Arend WP, Michel BA, Bloch DA, *et al.*
Arthritis Rheum 1990 33:1129–34.

American College of Rheumatology classification criteria for Wegener's granulomatosis

The American College of Rheumatology 1990 criteria for the classification of Wegener's granulomatosis.
Leavitt RY, Fauci AS, Bloch DA, *et al.*
Arthritis Rheum 1990 33:1101–7.

American College of Rheumatology classification criteria for giant cell arteritis

The American College of Rheumatology 1990 criteria for the classification of giant cell arteritis.
Hunder GG, Bloch DA, Michel BA, *et al.*
Arthritis Rheum 1990 33:1122–8.

American College of Rheumatology 1997 revised classification criteria for systemic lupus erythematosus

The 1982 revised criteria for the classification of systemic lupus erythematosus.
Tan EM, Cohen AS, Fries JF, *et al.*
Arthritis Rheum 1982 25:1271–7.
Updating the American College of Rheumatology revised criteria for the classification of systemic lupus erythematosus.
Hochberg MC.
Arthritis Rheum 1997 40:1725.

American College of Rheumatology/European League against Rheumatism 2010 classification criteria for rheumatoid arthritis

2010 Rheumatoid arthritis classification criteria: an American College of Rheumatology/European League against Rheumatism collaborative initiative.
Aletaha D, Neogi T, Silman AJ, *et al.*
Arthritis Rheum 2010 62:2569–81.

American Rheumatism Association 1987 classification criteria for rheumatoid arthritis
The American Rheumatism Association 1987 revised criteria for the classification of rheumatoid arthritis.
Arnett FC, Edworthy SM, Bloch DA, *et al.*
Arthritis Rheum 1988 31:315–24.

Bohan and Peter diagnostic criteria for inflammatory myopathies
Polymyositis and dermatomyositis.
Bohan A, Peter JB.
N Engl J Med 1975 292:344–7 & 403–7.

Brussels revision of Ghent criteria for the diagnosis of Marfan syndrome
The revised Ghent nosology for the Marfan syndrome.
Loeys BL, Dietz HC, Braverman AC, *et al.*
J Med Genet 2010 47:476–485.

Classification of Psoriatic Arthritis (CASPAR) criteria for diagnosis of psoriatic arthritis
Classification criteria for psoriatic arthritis: development of new criteria from a large international study.
Taylor W, Gladman D, Helliwell P, *et al.*
Arthritis Rheum 2006 54:2665–73.

Griggs 1995 diagnostic criteria for inclusion body myositis
Inclusion body myositis and myopathies.
Griggs RC, Askanas V, DiMauro S, *et al.*
Annals Neurol 1995 38:705–13.

International consensus criteria for diagnosis of anti-phospholipid antibody syndrome
International consensus statement on preliminary classification criteria for definite antiphospholipid syndrome.
Wilson WA, Gharavi AE, Koiki T, *et al.*
Arthritis Rheum 1999 42:1309–11.

Jones and Hazleman criteria for diagnosis of polymyalgia rheumatica
Prognosis and management of polymyalgia rheumatica.
Jones JG, Hazleman BL.
Ann Rheum Dis 1981 40:1–5.

Le Roy classification scheme for systemic sclerosis
Criteria for the classification of early systemic sclerosis.
LeRoy EC, Medsger TA Jr.
J Rheumatol 2001 28:1573–6.

Modified New York classification of ankylosing spondylitis
Evaluation of diagnostic criteria for ankylosing spondylitis. A proposal for modification of the New York criteria.
Van der Linden S, Valkenburg HA, Cats A.
Arthritis Rheum 1984 27:361–68.

Moll and Wright classification of joint involvement in psoriatic arthritis
Psoriatic arthritis.
Moll JMH, Wright V.
Sem Arthr & Rheum 1973 3:51–78

World Health Organisation definition of osteopenia and osteoporosis
World Health Organisation definition of osteopenia and osteoporosis
WHO (1994). "Assessment of fracture risk and its application to screening for postmenopausal osteoporosis. Report of a WHO Study Group".
World Health Organization technical report series 1994 843:1–129.

Index